£34.99

Assertive Outreach
in Mental Healthcare:
Current Perspectives

Assertive Outreach in Mental Healthcare: Current Perspectives

Edited by

Caroline Williams
Mike Firn
Simon Wharne
Rob Macpherson

Foreword by

Kim T. Mueser, PhD

WILEY-BLACKWELL

A John Wiley & Sons, Ltd., Publication

Library of Congress Cataloging-in-Publication Data

Assertive outreach in mental healthcare: current perspectives / edited by Caroline Williams ... [et al.] ; foreword by Kim T. Mueser.
       p.   ; cm.
   Includes bibliographical references and index.
   ISBN 978-1-4051-9865-3 (pbk. : alk. paper)   1. Community mental health services – Europe.
2. Community mental health services-Great Britain.   I. Williams, Caroline, 1971–
   [DNLM: 1.   Community Mental Health Services-Europe.   2. Community Mental Health Services –
Great Britain.   3. Community-Institutional Relations – Europe.   4. Community – Institutional
Relations-Great Britain.   5. Outcome and Process Assessment (Health Care) – Europe.   6. Outcome
and Process Assessment (Health Care) – Great Britain. WM 30]
   RA790.55.A87 2011
   362.2′2–dc22

                                          2010040967

A catalogue record for this book is available from the British Library.

This book is published in the following electronic formats: ePDF 9781444393293; ePub 9781444393309

Set in 10/12.5pt Times by SPi Publisher Services, Pondicherry, India
Printed and bound in Malaysia by Vivar Printing Sdn Bhd

1   2011

Contents

Contributors

Rory Allott
Clinical Psychologist
Greater Manchester West Mental
 Health NHS Foundation Trust
Salford, England

Tom Burns
Professor of Social Psychiatry
Department of Psychiatry
Oxford University
Oxford, England

Jo Coldwell
Clinical Psychologist
St Mary's Wrestwood Children's Trust
East Sussex, England

Tizzie Coleman
Carer
Sussex, England

Tom Edwards
Consultant Psychiatrist
Walsall Assertive Outreach
 and Recovery Team
Walsall, England

Mike Firn
Chair, National Forum for
 Assertive Outreach (NFAO)
Clinical Service Development Lead
 South West London & St. George's
 Mental Health NHS Trust
London, England

Robert Griffiths
Psychological Therapist
Greater Manchester West
 Mental Health
NHS Foundation Trust
Salford, England

Neil Harris
Mental Health Nurse Consultant
Manchester Mental Health & Social Care
 Trust / University of Manchester
Manchester, England

Sue Jugon
Community Services Manager
Assertive Outreach / Dual Diagnosis
 Northamptonshire Healthcare
NHS Foundation Trust
Kettering, England

Rob Macpherson
Consultant Psychiatrist
NHS Foundation Trust
Wotton Lawn Hosptial
Gloucester, England

Sara Meddings
Clinical Psychologist in AOT
Sussex Partnership
NHS Foundation Trust
East Sussex, England

Andrew Molodynski
Consultant Psychiatrist
Oxfordshire and Buckinghamshire
    Mental Health
NHS Foundation Trust
Oxford, England

Steve Morgan
Practice Based Evidence
Practice Development Consultancy
    for Mental Health
www.practicebasedevidence.com

Steve Onyett
Director, Senior Development
Consultant at Steve Onyett
    Consultancy Services Ltd.
Visiting Professor at the University of the
    West of England
Bristol, England

Neil Sanyal
Senior Social Work Practitioner and
    Approved Mental Health Professional
Hampshire County Council / Hampshire
    Partnership NHS Trust
Hampshire, England

Hannah Steer
Principal Clinical Psychologist
Psychological Therapies Service for
    Assertive Outreach & Inpatient Recovery
NHS Foundation Trust
Gloucester, England

Kamal Spilsted
Student and Former User of AOT Services

Simon Wharne
Committee Member, National Forum
    for Assertive Outreach (NFAO)
AOT Team Leader
Sussex Partnership NHS
Foundation Trust
East Sussex, England

Caroline Williams
Independent Mental Health Nurse
Consultant & Cognitive Behavioural
    Psychotherapist
User Friendly Psychiatry Ltd
(www.ufpmentalhealth.com)
Northwich, England
Past committee member, National Forum
    for Assertive Outreach (NFAO)
Programme Director
Lancaster University
Lancaster, England

Ian Wilson
Dual Diagnosis Nurse Specialist
Dual Diagnosis Service
Manchester Mental Health and
    Social Care Trust
Manchester, England

Foreword

Kim T. Mueser, PhD

Over 30 years ago, in the midst of the deinstitutionalization movement, it became increasing clear that significant numbers of people with serious mental illness were either unable or unwilling to access psychiatric services in the fledgling but ever-evolving United States (US) community mental health system, condemning them to either the proverbial 'revolving door' of relapse and re-hospitalization, severely impaired psycho-social functioning or both. To address this problem, Stein, Test and their colleagues proposed a bold new solution: if those clients who need community-based psychiatric services the most were also the least likely to seek them on their own, then why not bring the services to wherever they were in the community, be it their apartment, the home of a family member, a local coffee shop or even the street? Originally called the Training in Community Living (TCL) Programme, the name was changed to the Programme for Assertive Community Treatment (PACT, and then shortened to ACT) to underscore the novelty and importance of outreach into the community as the basis for their programme (Stein & Test, 1985; Test, 1992). Stein and Test developed a specific team structure, and operating principles and responsibilities that were characterized by the following: low clinician/client ratio (1:10); most services provided in the community rather than in the clinic; shared caseloads between clinicians; direct rather than brokered provision of services; team coverage provided 24 hours per day, seven days per week; and combined focus on providing both traditional psychiatric services (e.g. medication evaluations, case management) and practical assistance in meeting daily living needs (e.g. shopping, transportation).

To evaluate the TCL program, Stein and Test conducted a randomized controlled trial comparing clients who received TCL services with those treated with usual care (Stein & Test, 1980; Test & Stein, 1980; Weisbrod, Test & Stein, 1980). The study was a resounding success, and the field of mental health treatment has never been the same since. Not only were service users who participated in the TCL programme less likely to have relapses and to be hospitalized, but they also showed significant improvements in the quality of their lives, including their psycho-social functioning. Furthermore, reduced inpatient treatment costs for clients who received TCL more than made up for the higher outpatient costs of the programme, so that the overall TCL programme resulted in net savings of total mental health treatment costs.

In the decade following the publication of this classic experiment on ACT, many of the findings were replicated in research conducted in the US and abroad. More important than just stimulating research on ACT, however, was the broader impact of the model on standard clinical practice, and in particular on assertive outreach. No longer did case managers and clinicians wait for their clients with serious mental illness to not show up for their appointments; the inescapable logic, and empirical support, for assertive outreach for engaging challenging clients in treatment and helping them address their most pressing needs now made it the obvious choice, even for many mental health providers not working on formal ACT or assertive outreach teams. In addition, variations and adaptations of the assertive outreach model were developed, implemented and studied, especially in Great Britain, to suit the specific needs of particular client populations, and to fill critical gaps in the mental health treatment system.

Assertive Outreach in Mental Healthcare is a testimony to the clinical richness spawned by the development of the ACT model. This book is a treasure trove for anyone with an interest in the nature, impact and inner workings of assertive outreach teams. The book opens with an excellent update of research on assertive outreach, and also provides practical information about treatment fidelity and flexibility to the assertive outreach model, and the evaluation of treatment outcomes. However, the preponderance of chapters address important clinical, social, experiential and legal issues related to providing assertive outreach to people with a serious mental illness.

Many topics are addressed that have not previously been the focus of attention, and valuable light is shed on the nuances of how to provide assertive outreach effectively, with the utmost respect to service users, and consistently as guided by the long-term goal of recovery. Chapters with a useful 'hands on' approach to assertive outreach teams address how different professionals work together on teams, cognitive behaviour therapy, the treatment of co-occurring substance misuse, and collaboration with family members and significant other persons. Several chapters deal with very important, but hitherto neglected, issues related to the experience of service users receiving assertive outreach, including engagement and recovery, the question of whether assertive outreach stigmatizes or promotes social inclusion of services users, special concerns of Black and Ethnic Minority service users, and diversity. One critical chapter addresses the fundamental challenge inherent to the very nature of assertive outreach: how to foster the autonomy of the service user who is receiving services that could at times be perceived to be, or actually be, coercive. A final chapter concludes with a welcomed reminder that from the outset assertive outreach has involved bending or challenging some of the traditional rules that have governed the provision of mental health services, and calls for a vision of 'funky mental health' that is aimed at nurturing and encouraging creative solutions to specific problems by embracing the individual qualities of team members in order to meet the needs of the diverse range of service users.

Assertive outreach has moved beyond the point of being considered an experimental intervention, and it is now widely accepted as a variant to standard practice for service users who do not access or benefit from the usual services. Like all other mental health services, assertive outreach has evolved from its inception and will continue to change over time. This volume makes a valuable contribution to the field by addressing in depth a wide range of topics critical to the delivery of assertive outreach services that have previously received scant attention in the growing clinical lore on this approach.

References

Stein, L. & Test, M. (1985) *The training in community living model: A decade of experience* (Vol. 26). San Francisco: Jossey-Bass.

Stein, L.I. & Test, M.A. (1980) Alternatives to mental hospital treatment: Conceptual, model, treatment program and clinical evaluation. *Archives of General Psychiatry,* **37**, 392–397.

Test, M.A. (1992). Training in community living. In R. P. Liberman (ed.), *Handbook of Psychiatric Rehabilitation.* pp. 153–170. Boston: Allyn and Bacon.

Test, M.A. & Stein, L.I. (1980) Alternative to mental hospital treatment: III. Social cost. *Archives of General Psychiatry,* **37**, 409–412.

Weisbrod, B., Test, M. & Stein, L. (1980) Alternatives to mental hospital treatment: II Economic benefit-cost analysis. *Archives of General Psychiatry,* **37**, 400–405.

Preface

Assertive outreach practice is sufficiently mature to warrant a book which moves beyond a textbook description of the model to a level of analysis and debate of some of the more thorny issues. We have also set out to reflect on how assertive outreach is adapting to new ideas and challenges in society and in mental health provision. Earlier descriptive texts such as Keys to Engagement (SCMH, 1998) and manuals for implementation such as Allness and Knoedler in the US (1998) and Burns & Firn in England (2002) as examples, did not have the benefit of the last decade of diverse operational experience, new evidence and the value shift and literature of recovery oriented practice. Other texts have favoured a particular model, the strengths approach in assertive outreach (Ryan & Morgan, 2004), or been aimed primarily at a specific professions and psychological approaches (e.g. Cupitt, 2010). This book continues the evolutionary story, through an edited series of chapters from clinicians in the field. The book provides a current perspective on how the assertive outreach model is being applied in the UK and Europe. The book is designed to be used as a reference for anyone with an interest in assertive outreach and the reader can focus on chapters of interest or the whole book.

We have used descriptors for people who use services such as 'patient' or 'service user' interchangeably. We appreciate that the use of some terms (eg. Patient) may bring disapproval from people who experience such labels on a daily basis – the people who use mental health services. We would like to reassure the reader that we have tried our upmost to use contemporary descriptors and remain respectful, without distracting from the text.

This book describes assertive outreach as it is practiced in modern Western societies where personal freedoms are considered to be of the utmost importance. So, it is useful to consider the power that language has to either constrain or open up possibilities for us. Some practitioners, for example, are avoiding the use of the term 'schizophrenia', because they consider it to be an unhelpful and stigmatising label. However, any way of categorising or describing individuals will set up distinctions between people and in applying any form of professional knowledge we are exercising power. Working in multi-professional teams and coordinating care with partner organisations requires acceptance and negotiation in tolerating different perspectives. To some people, assertive outreach will mean nothing more than 'getting them to take their medication'. For others, it requires a willingness to set aside our assumptions and to understand the world as it is viewed by people who have endured very different life experiences from our own. This book presents 'assertive' as a persistent and patient form of caring, rather than an unthinking coercion. Assertiveness means clearly expressing our own views without diminishing the views of others.

We have also adopted the term 'assertive outreach' or 'AO', however, we recognise the term 'assertive community treatment' or 'ACT' is commonly used in some parts of Europe as well as North America and Australia. We, therefore, refer to assertive community treatment or ACT when referring to the North American experience/model or where it is necessary to the text.

This book includes contemporary themes within current assertive outreach practice, as well as cross cutting themes relevant to any area of community mental health practice. Themes include perspectives on the assertive outreach evidence base, team working, psychological therapies, substance misuse, user and carer perspectives, discrimination and diversity, working with Black and Minority ethnic groups, targets and outcomes, the perspective of those who deliver services as well as the perspective of those who receive assertive outreach services. We understand that we may have neglected some key areas, however, we have endeavoured to provide an inclusive text.

Many different areas of research are referred to in the following chapters and different kinds of understanding are promoted in multi-professional work, with diverse social groups. This is not, however, to imply a simple path from knowledge to action and many reflections focusing on real life experiences are included. Contributors speak of their attempts to engage, to understand, to help or simply to be with those who are beyond the reach of established knowledge. The dilemmas that these experiences create in us are important sources of feedback which we need to reflect on and use to guide our practice. We have provided 'reflection points' to encourage the reader to think in depth about some of the many complex ethical issues which arise in practice. Such exercises can be used as a part of the evidence base for the professional's continuing professional development.

Psychosis might be understood as an escape from intrusive meanings, experienced in a hostile and indifferent social world; an improvisation that expresses idiosyncratic meanings and thereby evades the rejecting or stigmatising words of others. The majority of us experience freedom much more tangibly most of the time; that freedom means being able to enjoy relationships, to engage in fulfilling activities, to live in secure accommodation and to have money to spend. The practice of assertive outreach is in the most part about these needs but in many other ways much more complicated. We hope that this volume will bring some light to these darker corners.

Acknowledgements

Much of the breadth of perspective in this book has been enabled by our active involvement with the National Forum for Assertive Outreach (NFAO) over many years, and by extension our American cousin the Assertive Community Treatment Association (ACTA). We would like to thank all those who gave up their time to provide their valued input into making the book possible and for those who provided us with practice based examples that didn't quite make it into the book. We would also particularly like to thank those non-credited reviewers for their time in reviewing key aspects of the book: Dr Christine Padesky, Dr Neil Thompson and Professor Kim Mueser. We would particularly like to thank Professor Mueser for providing the Foreword to the book. We would also to thank Professor Nick Tarrier, Dean Smith and our colleagues who provided some 'behind the scenes' assistance.

Caroline Williams, Mike Firn, Simon Wharne, Rob Macpherson

References

Allness, D. and Knoedler, W. (1998) *The PACT model of community based treatment for persons ith severe and persistent mental illness: A manual for start-up.* National Alliance for the Mentally Ill Anti-Stigma Campaign. Arlington, VA.

Burns, T. and Firn, M. (2002) *Assertive Outreach in Mental Health. A Manual for Practitioners.* Oxford University Press. Oxford.

Cupitt, C. (ed) (2010) *Reaching Out. The Psychology of Assertive Outreach.* Hove, Routledge.

Ryan, P. and Morgan, S. (2004) *Assertive Outreach. A Strengths Approach to Policy and Practice.* Churchill Livingstone, Edinburgh.

SCMH (Sainsbury Centre for Mental Health) (1998) *Keys to Engagement: Review of Care for People with Severe Mental Illness who are Hard to Engage with Services.* Sainsbury Centre for Mental Health, London.

Chapter 1

What does research tell us about assertive community treatment?

Andrew Molodynski and Tom Burns

Introduction

Assertive Community Treatment (ACT) is probably the most researched form of mental health service delivery. Over 90 randomised and non randomised trials have been published throughout the world over a timescale of more than 30 years, since its inception in North America (Marshall & Lockwood, 1998; Burns, 2007). There has also, particularly recently, been a good deal of qualitative research attempting to capture and examine the personal experiences of patients and families in an attempt to understand what it is about ACT that is attractive to many patients and leads to greater engagement.

It may be thought that this wealth of research has brought understanding and a degree of clarity to the area, but for a variety of reasons this has not been the case. The findings of much of the research have been contradictory or of sub optimal quality, reflecting the difficulty of this type of research and of assigning meaning to the findings. These issues are compounded by uncertainty about the terminology used, with Assertive Community Treatment (ACT) being used in the United States (US) and most of the research literature, and assertive outreach and intensive case management often being used interchangeably in the United Kingdom (UK) and the rest of Europe. More recently some consensus has begun to emerge about what may constitute the ingredients of successful care, judged in terms of acceptability and social and clinical outcomes. This chapter presents some of the most important research in the area and derives potential ways forward in both clinical practice and in research.

The rise of a new model

In the mid 1970s in Madison, in the Midwest of the US, a decision was made to close a psychiatric ward. The ward staff was trained to look after people in the community instead in a project labelled Training in Community Living (TCL). This was the first example of what has come to be called ACT. The programme aimed to address comprehensively the

Assertive Outreach in Mental Healthcare: Current Perspectives, First Edition. Edited by C. Williams, M. Firn, S. Wharne and R. Macpherson.
© 2011 Blackwell Publishing Ltd. Published 2011 by Blackwell Publishing Ltd.

Table 1.1   Requirements for community tenure

1	Material resources such as food, shelter, clothing, and medical care. Community treatment programs must assume responsibility for helping the patient acquire these resources.
2	Coping skills to meet the demands of community life. These are skills we take for granted, such as using public transportation, preparing simple but nutritious meals, and budgeting money. Learning these skills should take place in vivo, where the patient will need and be using them.
3	Motivation to persevere and remain involved in life. A readily available system of support to help the patient solve real life problems, feel that he or she is not alone and feel that others are concerned is crucial.
4	Freedom from pathologically dependent relationships. To break the cycle of dependency community programmes must provide sufficient support to keep the patient involved in community life and to encourage growth towards greater autonomy.
5	Support and education of community members who are involved with patients. An important factor that influences patient behaviours and, thus, community tenure are the ways in which community members (family, law enforcement personnel, agency people, landlords, etc.) relate to patients.
6	A supportive system that assertively helps the patient with the previous five requirements. Chronically disabled patients are frequently passive, interpersonally anxious and prone to develop severe psychiatric symptoms. Such characteristics often lead these patients to 'drop out' of treatment, particularly when they are becoming more symptomatic. Hence the programme must be assertive, involve patients in their treatment and be prepared to 'go to' the patient … and actively ensure continuity of care.

(Stein & Test, 1980)

various factors that led to an inability to manage in the community that conventional care did not address adequately. These factors are shown in Table 1.1.

The fledgling service that was based upon these admirably clear principles was the subject of a randomised controlled trial (RCT), with 126 patients assigned either to TCL or hospital based care and rehabilitation. Patients were followed up for 14 months in the TCL programme and then for a similar period after it ended. The results were remarkable (Stein & Test, 1980). Rates of psychiatric readmission (to become the measure of choice in ACT studies) were 58% in the control group and 6% in the TCL group, with average time spent in hospital 20 and 9 days respectively. The TCL group also spent less time unemployed and more time in independent accommodation, and rated higher on measures of self esteem and activities. An economic analysis was favourable and an examination of family and community burden showed no increase in the TCL group. Most gains were lost when the subjects were followed up some months after the end of the programme, highlighting a need for ongoing or indefinite intervention in some cases. As might have been expected, these findings stimulated much interest in North America and overseas. The introduction of teams, however, was far from rapid.

In 1983, these results were replicated in a further RCT in Sydney, Australia (Hoult et al., 1983). The community treatment was home based and offered 24 hour availability from a multi-disciplinary team. It included medication, support, counselling, and social and life skills training along with family support and education. Again results were impressive, with highly statistically and clinically significant reductions in hospital use. Those receiving hospital based care spent on average 53.5 days in hospital over the course of a year compared with just 8.4 days in the project group. In addition to this, patients reported positively about their experience of the community intervention as compared to standard care and there were no significant differences in measures of community burden such as police involvement. A costing study found average direct and indirect treatment costs of A\$4489 for intervention patients and A\$5669 for control patients. The authors concluded that the majority of psychiatric patients could be treated more effectively and more economically outside hospital.

Adoption of the model

Because these two influential studies both found such clear benefit with an assertive community focussed treatment built on basic principles they led to widespread clinical and research replication in several countries. There was extensive commissioning of ACT teams in the US and the introduction of mobile treatment teams in Australia, run along very similar principles. The UK led their introduction in Europe, though initially this was mainly limited to large urban areas. Researchers in South London reported that an intensive community support programme, the Daily Living Project, showed encouraging results early on in terms of symptoms, functioning and hospital use but most gains were lost towards the end of the study period (Marks et al., 1994). The study was compromised by a high profile homicide by an experimental group patient. Control over hospital discharges was withdrawn in the experimental group as a result, diminishing its flexibility.

A large multi-centre study in the US (Rosenheck et al., 1995), the largest ever conducted with 873 participants, showed that intensive psychiatric community care (IPCC) programmes reduced bed use by 89 days (33%) over a 2-year period. In contrast to the earlier studies, they found intensive community care to be marginally more expensive despite the reductions in bed use. This study lent further support to the adoption of ACT as a mainstay of the community care of the severely mentally ill.

Two Cochrane Collaboration systematic reviews (Marshall et al., 1998 and Marshall & Lockwood, 1998) concluded that, while case management was not effective and actually increased admissions to hospital, ACT was clearly superior to standard care in maintaining contact with services and reducing hospital use, while improving satisfaction with services. They concluded that ACT was 'a clinically effective approach to managing the care of severely mentally ill people in the community' (Marshall & Lockwood, 1998: 2). There were also significant improvements in subjects' accommodation and employment status.

These two reviews taken together had an important effect on policy makers and less than a year later ACT teams were specifically prescribed as an essential element of mental health services in the National Service Framework for England (Department of Health, 1999). Funding was provided to start up ACT services and NHS mental health trusts were penalised if they were not established. Targets were introduced for the size of teams and number of patients, but not the exact nature of practice or the quality of care (see Chapter 13).

The dawning of doubt

Despite their huge influence, there were significant limitations in the methodology of the Cochrane reviews that could have influenced their results. One problem was that the designation of what was or wasn't ACT or case management was largely based upon the description by the original study authors, rather than being determined independently. ACT teams were introduced in the UK through the 1990s. Around the time of the Cochrane review several studies were underway that would come to cast substantial doubt on the ability of ACT to improve symptoms and functioning while reducing hospital use.

The first of these to be published was the PRiSM study in London (Thornicroft et al., 1998), which attempted to differentiate between the efficacy and effectiveness of an assertive approach to managing those with severe mental illnesses. The authors defined efficacy as the measurable differences in experimental circumstances, and effectiveness as the usefulness in routine, large scale clinical services for real populations. The design was extremely ambitious and wide ranging and consequently some of the results are hard to interpret. PRiSM found a reduction in bed use in the experimental services compared to standard care, but of a much lower magnitude; their explanation was the dilution of research effects in real world settings with other pressures coming to bear. At the same time, a smaller RCT was conducted by Holloway in London which found no significant differences between standard and intensive case management (Holloway & Carson, 1998): however, numbers were probably too small to positively exclude an effect (35 patients in each group).

The UK700 study (Burns et al., 1999) was a large multi-centre study in which 708 patients in London and Manchester were randomly assigned to intensive case management (ICM, caseloads of 10–15) or standard case management (SCM caseloads of 30–35) and followed up for two years. The primary outcome measure, overall hospital use, was exactly equal in the two groups, a mean of 72 days over 2 years. The conclusion from the study was that reducing workers' caseloads to allow them to work more intensively with people did not affect outcome substantially. It was also suggested that the ability of ACT to reduce bed usage may not be as great in healthcare systems that were already community focussed and using relatively few hospital beds. These results were far from those expected by the authors and generated a vigorous debate.

These negative findings have continued to be replicated. The REACT study (Killaspy et al., 2006) found no reduction in bed use with ACT in standard UK settings. REACT randomly assigned 251 people with psychotic illnesses who were high users of inpatient care to ACT or continuation of Community Mental Health Team (CMHT) follow up and monitored outcome over an 18 month period. The authors concluded that standard UK community mental healthcare was generally capable of supporting people with severe mental illnesses, but that ACT may be better at engaging clients and may lead to greater satisfaction with services.

Further support for this now seemingly robust finding of no difference in bed use has come from a study examining bed usage in a large number of mental health trusts across the UK after the introduction of Crisis Resolution Teams (CRTs) and ACT teams (Glover et al., 2006). Admissions were compared over the time period 1998–2004. While the overall rate of admission declined in most areas (as would be expected) it fell significantly more in areas with early introduction of CRTs but not where these were introduced late. However, the introduction of ACT demonstrated no reduction in admissions. While there are clearly wider factors influencing bed use, the authors considered their findings robust enough to conclude that crisis services reduced bed use but that ACT did not. With the state of current findings it must be concluded (at least in a contemporary UK setting) that ACT does not reduce hospital bed use.

An alternative way of looking at ACT

While the UK700 study, along with the later studies above, found that ACT did not significantly affect outcome, it encouraged a different way of thinking about ACT (and indeed mental health services in general) in the UK. The key question seemed to be: If the overall service does not make a difference is it individual components of care, alone or cumulatively, that influence outcome? This prompted a second question: If this is the case, can we measure the effects of specific aspects of care in a robust and meaningful way?

These questions were not entirely new and in North America attempts to measure fidelity to the ACT model had been made for some years (McGrew, 1994; Teague, 1998). Such attempts were an explicit acknowledgement that specific components of care were important and that ACT teams were not uniform. Such variability is probably greater in the UK as contracting arrangements tend to be less specific. McGrew, in 1994, noted that both research in the field and the implementation of new programmes were being significantly hampered by a lack of information on ACT teams and what they did. He and colleagues were concerned that newly introduced services could 'drift' away from the original models in the successful early studies by Stein and Test and Hoult and, thus, not provide such effective treatment. His group attempted to identify the most important characteristics of ACT. They started by interviewing 22 recognised experts in the field and refined their answers to a list of criteria to judge fidelity. This Index of Fidelity of Assertive Community Treatment (IFACT) included such things as client to staff ratios, a psychiatrist on the team, daily team meetings, twenty four hour availability, home based care and a team approach. These could be operationalised and the score indicated fidelity to the theoretical model.

Later work by Teague and colleagues in New Hampshire (Teague et al., 1998) used a similar approach utilising expert opinion and literature reviews to identify potentially important components. Their final list of twenty-eight components comprised three domains, were operationalised and had a scoring system evolved. The three domains were the structure and composition of the team (H), its organisational boundaries (O) and the nature of what went on (S). They were made explicit to reflect the fact that important components lay in different areas. Table 1.2 shows the 28 final components of the Dartmouth ACT scale (DACTS) which has been widely used in service planning.

Despite general consensus amongst practitioners and researchers on the core elements of a successful assertive outreach service, variability persists in provision and in working practices. The Pan-London Assertive Outreach (PLAO) Study (Wright et al., 2003) undertook to characterise ACT teams across London, including measures of their fidelity to the models above. The PLAO study discovered wide variation in practice, particularly in services provided in the voluntary sector and those addressing groups such as the homeless or

Table 1.2 Dartmouth ACT scale (DACTS)

H1 Small caseload 10:1	O4 24 hour cover
H2 Team Approach	O5 Responsibility for hospital admissions
H3 Frequent programme meetings	O6 Responsibility for hospital discharge planning
H4 Practising team leader	O7 Time unlimited services
H5 Continuity of staffing	S1 In vivo services
H6 Programme operates at full staffing	S2 No dropout policy
H7 At least 1 full time psychiatrist per 100 patients	S3 Assertive engagement
H8 At least 2 full time nurses per 100 patients	S4 Intensity of service high if needed
H9 Substance abuse specialist on staff	S5 High frequency of contact
H10 Vocational specialist on staff	S6 Work with support system with or without patient
H11 Sufficient staff size to provide consistent cover	S7 Individualised substance misuse service
O1 Explicit entry criteria	S8 Dual diagnosis treatment
O2 Low intake rate to maintain stable service	S9 Dual disorders model, considering interaction of illness and substance misuse
O3 Full responsibility for services (Housing, employment etc.)	S10 Consumers of services on treatment team, providing direct services

(Teague et al., 1998)

those from ethnic minorities. They found that (out of 24 teams studied) four rated as 'high fidelity' and three as 'low fidelity' to the ACT model as measured by the DACTS, with the rest in between.

Such differences do not always seem to reflect the deliberate adherence to or deviation from a theoretical model but are more naturalistic and dependent upon external factors. There are variations in size of team and whether there is direct medical input, in working practices such as availability outside of standard office hours, the use of the team approach and the thorny issue of responsibility for inpatients. There are significant variations in the availability of support work, psychological input and family intervention between teams. It appears that, if anything, this variability is increasing with time in the UK. The reasons for this are unclear, but may reflect the fact that individual health trusts are more autonomous than previously and also that ACT services are less important for their ratings so that more flexibility of approach is permitted. This will lead to innovative solutions to local issues in some places but there is a danger that drift from successful models may reduce clinical effectiveness.

A way forward

It is perhaps more useful to consider the elements of ACT that may make it successful rather than focussing on the services, with all their heterogeneity. The IFACT and DACTS were first steps on this path, but more recent empirical work, both qualitative and quantitative, has advanced our knowledge further.

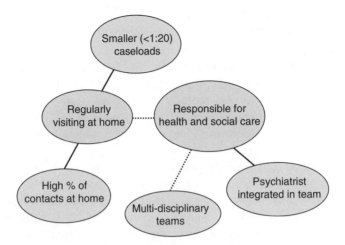

Figure 1.1 Components of care. Continuous lines represent statistically significant association ($p < 0.05$), broken lines association at trend level ($p < 0.10$).
Wright et al., 2004. Reproduced under the terms of the Click-Use Licence.

A Health Technology Assessment (HTA) for the Department of Health (Burns et al., 2001) and a systematic review by Catty and colleagues (Catty et al., 2002) examined the evidence for home treatment as a whole in contrast to the reviews by Marshall and Lockwood, which discriminated between different models prior to analysis. Marshall's approach could theoretically generate 'purer' results, but ran the risk of misidentifying services given the lack of evidence for their classification. By avoiding this potential pitfall, Catty and colleagues could examine a large body of evidence and investigate which components of care were most common and test which might make a difference (Wright et al., 2004). Hospital use, the most consistently reported outcome measure, was used as the benchmark for comparison. The analysis showed a group of related factors that characterised home treatment services and (using cluster analysis) their association (see Figure 1.1).

Using regression analysis the study demonstrated that there was a significant association between visiting patients at home and having joint responsibility for health and social care and reduced hospitalisation. Interestingly, the six components that were found to be associated did not reliably distinguish between service model labels, but were adopted to a greater or lesser extent in all types of home based care. This could both explain much of the heterogeneity in research findings and identify a way forward for service planning and further research.

All these potentially beneficial factors make sense. If we spend more time with our patients and attend to more of their needs (particularly those that cause them worry such as financial or housing problems) we will forge better relationships and be able to help more. Few probably doubt such an argument, yet we still don't really have the evidence to support it. This lack of evidence from research is compounded by the finding that only about a quarter of the experimental teams survived in their original form after the trials were over (Wright et al., 2004). Such findings cast further doubt as to how reproducible the effects are in routine clinical practice, particularly over the prolonged time periods that are often needed to help individual patients make lasting changes to their lives.

Qualitative research

The research examined above identifies what may help in improving outcome, but has not attempted to consider why. Such questions are extremely difficult to pose, never mind answer. However, over recent years there has been a substantial increase in the amount and sophistication of qualitative research in ACT, providing us with interesting and important information that underpins findings from the quantitative studies.

A good example is a study by Priebe and colleagues (Priebe et al., 2005) that explores the views of engagement and disengagement held by ACT patients. Forty selected patients were interviewed in depth. The sample purposively included a disproportionate number from African-Caribbean backgrounds known to be less satisfied with conventional services. There was a wide variety of views, but some themes were clearly identifiable, and these are shown in Table 1.3. The first column shows the most common reasons given by patients for their initial disengagement from mainstream services and the second column shows the reasons cited by them for their better engagement with ACT teams.

These results resonate with Stein and Tests' initial proposal that patients value being treated as individuals with a depth of character and some personal worth. This is perhaps not surprising, but may well be the most important factor in the increased engagement and retention in care of this disenfranchised group. Some quotes from those interviewed illustrate the point:

> *I felt like they never listened to me and they were just making choices for me and if they listened to me a bit more then I might have felt a bit more like I was. I just felt that my life was out of control and I didn't have a say in what I was doing.* (28 year old man talking about previous therapeutic relationships)

> *I talk to him about films and theatre and books and arts, and which balances it out because I don't really want someone coming to my flat making me feel mad.* (39 year old woman talking about relationship with an assertive outreach worker)

> *You don't talk to them purely about how I have taken my tablets and this. I mean it is broader than that.* (48 year old woman talking about lack of focus on medication)

Such quotes do not constitute evidence of causality, but they do back up the empirical evidence regarding engagement and have high face validity; such sentiments are commonly expressed by patients in clinical practice. Very few practicing clinicians in the field will not have heard something very similar. As the authors identify, however, this is not necessarily a 'win-win' situation in ACT. Not infrequently we are in a position where we have to choose between respecting our patient's wishes and accepting a course that may lead to relapse or alternatively following established evidence which can entail conflict with patient wishes. In the current risk averse climate, these dilemmas can be especially acute for individual practitioners and teams.

Table 1.3 Engagement and disengagement

Disengagement from mainstream services		Engagement with ACT services	
Theme	n (sample = 40)	Theme	n (sample = 40)
Desire to be an autonomous and able person.	26	Time and commitment (of staff).	22
Lack of active participation and poor therapeutic relationships.	22	Social support and engagement without a focus on medication.	31
Loss of control due to medication and its effects.	15	Partnership model of therapeutic relationship.	11

(Priebe et al., 2005)

Is there a consensus on the place of assertive community treatment?

The answer to this question is not a straightforward yes or no. However, it is becoming apparent that clinicians and researchers in the field can reach consensus on a number of points:

1 ACT does not harm people.
2 It does not significantly reduce bed use in contemporary UK systems.
3 It is neither cheaper nor more expensive than standard care.
4 It improves the engagement of hard to reach people.
5 It is appreciated by patients and their carers.

As regards what it is that may make it work, some themes are emerging from the meta analyses and qualitative work of recent years. The following five features are significantly associated with high quality home based care:

1 Multi-disciplinary working.
2 Smaller caseloads.
3 Responsibility for both health and social care.
4 A dedicated psychiatrist on the team (if possible dedicated in approach as well as availability!).
5 High rates of home visiting (rather than office contacts).

High rates of home visiting and responsibility for health and social care are associated with reduced bed usage even if the overall model is not, and it is worth considering all five features briefly in turn.

1. Multi-disciplinary working

Multi-disciplinary working is now established practice in most countries with developed healthcare systems. It is widely accepted to be the most effective way to provide support to the severely mentally ill. It is the bedrock of all UK community mental health services, albeit with some variability. The research evidence and practical experiences have taken us to the point where we no longer question it; it simply seems the right thing to do. However, it is important to keep trying to ascertain what it is about multi-disciplinary working that is successful; it is here that qualitative work has provided such valuable insights.

2. Smaller caseloads

There have been substantial shifts in our understanding of this issue, with the early land-mark studies showing huge apparent differences with reduced caseloads but later (prima-rily UK based) research showing that ICM with resulting smaller caseloads did not reduce the need for inpatient care. The much vexed question of caseloads is less settled, with the initial clear advantages of intensive (10–12 cases per worker) over standard (30–35 cases) case management becoming very much reduced with improved research. However, more recent studies, notably that of Wright and colleagues, have found good evidence that defined caseloads (<1:20) are an important feature of good quality home based care. This is an important finding as it shifts the focus of attention to something very practical and measurable, which is partly independent from the broad model of service delivery employed. For instance, a CMHT could be allowed to develop capacity for some staff to have a reduced caseload and work with people assertively, rather than pass people on to another service. Such an arrangement would be similar to the old 'bolt-on' ACT services, which by popular agreement were not felt to work well at the time, although some recent Dutch work does suggest they may have a place. Any move in this direction would require careful consideration.

Currently there are three types of service or 'team' that broadly fit into an assertive approach and that have reduced caseloads. These so-called 'modernisation teams' were prescribed by the National Service Framework (Department of Health, 1999) a decade ago and are now available in most areas of the UK. They are ACT, Early Intervention, and Crisis and Home Treatment Teams. All differ in their target popula-tion but all have limited caseloads and aim for an assertive and personalised approach to the care of the severely mentally ill. Caseloads in the UK vary between 10 and 20 for each care coordinator in ACT and early intervention teams, with more variability amongst crisis teams.

Defined caseloads allow a more individualised approach and it is this which patients and their families appreciate. They allow both practitioner and patient to develop a real-istic expectation of the level of contact which is no longer entirely crisis driven. This in turn may lead to greater engagement and retention in treatment. Where the boundary lies is uncertain in day to day practice. Some workers appear able to offer highly individual-ised support with fairly large caseloads while others are unable to do so even with limited caseloads. This may stem as much from the personality and drive of the worker, and from their appreciation of the others' feelings, as from any model of service delivery. It is a reminder of the need for effective management and supervision of all staff, along with a framework in which to do it (Burns & Firn, 2002).

3. Responsibility for both health and social care

Teams responsible for the broad range of care for individuals appear to be more effective at improving outcomes for their patients. The evidence supports a reduction in bed use and greater engagement and retention in treatment when the same core team can provide both health and social care. This may be due to their offering far greater continuity of care than traditional services where people are passed from team to team. Most generic mental health teams now operate along similar principles with attempts to provide care and support 'in house' first. This may include social support, occupational therapy or psychological input among other things. It reduces delays in help being given and inefficiency through repeated assessments. Both are often reported as being very frustrating for patients (and often staff!) and can lead to disengagement.

It makes common sense that disenfranchised people with adverse experiences of care in the past are far more likely to accept interventions from people they know and have worked with than if they are expected to attend appointments in far off buildings for further 'assessments' prior to anything being done. Effective interventions, such as family therapy for people with psychosis, improve outcomes and should, resource imperatives withstanding, be available in the team itself or be very easily accessible.

This principle also applies beyond the team in service level arrangements for resource allocation and structuring. Conflicting demands upon health trusts and social services departments may create an impasse that is not in the best interests of the patient. Progress requires that the barricades are taken down. Combined health and social care is experienced as holistic care by patients, they experience themselves being treated as 'people' rather than just 'patients'. The team attends to various needs in a coordinated way rather than focussing on a narrow spectrum of interest to professionals. Priebe's work (Priebe et al., 2005) strongly supports this view.

4. Dedicated psychiatric input

In some ways this may be the most vexed issue at a local level with much variability in practice. This is despite the research evidence and the commonly reported difficulties in ACT teams who have to relate to a number of different psychiatrists, many of whom have different ways of doing things. These psychiatrists will also have different levels of interest in, and commitment to, the ACT service and those under its care as they balance their differing priorities.

Having a psychiatrist on the team achieves a number of seemingly important objectives, both in terms of the care of individual patients and in a wider organisational context. Working as part of the team, attending meetings and talking with the other members regularly, the psychiatrist can easily keep abreast of the lives of patients. This enables them to take a much more personalised and knowledgeable approach when they see patients, often at times of great difficulty. It also enables them to get to know the team members well and respond to their requests intelligently. Care coordinators can have very different attitudes towards risk (for example) necessitating very different responses to seemingly similar requests. It is hard for an outsider to gain this type of knowledge and work in such a way with a team. The embedded psychiatrist fits well with the general principle of the team doing as much as possible and only out-sourcing when absolutely necessary, usually for some kind of specialised therapy or intervention or for physical healthcare.

Organisationally, a consultant can help to give the service a voice. This can provide security and help to maintain and develop the service. Rightly or wrongly it is much harder for a non-medical team leader to influence decisions as effectively. Assuming the psychiatrist is a reasonable individual, their presence usually improves working practices and relationships reducing turnover and burn out.

5. High rates of home visiting

In Stein and Test's original TCL programme home visiting was considered important on the grounds that psychotic patients had impaired transfer of skills learning. It has survived because of its impact on engagement. Visiting people at home increases contact. They might otherwise not come to appointments, either because they are too disorganised or because they lack understanding of their need for treatment. This can increase engagement and allow effective interventions. You cannot really help a person with their social anxiety or day to day budgeting, or persuade them to take medication, if you aren't seeing them consistently because they don't turn up. This holds whatever the reason for poor attendance and the remedy seems to be the willingness to go to the person physically, alongside the willingness to approach them as an individual with strengths as well as difficulties (Ryan & Morgan, 2004).

The evidence shows a significant association between home visiting and better outcome, but it could simply be that high rates of home visiting is a proxy measure for better quality services. Such services may have more motivated staff or increased investment and priority in local healthcare systems. It is unlikely that these factors could explain the research findings, but findings such as Glover's with crisis teams (Glover et al., 2006) remind us to consider them.

Where does all this leave us?

The effectiveness of ACT, as measured by careful research, depends on the criteria used to judge it. Using the fairly narrow criteria of hospital bed use and symptom levels, the early studies in the US and Australia showed striking improvements but these have not been replicated recently. There may be several reasons for this, but the contribution of improved standard care is fairly compelling. More broadly, the evidence from a number of studies (regardless of location) shows improvements in engagement and satisfaction, reductions in victimisation and improved social functioning in ACT teams. A recently published observational study in the Netherlands (Bak et al., 2007) demonstrated an increased probability of 'transition to remission' (getting substantially better) in ACT patients as opposed to those receiving standard care (31% versus 19%). However, there was also an associated reduction in hospital bed use which raises questions about the quality of standard care.

ACT is now well established as one of the cornerstones of community care for those with severe mental illnesses. It is likely to be around for some considerable time in the

UK. Interestingly, this is not the case across the rest of Europe, even in comparatively well funded mental health systems. UK services are now maturing and diversifying to meet local need. It is more important than ever for those involved in services, whether as clinicians or planners, to consider the evidence, in terms of what has been shown to improve patient outcome but also practices which are not supported by evidence.

It is likely that research will continue to focus on the individual elements of care to refine practice further. The days of large head-to-head trials are probably now over in the UK and US, but studies focusing on social and clinical outcomes may be of continuing use in service planning and delivery. In mainland Europe, where ACT services (and multi-disciplinary working generally) are less developed new trials may still provide important insights for UK practice. Perhaps the most important lesson from the rapid development of ACT, both in clinical practice and in research, is that to be successful it must take note of both international and very local issues. Above all it must be an interaction between individuals based upon clear and easily understandable principles that are effective in real world situations.

References

Bak, M., van Os, J. & De Bie, A. (2007) An observational, 'real life' trial of the introduction of assertive community treatment in a geographically defined area using clinical rather than service use outcome criteria. *Social Psychiatry and Psychiatric epidemiology*, **42**, 125–130.

Burns, T., Creed, F., Fahy, T., Thompson, S., Tyrer, P. & White, I. (1999) Intensive versus standard case management for severe psychotic illness; a randomised trial. *The Lancet*, **353**, 2185–2189.

Burns, T., Knapp, M., Catty, J., Healey, A., Henderson, J., Watt, H. & Wright, C. (2001) Home treatment for mental health problems: a systematic review. *Health Technology Assessment*, **5**(15), 1–139.

Burns, T. & Firn, M. (2002) *Assertive Outreach in Mental Health, a Manual for Practitioners*. Oxford University Press, Oxford.

Burns, T., Catty, J., Dash, M., Roberts, C., Lockwood, A. & Marshall, M. (2007) Use of intensive case management to reduce time in hospital in people with severe mental illness: systematic review and meta-regression. *British Medical Journal*, **335**(7615), 336–340.

Catty, J., Burns, T., Knapp, M., Watt, H., Wright, C., Henderson, J. & Healey, A. (2002) Home treatment for mental health problems: a systematic review. *Psychological Medicine*, **32**, 383–401.

Department of Health (1999) *The National service framework for Mental Health; modern standards and service models*. Department of Health, London.

Glover, G., Arts, G. & Babu, K.S. (2006) Crisis resolution/home treatment teams and psychiatric admission rates in England. *British Journal of Psychiatry*, **189**, 441–445.

Holloway, F. & Carson, J. (1998) Intensive case management for the severely mentally ill. *British Journal of Psychiatry*, **172**, 19–22.

Hoult, J., Reynolds, I., Charbonneau-Powis, M., Weekes, P. & Briggs, J. (1983) Psychiatric hospital versus community treatment: the results of a randomised trial. *Australian and New Zealand Journal of Psychiatry*, **17**, 160–167.

Killaspy, H., Bebbington, P., Blizard, R., Johnson, S., Nolan, F. & Pilling, S., et al. (2006) The REACT study: randomised evaluation of assertive community treatment in north London. *British Medical Journal*, **332**, 815–818.

Marks, I.M., Connolly, J., Muijen, M., Audini, B., Mcnamee, G. & Lawrence, R.E. (1994) Home-based versus hospital-based care for people with serious mental illness. *British Journal of Psychiatry*, **165**, 179–194.

Marshall, M., Gray, A., Lockwood, A. & Green, R. (1998) Case management for people with severe mental disorders (Review). *The Cochrane Library* 2009, issue 1.

Marshall, M. & Lockwood, A. (1998) Assertive community treatment for people with severe mental disorders (Review). *The Cochrane library* 2008, issue 4.

McGrew, J.H., Bond, G., Dietzen, L. & Salyers, M. (1994) Measuring the fidelity of implementation of a mental health program model. *Journal of Consulting and Clinical Psychology*, **62**(4), 670–678.

Priebe, S., Watts, J., Chase, M. & Matanov, A. (2005) Processes of disengagement and engagement in assertive outreach patients: qualitative study. *British Journal of Psychiatry*, **187**, 438–443.

Rosenheck, R., Neale, M., Leaf, P., Milstein, R. & Frisman, L. (1995) Multisite experimental cost study of intensive psychiatric community care. *Schizophrenia Bulletin*, **21**, 129–140.

Ryan, R. & Morgan, S. (2004) *Assertive Outreach, a Strengths Approach to Policy and Practice*. Churchill Livingstone, Edinburgh.

Stein, L. & Test, A. (1980) Alternative to mental hospital treatment. 1. Conceptual model, treatment program, and clinical evaluation. *Archives of General Psychiatry*, **37**, 392–397.

Teague, G.B., Bond, G.R. & Drake, R.E. (1998) Program fidelity in assertive community treatment: development and use of a measure. *American Journal of Orthopsychiatry*, **68**(2), 216–232.

Thornicroft, G., Wykes, T., Holloway, F., Johnson, S. & Smzukler, G. (1998) From efficacy to effectiveness in community mental health services; PRISM psychosis study 10. *British Journal of Psychiatry*, **173**, 423–427.

Wright, C., Burns, T., James, P., Billings, J., Johnson, S. & Muijen, M., et al. (2003) Assertive outreach teams in London: models of operation. Pan-London assertive outreach study, Part 1. *British Journal of Psychiatry*, **183**, 132–138.

Wright, C., Catty, J., Watt, H. & Burns, T. (2004) A systematic review of home treatment services; classification and sustainability. *Social Psychiatry and Psychiatric Epidemiology*, **39**, 789–796.

Chapter 2

Multi-professional working in assertive outreach teams

Hannah Steer and Steve Onyett

Introduction

The New Horizons consultation document on mental health services states:

> A key rationale for teams is that they can provide access to the range of specialist skills and expertise necessary to provide a comprehensive assessment of needs and a wide-ranging plan of treatment for people with multiple and complex problems. (Department of Health, 2009: 27)

Guidance for assertive outreach services states that:

> Assertive outreach services are best provided by a discrete, specialist team that has staff members whose sole (or main) responsibility is assertive outreach. (Department of Health, 2001: 19)

Fully-staffed multi-disciplinary assertive outreach teams include nurses, psychiatrists, social workers, occupational therapists, clinical psychologists and support workers. There may also be specialist workers in vocation and substance abuse, and consumers. They work together to provide a comprehensive range of intensive evidence-based services to clients with severe mental illness, in order to help them to achieve a life that is not driven by their mental illness (Stein & Santos, 1998; Burns, 2004). Typical interventions may focus on: treatment issues (medications, physical healthcare and symptom control); rehabilitation issues (employment, activities of living, interpersonal relationships and housing); substance abuse issues; practical assistance and crisis resolution; social issues; and family issues.

Many key attributes that define assertive outreach relate to multi-professionals working together (Test & Stein, 1976): for example, the team approach, multi-disciplinary staffing and integration of services. Team working is a product of personal skills and temperament (e.g. empathy), generic mental health skills (e.g. recognition of psychopathology) and professional training and skills (e.g. prescribing medication; mental capacity assessment). Assertive outreach teams should be designed to focus on motivation, and the need to match level of engagement with the way services are delivered. They are, thus, well suited

Assertive Outreach in Mental Healthcare: Current Perspectives, First Edition. Edited by C. Williams, M. Firn, S. Wharne and R. Macpherson.
© 2011 Blackwell Publishing Ltd. Published 2011 by Blackwell Publishing Ltd.

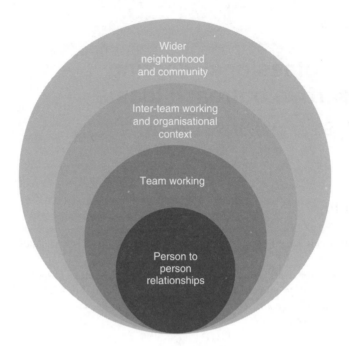

Figure 2.1   The team work holarchy.

to work with people who often have complex issues around dual diagnosis, physical health, social, criminal and vocational problems, in addition to their primary severe mental health issue.

Assertive outreach clients present with a diverse and complex range of health and social care needs that require the very best that effective team working can deliver. This chapter presents key features of multi-professional working within assertive outreach, prior to exploring some of the dilemmas and challenges associated with this way of working in everyday clinical practice.

Working as a team

When thinking of team working it is important to think of it as a whole that represents part of a wider system. It also crucially needs to have as its core the promotion of effective relationships between clients and staff. Without that, there is no platform for the assessment and wide range of interventions described above. Looking outwards it is also crucially important that the team connects well with other teams and the wider organisation and promotes connections with the wider range of neighbourhood resources which the client, as a local citizen, has a right to access.

Figure 2.1 describes team working as a 'holon' or 'whole-part' (Koestler, 1967; combining the Greek 'holos' meaning whole and the suffix 'on' which suggests a particle or part). Clearly the illustration is a gross simplification and this holarchy would need to connect horizontally with other holarchies that form part of ordinary life such as those concerned with work, education, leisure, the wider local community and society in general. However, the key message is that each level both transcends and includes the levels below and must work to support effective working in that level and the levels it transcends and forms part of.

Edwards (2005) describes how:

> Work teams include, but are more than (transcend), the sum of interactions between pairs of individuals (dyads); organisational departments include, but are more than, the sum of interactions between teams and dyads; organisations include, but are more than, the sum of interactions between departments, teams and dyads. (Edwards, 2005: 271)

It is crucially these interactions and how we make them more effective that is the concern in effective team working.

Key assertive outreach practices that are supported by team working

The central importance of the therapeutic relationship has been widely recognised in mental health since the 1950s (Burns, 2004). Assertive outreach crucially emphasises establishing effective working relationships between clients and staff to achieve agreed goals. This includes efforts to achieve effective engagement both with the team and other services. Other key practices may be defined in terms of what, how, when and where the work is done, as described in Table 2.1 (see also Gregory & Macpherson, 2006).

Key values and attitudes

Values and attitudes of the individual worker, the team and the whole organisation are important for any mental health worker to build effective relationships with clients and colleagues (Bleach & Ryan, 1995; Repper, 2000; Department of Health, 2001; Williamson, 2003) and so achieve effective team working. Indeed:

> Practitioners require more than a prescribed set of competencies to perform their role. Capability extends the concept of competence to include the ability to apply the necessary knowledge, skills and attitudes to a range of complex and changing settings. (SCMH, 2001: 2)

Research shows that users put values and attitudes before skills and knowledge as necessary attributes of services and staff (Institute for Healthcare Development, 1995). Key staff values and attitudes likely to promote effective multi-professional working include warmth, empathy, genuineness and respect, as well as having an approach that is friendly, non-judgemental, persistent and creative. Energy, reliability and commitment are qualities required for developing constructive and effective relationships over long time frames. Other qualities are especially important to cope with the dilemmas and challenges of this type of work. For example:

Table 2.1 Key practices and illustrations of these practices from the Gloucester assertive outreach team

	Assertive outreach key practices	Clinical illustration
What	• Providing services (education, support, treatment and therapy) that are relevant and individually focused. Bristol MIND's user-led study of assertive outreach teams highlighted that people were not intrinsically 'hard to engage' but rather simply did not see that what was on offer was relevant to them (Davies et al., 2009). • Holding knowledge about services in the community, covering both the range and quality of providers. • An understanding of the working of local authorities, benefits and housing agencies, health and social care provision and the voluntary sector. • Emphasis on monitoring and review.	Workers have strong links and regular communication with locality community mental health, substance misuse, child and adolescent and specialist rehabilitation services as well as with a range of residential units (including supported lodgings, respite care, council provision and non-statutory accommodation), the criminal justice system and children in need services. There is a regular system of multi-disciplinary review, where specific outcomes such as engagement and social functioning are monitored in addition to usual clinical indicators (e.g. number of contacts, hospital admissions).
How	• Having flexibility – of working hours, activities undertaken and length of time spent on activities together. • Being proactive in providing practical support and assistance – rather than just brokering referrals to other agencies. • Integrating different inputs for an individual rather than just collecting more – achieved through maintaining responsibility regardless of who else is involved. • An ability to work with or for users – rather than making plans on their behalf.	Workers are from five different professional disciplines as well as support workers, from a range of backgrounds with varying personal experience of mental health issues. Support for clients includes addressing psychiatric, psychological and physical health needs as well as social, financial, occupational, leisure and self-care aspects of individual's functioning. The team has developed an allotment with clients, in a local council allotment site. This combines skills from a number of different professions within the team, to help clients achieve not only exercise and healthy living goals, but also in terms of developing meaningful occupation; enabling socially inclusive ventures; relationship building; as well as providing support to cope with psychiatric symptoms such as paranoia, negative symptoms, anxiety and depression.

• Workers having the right 'style' – informed by their own life experience. Staff reflect the demographic characteristics of the locality, the life experience of clients, and promote choice for clients. 'New Horizons' (Department of Health, 2009) highlights the value of employing staff with experience as clients themselves as a way of promoting a service that is more responsive to need. • Having low expressed emotion – non-critical, non-judgmental and accepting, including accepting a certain level of risk. • Having limited caseloads.	The team operates an 8am–8pm seven day a week service, with caseload capacity limited to 75 (with 12 multi-disciplinary staff in the team). The team's approach incorporates a philosophy of assertive engagement and intensity of contact within a community setting. Some clients have been working with the team since it was set up in 2001, and are visited on a daily basis when their mental health difficulties so require (which sometimes involves crisis out-of-hours team support).
When • Available 24-hours a day, or at the very least having a very strongly coordinated and seamless approach to working with other out-of-hours teams. • Persistence is required to develop the therapeutic alliance – even up to 6 months. • Commitment to long-term relationships, over at least 12 months but often many years. • Working as intensively as required, with the capacity to visit several times a week if necessary. • Providing input that is not time limited – as long in terms of frequency, intensity, and duration as required.	
Where • Ability to work with users in informal settings including work in the client's own social environment where appropriate and where they and the practitioner feel safe to do so. By working as much in context as possible the individual's wider context is effectively considered in the work.	The majority of multi-disciplinary care programme approach reviews within the team are carried out in the client's home, underlining the commitment to outreach work with clients.

Reflection point

- Reviewing the bullet points above, how does the team that you know best compare? First of all run through the list highlighting from 1 to 5 how important that feature of team practice is in your opinion with 1 representing 'Not important at all' and 5 meaning 'Absolutely crucial'.
- Now run through again, this time rating where you feel your team is now from 1 to 5 where 5 is 'We are brilliant at this' and 1 is 'We don't do this at all'.
- Now subtract the second number from the first (you might get some negative numbers, e.g. 2–5 = –3). What does this tell you about where to direct some attention?

- Maintaining optimism (in the reality of relapse, setbacks and lack of change).
- Working with extreme views or where clients may have experienced feelings of discrimination or oppression from services in the past.
- Taking positive risks (workers need to enable clients to use their own resources and to do things that they may not agree with, or where there may be a risk of failure).
- Friendliness and informal helpfulness, whilst also managing professional boundaries.
- Ability to appropriately express and contain feelings that may be triggered in working in situations of high levels of emotional volatility.
- Tolerance (for example, of working in difficult and messy environments, with uncertainty and unpredictability).
- Tact and diplomacy (where liaising and advocating on behalf of clients with services that may have previously excluded or marginalised them).

Thus multi-professional team working is not just a combining of individual disciplines with professional training and skills. Team working represents multiple components of an individual client's care. All team members take responsibility for meeting together, jointly reviewing progress and making joint decisions about treatment plans – as well as allocating tasks.

Working appreciatively

Working 'appreciatively' describes an approach that gets played out at all the levels of a teamwork holarchy (Figure 2.1). It is about specifically focusing on appreciating the positive that individuals and groups bring to a situation. Guidelines on assertive outreach stress the need to focus on at least one aspect of the client that can be viewed positively and focused on, regardless of disturbed or challenging behaviour. This includes their personal strengths and resources, the value of what they have done already, and particularly actions that (either in themselves, or in the outcomes they produce) are in some way like the preferred future those individuals describe for themselves. In that this solution-focused approach appears to be effective at a clinical level (de Shazer et al., 2007) it seems fruitful to explore how such principles might play out at different levels within systems at clinical, team and inter-team levels.

For staff to exercise the non-judgemental approach that is required for effective work with people with psychosis, they also need to be able to exercise and receive such non-judgemental and affirming relationships from colleagues, managers and leaders. Part of taking a non-judgemental approach within the team includes working well with different ideologies of care (Coombes & Wratten, 2007). This is not just about being nice. There is considerable evidence that the creation of a 'positive emotional climate' at work is associated with better outcomes on a range of measures (Ozcelik et al., 2008). Jackson and McKergow (2002) have pioneered the application of solution focused thinking to organisations and 'appreciative inquiry' is another organisational intervention that consciously seeks out and expresses people's best resources, assets and intentions (Cooperrider et al., 2003; Hammond, 2008).

The desire to do good work with clients is usually at least one important shared value that transcends interpersonal differences. Giving voice to this, and consciously highlighting positive practice, creates a bedrock of appreciative working in the team that serves to prevent conflict becoming personalised or persecutory, or the exercise of illegitimate power relationships being played out within the team (Pelled, 1995). Conflict is important and necessary to team functioning. There is no reason why teams should adopt a uniform ideology and greater diversity means that a greater range of knowledge, skills and experience is brought to bear. Indeed, rather than focussing on areas of commonality which precludes new solutions emerging, the communications within the team should instead value diversity and, thus, the fuller universe of solutions which might therefore emerge.

At best, teams should aim for a deep dialogue (as formulated by Bohm, 1996) to emerge where team members are able to suspend assumptions and judgements, and promote active and attentive listening and individual and collective reflection on the thoughts and ideas that emerge. Contrary to popular wisdom, it is not always crucial to resolve 'relationship' conflicts, unless of course one party is subject to oppressive or bullying behaviour. Collaboratively managing new task conflicts while ignoring interpersonal annoyances may sometimes be beneficial in facilitating team working (De Dreu & Van Vianen, 2001).

The issue of generic and specialised roles

A generic approach was characteristic of the 'all things to all people' ideology of some community mental health centres of the late 1980s where valued notions of democratic team structures and flat hierarchies served to fudge the need to examine individual practice, skill mix within the team and individual team members' different levels of authority to make decisions (see Cupitt et al., 2010). In effect those with the most complex needs lost out (Patmore & Weaver, 1991).

Assertive outreach has moved on from this traditional view of 'generic' working. The Department of Health (2005a) states that: 'Assertive outreach teams should have a good mixture of mental health and social care disciplines' [and that] 'Individual competencies should be recognised and made best use of.' (Department of Health, 2005a: 6). In assertive outreach, clients have a designated care coordinator from within the team who takes on a lead role for coordinating care with allocated clients (Department of

Health, 1990), thus holding a 'generic' role that transcends traditional boundaries of professional expertise. Workers should possess at least a minimal competence across a range of areas (Kent & Burns, 2005), including:

- Motivational interviewing.
- Administering and monitoring medication in the community.
- Assessing medication side-effects.
- Diagnosing and managing substance misuse.
- Cognitive behaviour therapy.
- Family therapy.
- Life planning.
- Assessing activities of daily living.
- Vocational assessment and rehabilitation.

Although the care coordinator takes a lead role in 'coordinating' the client's health and social care, it is recognised that individual workers with different professional backgrounds and roles within the team, can offer different levels of specialist knowledge and skill. Care delivery is therefore shared between all workers within the team framework and workers hold 'specialist' roles where clinically indicated. This provides a depth and diversity of roles and fulfils a multi-professional team working approach (if these 'specialist' roles were not required, there would not be a need for the multi-professional aspect of the team functioning). For example, in many teams delivering medication (a shared team task) is seen as a means to enable exploration of other areas of the person's life than merely symptom control.

Nurses provide skills in mental state examination, medication management and delivery, direct personal care, and psychological interventions – nurses are trained in CBT and reviews showed most moved into assertive outreach teams following Thorn training programmes. Social workers have skills in addressing complex social care needs, addressing finances and appointeeship, Mental Health Applications, child protection issues, specialist residential provision, knowledge about local resources and funds, developing and monitoring tailor-made placements. Occupational therapists' skills involve evaluating the organisation of time and leisure, being specialists in vocational rehabilitation as well as in group work activities including family support groups or leisure groups. Clinical psychologists offer skills in psychological interventions (CBT for delusions, hallucinations, depression etc.), as well as behavioural analysis and specialist assessments for 'stuck' or 'challenging' clients. Medics have skills in prescribing, and organise involuntary treatment when needed. In addition to this, because of their status, they can also be instrumental in achieving action in relationships with the outside world where case manager or team manager input has failed. The skills that support workers offer are crucial in developing relationships with clients and engaging them in day-to-day activities within community settings.

There is, therefore, a need for core activities that are shared across the team, while at the same time diversity is maintained and wholesale 'generic' working is avoided. Even so this can present a challenge to professional boundaries (Wharne, 2005) with professionals fearing that they might lose their identities. There is also the risk that workers might rigidly follow their professional training and the team might not be able to develop an integrated approach. This leads to different and contradictory interventions (at the same time, or in consecutive periods of care). It is important that the balance between

> **Box 2.1**   Case discussion balancing multi-disciplinary working
>
> Bob has been supported by the assertive outreach team for some years. Prior to working with the team, he was compulsorily admitted to hospital, having no awareness of the ex-treme nature of his beliefs and the concern his behaviours caused. The first stage of team support involved low-key supportive nurse and medic contact, providing medication while genuinely listening to Bob's issues and concerns with empathy and not judging him as others from mental health services had done. Whilst delivering medication, conversations about issues to do with finances, family stresses, meaningful activity and accommodation began to take place. Relevant professionals within the team began to be able to provide specialist input to support Bob to fulfil his goals and aspirations in many areas of his life. Psychotic symptoms continued, but he began to achieve things despite these ongoing dif-ficult experiences, with continued support of the medic, nurse, social worker, occupational therapist and clinical psychologist within the team. Bob started an educational course, ap-plied successfully for a bus pass, moved to his own flat and began to explore and resolve significant psychological issues from his past. After seven years of assertive outreach working with Bob, his quality of life has significantly improved along with his level of en-gagement with mental health services and community activities.

specialised and generic work is thought through between team leader and each worker, and it is important that the whole team 'owns' this balance. This is part of the challenge of effective team working that characterises any clinical team as illustrated in the case discussion summarised in Box 2.1.

Advantages and challenges of a team approach

In a pure assertive outreach model there is value placed on a 'team approach' whereby all clients are expected to have a relationship with all members of the team, rather than a single worker in a care coordinator or key worker role. This is something quite specific and not the same as simply good team working. Some of the advantages claimed for this approach include:

- Opportunities for more intensive and flexible responses as different staff can be called upon to respond to changing need.
- Reliable weekly contact because workloads are shared.
- A better response to crises that is not reliant on one worker's availability.
- Preferences of the client can be accommodated within the team.
- Better access for users to staff who may share or be sensitive to their unique cultural and ethnic background.
- Improved continuity of care because strong relationships with individual staff have not come and gone.
- Reduced stress for staff, partly because of the greater containment of the emotional responses of staff to clinical work.
- Better peer support and consultation.
- Avoidance of 'pathological dependency' whereby the worker's ability to improve the mental health of the client paradoxically reinforces their low self esteem, and sense of inadequacy and personal failure.

A number of examples of assertive outreach team working approaches in the UK have been published: including teams in Croyden and Wandsworth (Firn, 2007), Gloucester (Gregory & MacPherson, 2006), Knowsley (Williams, 2005), East Sussex (Wharne, 2005), and North East Wales (Jones, 2002). These teams have evolved in their work, based upon different experiences (successes and difficulties) in trying out the 'team approach'.

Effective team working requires clear hierarchy; this builds role clarity within the team. There is also a need for a high frequency of meeting (although this can cause time management issues). There is some evidence for effective engagement among clients and good morale among staff in teams using this approach (Gauntlett et al., 1996). However, there are also major downsides:

- Some clients have a preference for individual relationships with fewer staff (ibid). Spindel & Nugent identified difficulties 'for any human being to establish warm, supportive, and trusting relationships with a "team"' (Spindel & Nuget, 1999: 7). Similarly, Burns & Firn (2002) found it problematic in working with people who were mistrustful.
- It can be difficult for all staff members to know all clients well enough to retain adequate knowledge of relapse signatures, risk indicators and social networks.
- Engaging individuals in treatment is more difficult if they have to deal with lots of staff instead of a few. Williams (2005), for example, found that a team approach can increase distress and anxiety as users have to meet new people and this can sabotage recovery.

Burns & Firn (2002) note that in reality many teams claiming adherence to the team approach operate more flexibly in response to need. The most pragmatic and sensitive response is usually to consider the individual and their social networks as the centre of the team and build the required supports and relationships around them on the basis of their preferences, needs and experience of what works. Far from always being 'pathological', periods of dependence on support from an individual are part of a normal pathway to independence. Burns & Firn (2002) advocated building up one relationship through time, commitment and consistency and only then working to expand the network of people involved so that at least three members of the team are fully familiar with them. Therefore, some individuals successfully engage with only one or two team workers, whereas others get to know all of the team over time. This is the pattern described in Knowsley by Williams (2005) where clients received the bulk of care from several individuals in a subgroup of the assertive outreach team (about three to five staff members, and never less than two) in a generic way. On occasion, however, other team members do provide specific elements of care such as dropping off a prescription or relaying messages about planned activities.

Reflection point

Based on your knowledge of this client group where do you feel that your team should be on this continuum from purely individual case working to a full blown team approach where individual more exclusive relationships are frowned upon? Where are you in practice? Do you need to make any changes?

Box 2.2   The key features of effective team working

1   Clear and achievable objectives.
2   Differentiated, diverse and clear roles.
3   A need for members to work together to achieve shared objectives.
4   The necessary authority, autonomy and resources to achieve these objectives.
5   A capacity for effective dialogue. This means effective processes for decision making, being able to engage in constructive conflict and if complex decision making is involved the team needs to be small enough (no larger than eight or nine people).
6   Expectations of excellence.
7   Opportunities to review what the team is trying to achieve, how it is going about it and what needs to change.
8   Clear and effective leadership.

The challenge of effective team working

The overall state of team working in health and social care is fairly parlous when considering the potential. For example, The Healthcare Commission (HC, 2006) NHS National Staff Survey revealed that 89% of staff responded positively when asked: 'Do you work in a team?' However, this shrunk to only 41% when the survey explored whether the team in question fulfilled criteria for a clearly defined team. These findings have been consistent every year since 2003. These are described in Box 2.2 (summarised from Onyett et al., 2007), pertaining to any kind of team (and are similar to the team definition used in the Healthcare Commission surveys).

In effective teams, each worker can see the contribution that they make to the aims of the team as a whole, whilst also working together to achieve team objectives (Carter & West, 1999). If this interdependency is not there to meet the complex range of presenting needs in assertive outreach, then it is questionable whether a team is needed.

In addition to the core features above, Allred et al. (2005) suggest that an effective assertive outreach team:

- Operates as a 'unit of expertise'. Maintaining the team as a unit is particularly challenging where workers are geographically dispersed or work on their own in the community away from close supervision supported by the traditional office setting.
- Constantly organises and reorganises itself in response to client needs. This really requires that the team is able to make the very best use of the diversity within the team described above.
- Works across professional boundaries in an interactive and integrated fashion.

It is important to acknowledge that while a team may be thinking about long term goals with respect to work with clients, the client themselves may be living, deciding and choosing minute by minute. Nonetheless a good working formulation of how the client's current issue emerged and what precedes and maintains problematic behaviours will be needed (see Johnstone & Dallos, 2006). This forms the basis of collaborative work both within the team and with the client on small next steps to a preferred future.

Team practice and process

The process of assertive outreach team working in supporting clients, according to Gold et al. (2003), includes the following:

- Both clients and the assertive outreach team, in their joint efforts, are primary agents of change.
- Workers take responsibility to engage clients into working alliances by gently instilling hope for relief, fostering a sense of safety and personal control, motivating taking on the tasks of healing, respecting and ensuring self-determination on the pathway to healing, and restoring of self-identity as a 'whole' person.
- Workers learn more about clients' patterns for response to internal and external factors impinging on their symptomatology.
- Workers and clients collaboratively develop intervention plans (this empowers client decision making and specifies goals and tasks for each worker and client).
- These interventions are constantly reviewed and adapted in the context of clients' preferences, interests, illnesses and disabilities fluctuating over time.

In addition to maintaining up-to-date clinical knowledge, Kent & Burns (2005) highlight other important clinical skills and attributes:

- Competence in assessment and management of risk (either to self or others) and the related skills in positive risk taking, boundary setting and risk minimisation.
- Managing the dilemmas of what constitutes 'success' in assertive outreach – this may vary from client (e.g. sorting out my benefits) to workers (e.g. maintaining contact with a previously disengaged client) to purchasers/planners (e.g. reducing hospital admissions and improving medication concordance). Managing the dilemmas and tensions associated with varying targets are important.
- Awareness of recent policy changes and implications for care provision.

Finally, there needs to be a recognisable and agreed process for communication and decision making. Although diversity is key, team members must have shared social reality about what they are doing, and a shared language with which to describe this reality. Building this shared reality should start with the experience of the client, and use language that promotes their inclusion. A mature team with stable membership is better placed to develop members who can take the perspective of others into account in relation to both their emotional and cognitive position. In these circumstances the team is better able to recognise the source of communication difficulties when they arise. Ideally, decision making is visible, inclusive and coherent, and it is afforded time and substance (see 'To learn more' below).

Inter-team working

Effective multi-professional assertive outreach teams have a good understanding and connect well with other teams, the wider organisation and the range of community resources which the client has a right to access. This helps to address the social inclusion and wide ranging needs of clients over long periods.

'Warm networking' describes the connecting that assertive outreach teams engage in with other teams: being well connected and inter-relating well with other parts of the system

(Bowles & Jones, 2005). This is not simple. Most team members will be familiar with the criticism and stereotyping of other parts of the system that characterises local inter-team working. Classically, for example, acute inpatient staff can be stereotyped as oppressive 'medical model' pill pushers, and CMHT staff as reactionary, burnt out and passive-aggressive. In return, assertive outreach workers are seen as spoilt prima donnas over concerned with their team boundaries and special identity. It is the unfortunate client who, on top of any existing stigma and disaffection with services, has to navigate these troubled waters. This negative team stereotyping is part of a natural and universal tendency to form groups partly through denigration of other groups. Nonetheless it has to be actively tackled.

Richter et al. (2006) highlighted the role of boundary spanners (e.g. staff who work across team boundaries), often the team managers, who have a dual identity – a positive sense of belonging to both the team and the wider organisation or service. They found this dual identity was positively related to effective inter-group relations, particularly if they had frequent contact with other groups. Their identification with the bigger picture appeared to function as a buffer against the detrimental effects of group identification by shifting the focus to the larger group without blurring team boundaries. Whilst appreciating the bigger picture it was important that the team could see how it made its own particular contribution to the aims of the service as a whole, and the values that underpinned it. This is another good reason for taking time to articulate why the service as a whole is there.

Richter et al. (2006) concluded that managers could combat ineffective inter-group relations by enhancing employees' identification with their organisation while acknowledging teams for their individual performance. Measures for enhancing organisational identification could include communication of organisational successes, values and goals; rotation of individual boundary spanners into key roles; promotion into boundary positions of employees with dual identification; ensuring that inter-group working is on the team's agenda, frequent inter-group meetings and inter-group social gatherings. Some assertive outreach team staff have 'split posts' within assertive outreach and generic adult mental health teams. This enables connection between teams. This also embeds interventions within a wider access of larger team resources. For example, shared group leisure or sports activity provide opportunity for peer support and self-help.

Reflection point

Think about the team that you have most difficulty working with and that you feel your team needs to work more effectively with in the interests of clients. How could you go about getting to know that team better?

Team leadership

Effective multi-professional team working – within the team, across teams and with clients of the team – is promoted by effective team leadership. Gowdy & Rapp (1989) noted that effective managers of community mental health teams constantly modelled good practice. They tended to focus less on traditional features of management such as attending

---

Box 2.3 Team leader activities that promote effective inter-professional team working

- Appropriate selection of staff – who are mindful (bring themselves into the present and are attentive to detail, alert, caring, notice changes, sense danger and coordinate actions); have diverse expertise and life experience; have expertise in a specific area as well as understanding how their expertise relates to that of other team members.
- Create opportunities for team members to discuss professional identities and values, as these are often a source of tension that can prevent team members from connecting and relating (for example, through team reflective practice sessions).
- Increase the number, variety, frequency and ways that team members participate in decisions.
- Encourage informal leaders so the team can learn that their fellow team members are working toward team goals rather than personal goals, and that they have the competencies to complete critical tasks.

- Create a work climate that makes open communication, questioning, exploring, experimenting and learning feel safe.
- Encourage team members to learn what other team members are doing by creating overlapping knowledge bases, because roles may disintegrate under pressured or novel conditions, but the knowledge necessary to act in a coordinated fashion can remain alive.
- Encourage rich, frequent personal interactions among team members (communication is a crucial source of coordination and groups that cannot interact easily are likely to malfunction in times of uncertainty).
- Support the goal of combining insights of different team members (who represent different areas of expertise/viewpoints) in ways that produce a new and/or shared understanding of what is currently happening.

---

meetings, preparing reports and proposals and instead spent most of their time helping clients or staff to achieve their goals. Recent research on team management found that the single most important factor in leadership in both predicting staff productivity and service outcomes was the leadership capacity to engage with others and, in particular, showing personal concern for the welfare and aspirations of the people they line managed (Alimo-Metcalfe et al., 2008). Making the most of the individual contributions that workers bring to the team is a key task for the team leader in effective multi-professional team working. The table in Box 2.3 summarises tasks and goals that go some way toward achieving this (as suggested by Allred et al., 2005).

There are some very practical contextual issues concerning the wider service that only leaders and managers at team level and above can address. Assertive outreach clients need fair access to the care programme approach and effective risk management processes. It is also important that client pathways to, through and from team-based provision have clear and dedicated capacity to work with this group and so demand and capacity need to be mapped locally. Inclusion and exclusion criteria that teams adopt when looked at holistically within a locality should not create gaps for people to fall into. Otherwise they are likely to find themselves 'bounced' around the local service, which is devaluing, creates further disaffection and works against effective engagement with local services. Where people are 'bounced' this should be audited and reported to service commissioners (Clark, 2008). Managers above team level also have particular responsibility for avoiding the 'trip wires' (Hackman, 1994) that impede effective team working such as:

- Describing the performing unit as a team but continuing to manage members as individuals.
- Failing to exercise appropriate authority over the team – leaving it to clarify its own aims and boundaries regardless of what is happening around it.
- Failing to provide organisational supports in the form of rewards, training, information and the material resources required to get the job done.
- Assuming that team members already have all the competence they need to work well in teams.

Team leadership is about creating a supportive environment for creative thinking, for challenging assumptions about how the service should be delivered. It is also about sensitivity to the needs of a range of internal and external stakeholders, inside and outside the team and the organisation. Managers of front-line staff must be visible and available to staff and accountable for service delivery (SCMH, 1998). Whoever holds the team leader position requires an open, transparent and equitable approach in order to manage diverse staff and disciplines. The 'New ways of working for psychiatrists' report states:

> Clearly no discipline can claim to have exclusive competences for [team leadership] as a consequence of their professional training. Individuals from all professional backgrounds need to be developed and selected with care to fulfil these crucial team management/leadership roles (Department of Health, 2005b: 46, see http://www.newwaysofworking.org.uk).

Ultimately the job of the leader is to create an environment wherein everyone can exercise leadership to the full extent of their power and authority, including clients themselves. It is, however, important that formal leadership roles are clear and that there is an absence of conflict about leadership. This is associated with leadership clarity which in turn is associated with clear team objectives, high levels of participation, commitment to excellence and support for innovation (West & Markiewicz, 2004).

Multi-professional team working and managing boundaries

In assertive outreach team working, ethical and professional dilemmas abound. A number of these relate to boundary issues. Gutheil & Brodsky (2008) describe a boundary as 'the edge of appropriate behaviour at a given moment in the relationship between a client and worker.' (Gutheil & Brodsky, 2008: 4).

Examples of such dilemmas are visible from the moment a request is made to the team to accept a client onto their caseload, to the point the assertive outreach team completes their involvement in that person's care:

- Managing referrals and discharges to the team. As in all parts of the health service, it is important that assertive outreach teams work with appropriate clients, and are able to hand care over to other teams when work with the client has been completed. The team leader holds a crucial role in regulating this, supporting the team to be clear about who to work with, for how long, and communicating with services outside the team to help regulate these processes. For example, since regularly meeting with community mental health team leaders, the assertive outreach team in Gloucester has been able to joint-work and discharge clients to those services in a timely fashion, whilst also maintaining awareness of the most appropriate referrals to be made to the team.

- Navigating the challenges of 'therapeutic engagement'. The central aim of working with a client in assertive outreach is to engage that person in a meaningful relationship in order to achieve therapeutic goals. In addressing social inclusion goals, it may be more acceptable for the worker to take on the role of a professional who is being friendly in order to support the person to join in community life; for example, both client and worker joining a snooker club or walking group. In addressing substance misuse and money management issues, taking the stance of supporter is important. However, it's also relevant to evaluate carefully the client's request for '20 quid to tide me over' because they've just spent all their benefit on crack cocaine leaving them no money for the rest of the week. In such a situation, supplying an emergency food ration (loaf of bread and tin of beans) could be a powerful therapeutic tool. Role clarity helps to maintain firm yet fair boundaries, to offer support in a way that doesn't directly collude with illegal and health-risking behaviour.

- Managing the expectations and consequences of frequent, informal and often lengthy time spent with the client as part of therapeutic contact. For example, meeting in cafés and pubs for 'clinical' interventions, the accepting or giving of gifts, providing a social life or sharing personal information.

- Attending to issues around dependency which develop as client and workers' attachment processes play out. This requires thoughtful reflection as dependency can vary in its level of helpfulness to the client, worker and therapeutic task.

- Managing the balance between collaboration and coercion. A study exploring client experiences of assertive outreach support (Krupa et al., 2005) indicates that there is a fine line between assertiveness and being controlling. Respondents saw that the assertive approach used by staff was helpful in engaging them in treatment and in encouraging the persistence necessary to manage community struggles. However, the relationship was not always ideal. They saw some workers as stepping over 'the line' and becoming authoritative and intrusive, largely around choices regarding medication and finances. Supportive elements of the relationship seemed at times inhibited by workers who maintained strict professional–client relationship boundaries, or by a worker's lack of familiarity with a client. The introduction of the new Mental Health Act (Department of Health, 2007) which includes the provision of Compulsory Treatment Orders highlights this dilemma, producing pressure for workers to become potential agents of social control.

Generally for any worker in the team, an awareness of the differences between friendships, therapeutic relationships and being a carer are important to hold in mind. These boundary issues and dilemmas will be more or less relevant for different professionals and workers within the team, depending on their roles and responsibilities. Ethics (the theory of moral conduct), NICE guidelines, professional codes of conduct and operational policies all provide guidance for workers and teams in providing appropriate assertive outreach interventions. See Gray & Johanson (2010) for further exploration of some of these issues. The opportunity to reflect on these challenges (in shared or individual reflections) helps the assertive outreach team to maintain a healthy, ethical stance in its care provided.

> ### Reflection point
>
> Think about the client that you met with most recently. What boundary issues were you navigating during that meeting, and that maybe have arisen at other times during that person's care? Can you identify how these issues are being managed by you as an individual and as a team? What pressures do you feel and are they legitimate? What might the client say about it?

Taking positive risks

One particular dilemma for workers is how to work with clients in therapeutic ways, whilst also ensuring safety and risk minimisation. Effective teams are more likely to be able to deal with unusual, risky or complex situations (which are likely to challenge the team's ability to respond to need). This is helped by having a system that can handle risk and manage each worker's anxiety (Bowles & Jones, 2005), such as shared assessment and collective decision making.

For assertive outreach teams, it is common for positive risks to be taken in many areas of a client's care. Here are a number of clinical examples of taking positive risks with individual clients:

- Accommodation – supporting someone to move to an independent flat, where they may never have managed to live on their own before.
- Changing medication – supporting someone to change or reduce their psychiatric medication, where in the past they have become unwell.
- Managing symptoms – supporting someone to be in charge of collecting and taking their own medication, when compliance has been an issue in the past.
- Treatment – supporting someone to apply for a review of their Compulsory Treatment Order, even though the team has mixed views.
- Illicit substance use – supporting someone to minimise their use of drugs or alcohol, where abstinence has been impossible for them in the past.
- Relationships – supporting someone to find and make contact with their family, who've lost contact through the consequences of their mental health problem.
- Education and work – supporting someone to return to university, when their first episode of psychosis occurred during their university studies.
- Meaningful occupation – supporting someone who is keen to volunteer at the local library, even though at times they are suspicious of people.
- Social inclusion – supporting someone to join water aerobics classes, even though they find it difficult to get up in the daytime.

Box 2.4   Clinical illustration

The assertive outreach team always takes a shared risk in moving a client from hospital to an individually-tailored independent care placement in the community. For one client with major physical and mental health problems and regular aggressive behavioural outbursts, her preference was to live near her family in her local community as opposed to an out-of-county nursing home. This goal involved specialist input from the psychiatrist and social worker to liaise with and bring together multiple teams from physical and mental health statutory services, the independent sector, together with client and family (who had already experienced some traumatic and negative experiences of services). Through listening to all parties, making objective judgements, with support of professional and team supervision, the workers managed to reach an agreed plan with all parties for the move. With much support, the client moved and has now been settled in local accommodation for over a year without the need for hospital readmission.

Risk taking is an important part of enabling clients to make informed choices about their own lives, with safe support for their intended actions. Workers in the team need to share and contain their own anxieties, acknowledge and learn from mistakes, and work together to support whatever appropriate clinical decisions are made (see Box 2.4).

Staying effective

Being able to acknowledge and handle ethical and professional issues, and also having personal attributes that clients find helpful, are all part of being an assertive outreach worker. Multi-professional working within assertive outreach services allows for sharing of responsibility and expression of different professional viewpoints, in an attempt to resolve some of the ethical dilemmas. However, competing demands (such as engaging with a chaotic client group and ensuring the continued safety of the public) can place stress on individual workers. Workers and the team need to commit to training, supervision and support in order to help sustain effective practice in the long term.

A key feature of team working that should be particularly highlighted is the need for participative safety, in other words the capacity of the team to welcome contributions from all team members (e.g. in meetings) without their being any fear of ridicule or abuse (West & Markiewicz, 2004). The work is stressful not only because of the nature of the clients' presentations but also because of organisational issues such as such inter-team difficulties, funding issues, lack of services to refer on to and lack of training and support. It is therefore crucial that the team defends time to look at its internal processes, including (as referred to above) maintaining awareness of all its strengths and assets, and particularly the ways in which energy and creativity can be maintained through people feeling able to contribute to their best even when ideas may seem a bit tentative or 'half-baked'.

The usual format of these support structures are in the form of supervision or reflective practice groups. Reflective practice is 'a process by which the practitioner should stop and think about their practice, consciously analyse their decision making processes, and

---

Box 2.5   Aspects of a successful staff support group

Setting up the group
- There is mutual agreement on the choice of facilitator (seen as neutral in terms of their relationship with the team, and there is sufficient common ground to work with the team).
- Room and time arrangements are appropriate.

Aspects of the group itself
- Based on realistic and agreed expectations.
- Deals with important issues.
- A sense of safety is established and maintained.

Aspects the facilitator brings to the group
- He or she sets up the group with clarity, transparency and full staff involvement.
- Style and technique are appropriate to the needs of the group.
- He or she helps the group stay 'on task'.
- Aware of his or her own responses and takes care not to let them interfere with their role as facilitator.

Review processes
- There are arrangements for monitoring the group's success in meeting the needs of members and the organisation.

Box 2.6   Clinical illustration

A reflective practice group has been running in the Gloucester Assertive Outreach Team for several years. Meetings are held on a fortnightly basis with the usual multi-disciplinary team meeting being shortened to allow time for the group to run (for an hour). The group is facilitated by the team's clinical psychologist, who has responsibility for keeping the group planned, structured and boundaries in place. The goals, purpose, timing and regularity of the group were agreed as the group was set up. The focus of each meeting is negotiated with the team in advance, and usually the care coordinator introduces a client for reflection – usually someone causing concern to the team, or a 'new' person to the team's caseload (although the team has also effectively used the space for reflecting on team or organisational dilemmas). Regular feedback helps the group maintain its focus and evolve. Reflective practice is well attended by all staff disciplines and valued highly by the team – demonstrated by the team being very pro-active in attending to gaps in reflective practice provision (during facilitator absence or staff re-allocation).

---

relate theory to what they do in practice' (Kennard & Hartley, 2009: 14). Reflective practice groups provide an agreed time and place to step outside the work with clients, to reflect on what was done and the feelings aroused. Experiences are shared and learned from. They are led by a facilitator who maintains structure and timing issues, and encourages members to maintain a degree of emotional detachment. Hartley & Kennard (2009) propose and elaborate on a number of key ingredients that contribute to a successful staff support group, outlined in Box 2.5. These are helpful for any assertive outreach team considering their own support needs (see clinical illustration in Box 2.6).

The more formal support mechanisms help the team as a whole work well together as well as helping team members as individuals to cope with the stresses of the job. In other words, according to Hartley & Kennard (2009), they help to:'

- Promote the value and the practice of open communication.
- Provide a protected time and space in which staff can get support from colleagues and learn from each other.
- Sustain staff well-being (which enables better client care and smoother team functioning).
- Enable staff to express, discuss and manage difficult or painful emotional responses (such as guilt and anxiety) to people and situations in their work.
- Enable staff to be sensitive to others' feelings and emotional states (clients and colleagues).
- Acknowledge and normalise the experience of vulnerability.
- Enable the team to discuss and address obstacles to team working that may arise from issues between individuals, within the team as a whole, or between the team and the wider organisation.

Reflection point

What one thing could you consider with your team in order to help stay effective?

Final thoughts and where to find out more

Ultimately team design and process needs to be shaped by individual and collective need as assessed locally. The ideal is to start with the individual (see Figure 2.1) and let form follow function. Effective management of team processes, good team work and supervision contribute to team satisfaction in their work and, hence, the ability to develop good, flexible therapeutic relationships (Department of Health, 2005a). What works well at a clinical level, is likely to work for all of us, wherever we are in the local service system. And in terms of clinical governance for multi-professional team working, this encompasses supervision and critical reflection on how the team and individuals are working. The Department of Health (2005a) stipulates that teams should routinely monitor what they do, and this is bringing a number of initiatives led by the Department of Health to measure outcomes: they are already using this to commission services for the future.

This chapter has only been able to scratch the surface of a very wide ranging subject. In addition to the texts in our reference list, a comprehensive **review of some of the key issues with respect to team working** may be found in the 'Working Psychologically in Teams' document at http://www.bps.org.uk/the-society/organisa tion-and-governance/professional-practice-board/new_ways_of_working_for_ applied_psychologists.cfm.

For more detail of team work issues, including team design, process and leadership see Onyett (2003).

For an immensely scholarly review of a range of team work issues see Byrne (2006). See also the same author's forthcoming guidance on team working written for the Irish Mental Health Commission.

For recent guidance on **responsibility and accountability issues** see the National Institute for Mental Health in England (NIMHE) National Workforce Programme (NWP; 2009).

For issues concerning **team training** see the Creating Capable Teams Approach (CCTA) at http://www.newwaysofworking.org.uk.

Or for the 'Effective Teamworking and Leadership Programme' see Onyett et al. (2009); see http://www.innovation.cc/scholarly-style/onyett6.pdf.

For tools for **evaluating the effectiveness of your team working**, see:

The Integrated Team Monitoring and Assessment (ITMA). However, using such tools outside of an affirming solution-focused development process is not advocated. Otherwise people may merely assess their team as poor and become demoralised.

The Aston Team Performance Inventory (ATPI) http://www.readiness-tools.com/tool-full.aspx?toolguid=0d6382ad-f017–4623–8d10–93f2f314e346.

The Aston Team Performance Inventory (ATPI) http://www.astonod.com/atpiView.php?page=1.

The Community Mental Health Team Effectiveness Questionnaire (CMHTEQ). See Rees, et al. (2001), The Productivity Measurement and Enhancement System (ProMES). http://promes.cos.ucf.edu/index.php.

For more on **working appreciatively and with a solution focus**:

The Centre for Solution Focus at Work. hppt://www.sfwork.com.

A very rich source of SF papers and presentations from around the world. http://www.solworld.org.

Home of the work of Cooperrider, the founder of Appreciative Inquiry. http://www.appreciativeinquiry.case.edu/.

Good source of publications on Appreciative Inquiry at University of Virginia. http://www.appreciativeinquiry.virginia.edu.

References

Alimo-Metcalfe, B., Alban-Metcalfe, J., Bradley, M., Mariathasan, J. & Samele, C. (2008) The impact of engaging leadership on performance, attitudes to work, and well-being at work: a longitudinal study. *Journal of Health Organization and Management*, **22**(6), 586–598.

Allred, C.A., Burns, B.J. & Phillips, S.D. (2005) The assertive community treatment team as a complex dynamic system of care. *Administration & Policy in Mental Health*, **32**(3), 211–220.

Bleach, A. & Ryan, P. (1995) *Community Support for Mental Health*. Sainsbury Centre for Mental Health, London.

Bohm, D. (1996) On Dialogue. In: *On Dialogue*, (ed. Nichol, L.). pp. 6–47. Routledge, London.

Bowles, N. & Jones, A. (2005) Whole systems working and acute inpatient psychiatry: an exploratory study. *Journal of Psychiatric & Mental Health Nursing*, **12**, 283–289.

Burns, T. & Firn, M. (2002) *Assertive Outreach in Mental Health: A Manual for Practitioners.* Oxford University Press, Oxford.

Burns, T. (2004) *Community Mental Health Teams: A Guide to Current Practices.* Oxford University Press, Oxford.

Byrne, P. (2006) A response to the Mental Health Commission's discussion paper 'multidisciplinary team working: from theory to practice' (January 2006). *The Irish Psychologist,* **32**(12), 323–339.

Carter, A.J. & West, M.A. (1999) Sharing the Burden – Teamwork in HealthCare Settings. In: *Stress in Health Professionals: Psychological and organisational causes and Interventions,* (eds. R. Payne & J. Firth-Cozens) pp. 191–202. John Wiley & Sons, Chichester.

Clark, J. (2008) *'On the Bounce.' Understanding Mental Health Systems in the NW.* Care Services Improvement Partnership.

Coombes, L. & Wratten, A. (2007) The lived experience of community mental health nurses working with people who have dual diagnosis: a phenomenological study. *Journal of Psychiatric & Mental Health Nursing,* **14**(4), 382–392.

Cooperrider, D.L., Whitney, D. & Stavros, J. (2003) *Appreciative Inquiry Handbook: The First in a Series of AI Workbooks for Leaders of Change.* Lake Shore Communications, Bedford Heights, OH.

Cupitt, C. (2010) *Reaching Out: The Psychology of Assertive Outreach.* Routledge, London.

Cupitt, C., Gillham, A. & Law, A. (2010) The Whole Team Approach: Containment or Chaos? In: *Reaching Out: The Psychology of Assertive Outreach,* (ed. C. Cupitt) pp. 43–63, Routledge, London.

Davies, R., Shocolinsky-Dwyer, R., Mowat, J., Evans, J., Heslop, P. & Onyett, S.R. (2009) *Effective Involvement in Mental Health Services: Assertive Outreach and the Voluntary Sector.* Bristol Mind: Bristol. Available to download at http://www.bristolmind.org.uk

De Dreu, C.K. & Van Vianen, A.E. (2001) Managing relationship conflict and the effectiveness of organisational teams. *Journal of Organisational Behavior,* **22**(3), 309–328.

Department of Health (1990) *The Care Programme Approach for People with a Mental Illness Referred to the Specialist Psychiatric Services.* Department of Health, London.

Department of Health (2000) *NHS Plan: A Plan for Investment, a Plan for Reform.* Department of Health, London.

Department of Health (2001) *Mental Health Policy Implementation Guide.* Department of Health, London.

Department of Health (2005a) *Assertive Outreach in Mental Health in England. Report from a Day Seminar on Research, Policy and Practice.* Department of Health, London.

Department of Health (2005b) *New Ways of Working for Psychiatrists: Enhancing Effective, Person-Centred Services Through New Ways of Working in Multidisciplinary and Multi-Agency Contexts.* Department of Health, London.

Department of Health (2007) *Mental Health Act.* Department of Health, London.

Department of Health (2009) *New Horizons: Towards a Shared Vision for Mental Health.* Consultation, Department of Health Mental Health Division, London.

Drake, R.E., McHugo, G.J., Clark, R.E., Teague, G.B., Xie, H. & Miles, K. (1998) Assertive community treatment for patients with co-occurring severe mental illness and substance use disorder: a clinical trial. *American Journal of Orthopsychiatry,* **68**(2), 201–215.

Edwards, M.G. (2005) The integral holon. A holonomic approach to organisational change and transformation. *Journal of Organizational Change Management,* **18**(3), 269–288.

Firn, M. (2007) Assertive Outreach: has the tide turned against the approach? *Mental Health Practice,* **10**(7), 24–27.

Gauntlett, N., Ford, R. & Muijen, M. (1996) *Teamwork: Models of Outreach in an Urban Multi-cultural Setting.* Sainsbury Centre for Mental Health, London.

Gold, P.B., Meisler, N., Santos, A.B., Alberto, B., Keleher, J. & Becker, D.R., et al. (2003) The program of assertive community treatment: implementation and dissemination of an evidence-based model of community-based care for persons with severe and persistent mental illness. *Cognitive and Behavioural Practice*, **10**, 290–303.

Gowdy, E. & Rapp, C.A. (1989) Managerial behaviour: the common denominator of effective community-based programs. *Psychosocial Rehabilitation Journal*, **13**(2), 31–51.

Gray, A. & Johanson, P. (2010) Ethics and Professional Issues: The Universal and the Particular. In: *Reaching Out: The Psychology of Assertive Outreach*, (ed. C. Cupitt). pp. 229–247, Routledge, London.

Gregory, N. & MacPherson, R. (2006) The Gloucester Assertive Community Treatment Team: a description and comparison with other services. *Irish Journal of Psychiatric Medicine*, **23**(4), 134–139.

Gutheil, T.G. & Brodsky, A. (2008) *Preventing Boundary Violations in Clinical Practice.* Guilford Press, Guilford.

Hackman, J.R. (1994) Trip wires in designing and leading work groups. *The Occupational Psychologist*, **23**, 3–8.

Hammond S.A. (1998) *The Thin Book of Appreciative Inquiry* (2nd edn). Thin Book Publishing Co., Oregon.

Hartley, P. & Kennard, D. (2009) *Staff Support Groups in the Helping Professions: Principles, Practice and Pitfalls.* Routledge, London.

Healthcare Commission (2006) *Mental Health and Learning Disability Trusts, the Views of Staff: Key Findings from the 2006 Survey of NHS Staff.* The Healthcare Commission, London.

Institute for Healthcare Development (1995) *Core Competencies for Mental Health Workers.* NHS Executive North West Office, Manchester.

Jackson, P.Z. & McKergow, M. (2002) *The Solutions Focus.* Nicholas Brealey Publishing, London.

Johnstone, L. & Dallos, R. (2006) *Formulation in Psychology and Psychotherapy: Making Sense of People's Problems.* Routledge, London.

Jones, A. (2002) Assertive community treatment: development of the team, selection of clients, and impact on length of hospital stay. *Journal of Psychiatric and Mental Health Nursing*, **9**, 261–270.

Kennard, D. & Hartley, P. (2009) Ten Keys to a Successful Staff Support Group. In: *Staff Support Groups in the Helping Professions: Principles, Practice and Pitfalls*, (eds. P. Hartley & D. Kennard). pp. 26–33. Routledge, London.

Kent A. & Burns, T. (2005) Assertive community treatment in UK practice: revisiting … setting up an assertive community treatment team. *Advances in Psychiatric Treatment*, **11**, 388–397.

Koestler, A. (1967) *The Ghost in the Machine.* Arkana, London.

Krupa, T., Eastabrook, S., Hern, L., Lee, D., North, R. & Percy, K., et al. (2005) How do people who receive assertive community treatment experience this service? *Psychiatric Rehabilitation Journal*, **29**(1), 18–24.

National Workforce Programme (2009) *Moving On: From New Ways of Working to a Creative Capable Workforce – Guidance on Responsibility and Accountability.* The National Institute for Mental Health in England. http://www.newwaysofworking.org.uk/pdf/0330_randaguidanceconf.pdf

Onyett, S.R. (2003) *Teamworking in Mental Health.* Palgrave, London.

Onyett, S.R. (2007) *Working Psychologically in Teams.* British Psychological Society/National Institute for Mental Health in England.

Onyett, S.R., Rees, A., Borrill, C., Shapiro, D. & Boldison, S. (2009) The evaluation of a local whole systems intervention for improved team working and leadership in mental health services. *The Innovation Journal*, http://www.innovation.cc/scholarly-style/onyett6.pdf

Ozcelik, H., Langton, N. & Aldrich, H. (2008) Doing well and doing good. The relationship between leadership practices that facilitate a positive emotional climate and organizational performance. *Journal of Managerial Psychology*, **23**(2), 186–203.

Patmore, C. & Weaver, T. (1991) Unnatural selection. *Health Service Journal*, **10** Oct, 20–22.

Pelled, L.H. (1995) Demographic diversity, conflict, and work group outcomes: an intervening process theory. *Organization Science*, **7**, 615–631.

Rees, A., Stride C., Shapiro, D.A., Richards, A. & Borrill, C. (2001) Psychometric properties of the Community Mental Health Team effectiveness questionnaire (CMHTEQ). *Journal of Mental Health*, **10**(2), 213–222.

Repper, J. (2000) Adjusting the focus of mental health nursing: incorporating service users' experiences of recovery. *Journal of Mental Health*, **9**, 575–587.

Richter A.W., West, M.A., Van Dick, R. & Dawson, J.F. (2006) Boundary Spanners' identification, intergroup contact, and effective intergroup relations. *Academy Of Management Journal*, **49**(6), 1252–1269.

SCMH (1998) *Keys to Engagement*. Sainsbury Centre for Mental Health, London.

SCMH (2001) *Capable Practitioner: A Framework and List of Practitioner Capabilities Required to Implement the National Service Framework for Mental Health*. Sainsbury Centre for Mental Health, London.

de Shazer, S., Dolan, Y., Korman, H.T., Repper, T., McCollum, E. & Berg, I.K. (2007) *More than Miracles: The State of the Art of Solution Focused Brief Therapy*. Haworth Press, New York.

Spindel, P. & Nugent, J.A. (1999) *The Trouble with PACT: Questioning the increasing use of assertive community treatment teams in community mental health*. http://www.peoplewho.org/readingroom/spindel.nugent.htm

Stein, L.I. & Santos, A.B. (1998) *Assertive Community Treatment of Persons with Severe Mental Illness*. WWNorton, New York.

Test, M.A. & Stein, L.I. (1976) Practice guidelines for the community treatment of markedly impaired patients. *Community Mental Health Journal*, **12**, 72–82.

West, M.A. & Markiewicz, L. (2004) *Building Team-Based Working: A Practical Guide to Organizational Transformation*. Blackwell, Oxford.

Wharne, S. (2005) Assertive outreach teams: their roles and functions. *Journal of Interprofessional Care*, **19**(4), 326–337.

Williams, C. (2005) Assertive Outreach: the team approach. *Mental Health Practice,* **9**(2), 38–40.

Williamson, T. (2003) Enough is good enough. *Mental Health Today*, Apr., 24–27.

Chapter 3

Fidelity and flexibility

Caroline Williams, Rob Macpherson and Mike Firn

With contributions from Nigel Spencer, Ged Haresnape, Kate Dunne, Suzanne Wyatt, Maggie Mason, Andrea Clarke and Robert Higgo

> From the outset, the strength of the ACT model has been its foundation on empirical data rather than ideology. Adaptations may be intuitively appealing, but they require careful research before they can be recommended. (Bond et al., 2001: p. 151)

Introduction

The above quote from Bond and colleagues illustrates the tension between striving for an empirical, evidence based approach and an evolutionary approach to service development. Assertive outreach teams were developed to provide a flexible approach to engaging and maintaining contact with individuals estranged from mental health services. The assertive outreach approach is an evidence based method of service delivery (Bond et al., 2001) which was founded on the demonstration of improved outcomes for people with the most severe illness, in teams with a specified set of professionals providing a defined range of skills. In the United Kingdom (UK), the development of assertive outreach has been one component (alongside crisis teams and early intervention teams) of a range of mental health service reforms which have radically changed the face of UK community psychiatry since 1999.

Assertive outreach has its roots in a North American model of service delivery known as the Program of Assertive Community Treatment (PACT), also known as Assertive Community Treatment (ACT), which was developed in response to the challenges of the United States (US) mental health system in the 1970s. Following the classic research paper demonstrating highly favourable outcomes of the PACT programme by Len Stein and Mary Ann Test (Stein & Test, 1980), replications of the model followed in a number of healthcare systems around the world, including the UK and mainland Europe.

The validity of the assertive outreach model has been extensively debated in the literature and it has often been argued that fidelity to the model is important (Lachance & Santos, 1995; Teague et al., 1998; Bond et al., 2001) in recreating the outcomes seen in the Stein & Test (1980) paper. However, it has become apparent that within the UK healthcare system very different strengths and challenges exist in contrast to the North

Assertive Outreach in Mental Healthcare: Current Perspectives, First Edition. Edited by C. Williams, M. Firn, S. Wharne and R. Macpherson.
© 2011 Blackwell Publishing Ltd. Published 2011 by Blackwell Publishing Ltd.

American healthcare system and, as discussed in Chapter 1, the positive findings from the US and Australia have not been replicated in research evaluating the outcome of assertive outreach teams in the United Kingdom (UK) (Killaspy et al., 2006; Burns et al., 2007). This has led to a real debate about whether it is possible to justify the continuing provision of high fidelity assertive outreach teams in the UK, or whether models with greater flexibility and perhaps provided in different ways may be more appropriate.

This chapter considers further the UK context in this regard and looks at components of assertive outreach teams which may be core and essential elements of the model. We look at how assertive teams will adapt to changing healthcare policy in the new, plural, mixed economy of healthcare provision in the twenty-first century. We discuss how some UK assertive outreach teams have, in the face of complex clinical challenges, adapted, innovated and developed service models which meet need and demonstrate positive outcomes for their service users.

Dr Robert Higgo, Liverpool Assertive Outreach Team

'Our own survey of service users showed immense preference for the Assertive Outreach model as compared to care as usual. We found a reduction in bed usage of 49 days per service user per year when we compared their bed use pre and post AOT'

Early variations of the assertive outreach approach

In the paper 'Variations in an Assertive Outreach Model', Gary Bond (1991) charted the development of assertive outreach in the US and the variations in approaches up to the end of the 1980s. Bond provided a description of the variations in teams and identified teams in two ways – 'Growth Orientated' and 'Survival Orientated' programmes (Bond, 1991: 69). He described growth orientated programmes as aiming to improve quality of life, providing vocational and social support, with skills training and management of key community resources as key interventions; he also described these programmes as having a focus on any service users with a severe mental illness. Growth orientated teams were described as time unlimited, multi-disciplinary, open 24 hours a day/7 days a week with a team approach and accruing high costs.

Case study 3.1   'Flexibility vs Fidelity'
Working in different assertive outreach team configurations – a professional's view of a hub and spoke model and a small rural assertive outreach team

I first worked in assertive outreach with a new service designed using the 'Hub and Spoke Model', which consisted of a small full-time core team (team leader, social worker and two support workers) and generic link workers who were employed half-time within a large CMHT and half-time with the assertive outreach team. We had initial difficulties establishing this approach which had an impact on the start up of the team and implementation of the team approach. The assertive outreach team included specialist workers such as a court liaison CPN, a substance misuse CPN, and had input from specialists in psychosocial therapies. This accessible mass of specialist knowledge and experience was invaluable, not only in supporting the clients but also in sharing practice, team training and supervision. Problems within the model included access to and liaison with psychiatrists as we worked across a number of different consultants.

I now manage a stand alone service assertive outreach team, which maintains a 'high fidelity' assertive outreach approach, with its own medical lead and a full multi-disciplinary team, as would be expected from a team maintaining high levels of fidelity to the model. We are based in a resource centre which is centrally located for our large geographical area and are able to maintain individual caseloads of ten clients. We have range of highly trained staff, including staff trained in psychosocial interventions, non medical prescribers and an Approved Mental Health Practitioner (AMHP). We have regular team meetings, colleague support and clear communication.

Comparing the two approaches, a small team was more easily affected by staff absences and cannot absorb the increased workload, whereas a larger team can cope better with the work. In the rural assertive outreach team we have had to work flexibly and when link workers were absent, colleagues in CMHT sometimes stepped in. Referrals from our colleagues have not been as high as expected and not always appropriate, this was not an issue in my previous team as link workers knew their CMHT caseloads well and screened appropriate referrals. In the stand alone team, I have been able to provide a higher standard of care and consistency to my clients.

Andrea Clarke,
Stroud and Cirencester Assertive Outreach Team Leader.

Bond (1991) described staff in 'Survival Orientated Programs' as more 'generalist' rather than multi-disciplinary fragmentations; furthermore these types of programmes were said to be different to 'Growth Orientated' in that they were open 9am–5pm weekdays with additional crisis response. Bond (1991) stated the prototype for the Growth Orientated Approach was the Training in Community Living (TCL) model developed by Stein & Test (1980) and the Survival Orientated Approach was based on the Bridge Project in Chicago. The Stein & Test model is the model in which most teams base their project plan on when developing their team; highly quoted in the literature it is considered to be a classic paper and the standard template for assertive outreach. However, the Bridge is seldom referred to in the wider literature or when discussing assertive outreach with UK based teams. However, teams in the UK seem to mirror aspects of both survival orientated and growth orientated approaches, but the emphasis of teams working within community mental health today is to adopt a 'Recovery Focussed' approach. It is apparent from this early paper that teams in the US were never static and homogeneous, as also highlighted by Lachance & Santos in 1995.

When writing about the development of the Bridge Project in Chicago, Witheridge et al. (1982) describe the Bridge project as existing within a plethora of community mental health providers (unlike the early ACT provision), developed in 1978 and with different challenges to the early implementation of ACT in Madison Wisconsin (Witheridge, 1990). Witheridge et al. (1982) write:

Unlike the Madison Group, (1) we would be working with a sample of the most frequent recidivists we could find; (2) we would be operating in an exceedingly complex inner city environment; (3) we would have no formal control over the channels of readmission or the course of inpatient treatment; and (4) we would be constrained by a severely limited budget. (Witheridge et al., 1982: 10)

When reading this passage, one cannot help but compare this context and experience with that of assertive outreach development in the UK. Teams that were developed in the UK after the introduction of the National Service Framework for Mental Health in England (Department of Health, 1999) shared very similar challenges to that of the Bridge in the late 1970s when trying to replicate the assertive outreach model, as described by Stein & Test (1980). Variations to the ACT model provided by the Bridge project were (1) to provide a flexible duration of service, so people could step down; (2) a liaison worker was provided to be based at the local State hospital, which helped to identify revolving door clients and helped with discharge arrangements and general inpatient relations; (3) a team psychiatrist provided in vivo intensive medication monitoring seven hours a week; (4) the provision of extended meetings for all team members to discuss the direction of the team and an oversight of cases (Dincin et al., 1993).

In the early development of assertive outreach and ACT programmes, it can be seen that early implementers also struggled to find the best fit for their local needs and modified elements of their service to fit. This has been the case for most teams in the UK over the last ten years or so, but there seems to be insecurity about variation and development and concerns that variation may be spells the death knell for the assertive outreach approach; however, is this a true reflection of model implementation? Do teams fail if they do not meet model fidelity items or do they just provide a different experience, also valued by service users? Does the policy context govern how assertive outreach is implemented? Also, can a national health service provide a consistently high level of model fidelity no matter where in the country assertive outreach is delivered; and is this always necessary? These are examples of the questions teams in the UK are currently asking.

How useful are fidelity markers?

Reflection point

Fidelity scales are commonly used to measure whether a team is fully adherent to the assertive outreach model. Expert reviews (Marshall & Lockwood, 1998; Bond et al., 2001) have highlighted caution in adapting the approach. How rigidly should teams stick to such scales and are fidelity scales useful in planning a service?

Fidelity scales are useful in measuring the extent to which evidence based interventions are implemented (Drake et al., 2001); otherwise, how can researchers and clinicians ever be sure that the same approach is being replicated across a number of teams in different sites and, thus, evaluate the approach consistently and reliably? Furthermore, how can commissioners and providers be sure that evidence based approaches and services, such as assertive outreach, are consistently replicated in practice? Fidelity scales, such as the Dartmouth Assertive Community Treatment Scale (DACTS) (Teague et al., 1998) or the Index of Fidelity to Assertive Community Treatment (IFACT) (McGrew et al., 1994) allow the measurement of team characteristics which are considered essential in delivering evidence based interventions. Researchers can be transparent in reporting the service model they are evaluating and this may allow service planners and commissioners to ensure provision of the right service model.

Fidelity to the assertive outreach model is a contentious and fiercely debated issue. Although fidelity scales have been in existence for some time, the delivery of assertive outreach teams is anything but consistent. Teams across the UK and US vary in their level of model fidelity (Burns et al., 2001a; Williams, 2006) and evidence from England suggests that UK teams are struggling to meet government guidance in providing evidence based interventions and attracting staff quotas (Chisholm & Ford, 2004).

In practice, problems may arise from attempting to apply a rating scale of this type in the same way, across a range of different geographical and cultural boundaries. There is a risk that services could become 'slaves to fidelity', and neglect local priorities. The needs in inner city areas, such as Tower Hamlets in London, are likely to differ from those in communities with particular geography, such as the Isle of Wight. There may also be a range of important local issues which lie beneath the 'broad brush stroke' of the fidelity score: fidelity markers advising that the team leader should be clinically active and provide services at least 50% of the time may seem laudable, but in a team of 24 staff covering 160 assertive outreach service users, this may be unrealistic. Similarly, continuity of staffing may seem ideal, but may be impossible to achieve in a climate of service reorganisation, and may be undesirable where a team is dysfunctional. Low intake rates may be desirable in an ideal world, but in reality relate to other factors such as team boundary changes and even hospital closure programmes.

Arguably, there may be a conflict in philosophy between the fidelity marker of time-unlimited services (with an expectation of fewer than 5% of the team caseload being discharged annually), and models of recovery which favour a more acute, episode-of-care model, with an expectation of referral back to primary care. Similarly, although a no-drop-out policy seems a good idea in theory, if the reality of this means that cases are being kept on the caseload of an assertive outreach team, despite a lack of progress towards recovery or active engagement, this raises serious concerns about use of resources.

The question of responsibility for crisis and inpatient treatment is a particular challenge for many smaller teams, who in reality have no choice but to work alongside the other functional teams and develop positive collaboration. One of the drivers for crisis/inpatient specialist teams was to try to improve the quality of service for acute inpatients and ensure they had good access to psychiatric support as needed. While service users under the care of assertive outreach teams may benefit from continuity of care, they may be disadvantaged by the lack of access to regular input from the psychiatric team while they are inpatients (assertive outreach psychiatrists and teams focusing primarily on community responsibilities).

A further challenge arises through the expectation in fidelity markers of tightly defined assertive outreach caseloads. Most teams have an operational policy, describing clear inclusion criteria which relate to diagnosis of severe mental illness and exclude service users with primary diagnosis of borderline personality disorder or learning difficulties. This team boundary persists even where the problems of these service users are associated with the kind of clinical challenges which might otherwise be expected to require assertive outreach. The exclusion of all non-psychotic mental disorders from the assertive outreach approach relates largely to the historical development of the model (in poorly developed community services in the 1970s and 1980s), rather than to comparative studies which have examined the effectiveness of intensive case management (ICM) in different groups, such as learning disability (LD) and personality disorder.

Despite concerns about their validity, there are risks inherent in the abandonment of fidelity markers. These have been used to support the development of clearly defined teams with a clear definition of purpose and activity. It is reported that mental health service users seldom receive adequate evidence based services (Rowlands, 2004) or evidence based treatments (Drake et al., 2001; Mueser et al., 2003). However, assertive outreach can offer service users an empirically based service delivery model which relates to a strong evidence base (NICE, 2009): are service providers cheating service users by adapting the model? Service managers and commissioners may be reluctant to dedicate resources to provide the effective components of a particular evidence based model and service reconfigurations and the erosion of assertive outreach services may also be a reality for services (Firn, 2007). However, are adaptations to the model reckless experiments or sensible adaptations to local need? Clinicians often intuitively resist the rigid acceptance of models of care, in favour of a pragmatic and eclectic approach: reification of any system risks diverting attention from the ultimate goal, which is of course to try to provide the best service to those service users who are in greatest need and who are most likely to benefit from it.

Assertive outreach and risk

There is a need within mental health research for attention to the broader aspects of assertive outreach work such as working with the criminal justice system, risk and forensic issues. Assertive outreach teams often assume the role of community forensic teams, which tend to be available only in large urban centres. Although careful research has tended not to show evidence of greater rates of serious violence by those with severe mental illness in the community (Shaw et al., 1999), society's attitudes to risk containment may be in part responsible for changes in service provision, with evidence of a shift towards greater use of secure inpatient psychiatric services over the last two decades. There is increasing concern about the plight of service users in forensic units, often remote from the individual's home and receiving poor quality care (Ryan, 2004). Assertive outreach teams have an obvious role in supporting the rehabilitation of individuals in costly secure care packages, into community placements. The case of Christopher Clunis (Ritchie et al., 1994) taught services valuable lessons, in particular the need for an approach which maintained contact and engagement even in the face of an individual who moved around the local community and had repeatedly been lost to follow up. Along with the introduction of the Care Programme Approach (CPA), new teams such as assertive outreach were seen as a way to keep users in contact with their mental health team and also provide a flexibility not seen previously; it would encourage social inclusion and would enable people to reconnect with their community. A similar argument can be advanced for the specific role of assertive outreach in implementing and effectively using the Community Treatment Order, which became available in November 2008, in England and Wales in the 2007 amendment to the Mental Health Act (1983).

Assertive outreach practitioners would wish to be reassured that the practice of their teams is guided by logical principles and more importantly, sound evidence. However, is there a risk that if we do not strive for progressive, innovative practice, we may remain stuck on orthodoxy and confined by model fidelity scales? Is it possible to innovate and adapt an already innovative approach? The development of assertive outreach teams in the UK has come a long way since the early implementers in London (e.g. Audini et al., 1994; Marks et al., 1994; Muijen et al., 1994; Ford et al., 2001; Burns & Firn, 2002), Norfolk, East Anglia (Hemming et al., 1999), Dewsbury, West Yorkshire (Gibson & Leggett, 2000) and North Birmingham (Tasker, 1998) – to name but a few of the early UK teams. A systematic review of the literature (Marshall & Lockwood, 1998) recommended sticking closely to the prescribed model of care, and stated 'the research evidence supports only the practice of the whole ACT model, not the selective adoption of any of its particular elements.' (Marshall & Lockwood, 1998: 10). However, as discussed in Chapter 1, the results of recent meta analyses (Burns et al., 2001a; 2007) has challenged this view and suggested that other components of assertive outreach team working, which are not exclusive to these teams, were equally important in achieving significantly improved outcomes.

It is fair to say from the empirical literature that major studies of assertive outreach in England and Europe have generally failed to replicate the outcomes demonstrated in earlier US studies. As discussed, it would seem that teams based in the UK and mainland Europe have experienced different challenges within their health economies. Implementing assertive outreach services within an established UK community mental health case management structure, which was already delivering effective community services (Tyrer et al., 2007), was evidently a different process from implementation against the US background of largely private outpatient psychiatry and State hospital services. In the UK context, the place of assertive outreach within the wider context of community mental health services has been described as a form of evolutionary development of the 'fittest teams', with the need to adapt to its environment as highlighted by Tyrer et al., (2007) – 'assertive treatment shows many of the principles of plant succession in botany, where highly specialised plants do very well in alien environments, but in naturally improving these, become themselves redundant unless they can adapt to the new situations.' (Tyrer et al., 2007: 499). Therefore, are assertive outreach services under threat if they do not innovate and adapt to their local health contexts and health needs of the local communities in which they ultimately serve?

Case study 3.2   'Fidelity' South Staffordshire AO team

The assertive outreach service across South Staffs is constantly striving to improve service delivery and respond to the changing needs of their service users, research and evidenced-based practice and audit and constantly reflect on their philosophy, values model of care delivery and innovation to ensure a quality based service. They have employed a full time Clinical Audit Officer who is part of the team and is central to the development of their service. They have developed a set of routinely used structured assessments and outcome measures that inform their practice and service development.

At the core of this is a values based clinical practice philosophy of assertive outreach. This audit tool has been piloted to provide a position statement for the team to be measured against and makes then accountable to their service users. This ongoing process ensures that we work in partnership with our service users to help us develop our service. The values based statement enables us to measure fidelity to the principles of our operational policy and philosophy of delivering a recovery-focussed service.

Clinical Audit Project Manager, Maggie Mason:

'Based within the teams, my post is central to the development of assertive outreach teams across the Trust, enabling improvement of services in line with recommended national guidelines. I support the team in developing policies / protocols for auditing the service, providing information, training and audit of current services to prove effectiveness and highlight deficiencies. I ensure implementation of proven projects and communicate to statutory and non-statutory agencies when completing audits and feedback on clinical service outcomes. I coordinate, facilitate and manage all projects within the Assertive Outreach Team, whilst linking in with the Trust's Clinical Audit Team using their protocols and systems.'

Team Leader, Suzanne Wyatt:

'As a team leader and clinician, I see the post of Clinical Audit Project Manager invaluable in enabling us to evaluate our service in a structured way, keeping service evaluation a high priority within the team and maintaining fidelity to the AO model.'

Innovation or extinction?

It is argued that rural or smaller assertive outreach teams may require modification – as long as caseloads are managed effectively (Lachance & Santos, 1995). Rural and semi rural settings have different challenges, such as a disparate and isolated population, a reduced critical mass of people with severe mental illness, and possibly disparate access to community resources. Such teams in the UK have developed different solutions to this problem. We were aware of an 'assertive outreach team' in Snowdonia, Wales which was just one man (attached to a mental health team) (see case study 3.3), and we are aware of other similar models operating in the UK and in fact adaptations with lower staff numbers and different methods of operating have been reported in the literature (Chisholm & Ford, 2004). The model of one or two workers attached to a community mental health team (CMHT) seems to be favoured in some rural settings, however it is argued by those in the field of AO that this does not constitute 'assertive outreach'. This subset of practitioners target the most severely disabled individuals after the CMHT has identified them and intensive support is provided, using a brokerage model. Care then goes back to the CMHT when the service user no longer requires intensive support. This approach is most definately 'assertive' and provides community outreach; however this is not delivered by a discreet team which is where those working in urban teams may struggle with this approach.

There is a paucity of literature of this approach; however without it many isolated service users would not receive an intensive service. There are variations to rural models in the UK (Chisholm & Ford, 2004), with other teams operating a full team approach and remaining consistent with the assertive outreach team model (Wane et al., 2007). The model described by Wane et al. (2007) demonstrated that an assertive outreach model can be effective in reducing bed occupancy in rural and semi rural settings.

Case study 3.3   'Flexibility' A one man assertive outreach team in Snowdonia, Wales

The essence of assertive outreach is the team approach but in North Wales a single individual organises the service from within a community mental health team. The clients receiving this service are the same individuals who would be eligible to an assertive outreach service elsewhere. However because of limited resources funding a whole team has not been an option at this time. Interestingly the sole worker has not become burnt out as is often suggested. In time, 'difficult to engage' service users have been won over to receiving a service from the clinician. Although this approach is recognised as being removed from assertive outreach orthodoxy, the service users have later emerged from the relationship agreeable to return to work with members of the community mental health team (CMHT) and engage with community support.

Importantly CMHT staff have found more time for clients who turn up for appointments and don't create turmoil as revolving door patients. Clearly a win-win situation for all! The worker has found all the helpful components of an assertive community home treatment team in the CMHT – supervision, guidance and support. The clinician has a reduced caseload and this allows more time to meet and become meaningfully engaged with clients, as well as step up care for CMHT clients requiring an assertive approach.

Ged Haresnape
Assertive Outreach Team Practitioner

Although it can be argued that the effectiveness of the assertive outreach approach is established, there is an emerging anecdotal trend that some UK National Health Service Trusts are moving away from the traditional assertive outreach model. In recent years a number of service providers in England have displayed their ambivalence to assertive outreach by decommissioning their dedicated team and moving the function into a generic secondary mental health team predominantly with an individual case management approach. Some of the teams that have been lost were poorly functioning or poorly resourced teams with high bed use and low fidelity that had failed to make themselves indispensable. The stated reasons for local executives' decision to no longer demonstrate their value provide assertive outreach are summarised in Box 3.1.

The assertive outreach practitioners network in England, The National Forum for Assertive Outreach (NFAO), produced a written response to the decommissioning of services (Firn, 2007) that intended to present a balanced and realistic argument outlining the advantages and disadvantages when considering integrating the assertive outreach function back into standard care (see Table 3.1).

In tough economic times, health services have to be seen to be using public money efficiently. Although UK research focusing on bed usage has generally failed to demonstrate improved outcomes compared to controls or 'treatment as usual' (Killapsy et al., 2006), service user and staff evaluations of the assertive outreach approach have generally reported

---

Box 3.1   Stated rationales for decommissioning assertive outreach teams

- Local evidence has shown that the service has not reduced hospital usage.
- National evidence has confirmed that assertive outreach does not reduce bed use (Killapsy et al., 2006).
- Assertive outreach is a more intensive and, therefore, an expensive team to provide unless it reduces bed use.
- We have to reduce our costs and this means that even services protected by targets and preferred by service users and carers are not immune to the recession.

Table 3.1   Integrating ACT workers into existing CMHTs (from Firn, 2007)

Potential disadvantages	Potential advantages
• Loss of programme fidelity. • Secondment of key workers to other (non – ACT) tasks. • Inefficient use of time (e.g. multiple meetings). • Professional isolation. • Reduced control over inpatient stays.	• Perhaps fuller multi-disciplinary support from more disciplines. • Vertical and horizontal service integration. • Avoids fragmentation of sectorised community mental health services. • Retains CMHT focus on people with severe mental illness.

Reproduced with permission from the RCN

positive findings, particularly as regards service user satisfaction and staff satisfaction, retention and 'burnout' (McGrew et al., 1996; Minghella et al., 2002; Priebe et al., 2005). The increasing influence of the recovery movement, which focuses on the empowerment and recognition of service user strengths, may be in favour of services which work extensively around positive engagement and social/occupational outcomes. Similarly, the rise of the personalisation agenda may give the service user greater ability to influence services and to choose the preferred style of service. The emphasis on continuity inherent in the assertive outreach model (even across the community/inpatient divide) makes it attractive to many service users and carers.

Variations to the assertive outreach approach in Europe

A European context to model variation

Variations in the provision of mental healthcare exist within a Pan-European context; however, there exists a wider drive for community based care (Muijen, 2006). The assertive outreach model has been adapted for use in Europe and it has been documented that adaptations to the ACT model have taken place in England, Italy, Germany, Sweden (Burns et al., 2001b), Spain (Morago, 2006) and Lithuania (Tyrer et al., 2007). Outcomes from the provision of assertive outreach within some European countries vary widely (Burns et al., 2001b) and possible reasons have been cited as:

- The focus on 'services' rather than distinct focussed 'programmes' (as seen in the US) – in Europe, teams exist within a wider service and, therefore, do not exist within a vacuum.
- The role of mental health professionals and their clinical responsibilities vary – for instance in Italy the psychiatrist assumes greater professional responsibility, whereas in the UK, nurses have greater professional responsibility. It is reported that in German speaking countries, social workers carry considerable professional responsibility in assertive outreach teams.
- Evidence based psychosocial interventions are regarded differently across different European countries and, thus, prioritised differently.
- Health and social care integration differs across Europe and, therefore, this possibly cascades down to the generic working of assertive outreach teams.
- European teams rarely provide 24 hour cover as a self contained team and cover is usually sought via the wider community mental health service.
- There are wide cultural variations in the organisation of community mental health services across Europe.

Consistent and homogenous assertive outreach implementation across Europe is a tall order, considering the variation in the cultural and historical contexts of community psychiatry in Europe. It would seem naive to suggest that one model will fit all contexts and cultures equally and will meet local need adequately. The way in which services are organised in Europe provides a different platform for assertive outreach in which to operate and organise itself. This is particularly the case in respect of integration or non integration of health and social care and the role of different professions in providing clinical leadership and responsibility (Burns et al., 2001b). Such variables are likely to interact when implementing the ACT model in a European health economy and variation to the model is likely to be an outcome.

Assertive outreach in England: current perspectives in model variation

The UK operates a national health service (NHS) in which all services are nationally standardised and delivered. Budgets are devolved from government and mental health services are mandated to work within the CPA (see Box 3.2). From 2001 onwards, the Department of Health published the 'Mental Health Policy Implementation Guide' (MH-PIG), to guide the development and implementation of assertive outreach teams, early intervention teams (EITs) and crisis resolution teams (CRTs). In the MH-PIG service models were described in some detail in order to provide a blueprint for service commissioners to provide standardised services, no matter where in the country these services were based and delivered.

The vision was to allow individuals to receive the same standard of care, addressing issues of inadequate provision in some areas and to ensure that all service users could be ensured a consistent and predictable care pathway through services from referral to discharge. The MH-PIG included key components, which were essentially team fidelity markers and these were translated into operational policies, as a way of identifying the

---

Box 3.2   The Care Programme Approach (CPA)

The Care Programme Approach (CPA) was introduced in 1990 to provide a framework for effective mental healthcare for people with severe mental health problems. Its four main elements are:

- Systematic arrangements for assessing the health and social needs of people accepted into specialist mental health services.
- The formation of a care plan which identifies the health and social care required from a variety of providers.
- The appointment of a key worker (care coordinator) to keep in close touch with the service user and to monitor and coordinate care.
- Regular review and, where necessary, agreed changes to the care plan.

Department of Health (2006) *Reviewing the Care Programme Approach*, London, DH.

---

structural aspects of teams and their organisational boundaries. This process has enabled teams to have clearer operational definitions, and it has helped the commissioning process, by identifying the services which should be available within these teams.

There is an emerging awareness of possible tensions that exist between policies aiming to implement the care programme approach and the assertive outreach team approach. This tension is evident in an assertive outreach service (operating three teams) in Manchester, England which operated a full team approach for a number of years, but recently and following a review of their services opted to introduce a case management approach (see case study 3.4).

ICM has been seen as the focus for delivering mental health services in the UK (Brooker & Repper, 1998) and is a central tenet of the CPA. This model of service delivery has been widely described and there is extensive experience of the approach in UK psychiatry. However, in assertive outreach and other functional teams such as CRTs, there is an explicit rejection of the ICM approach, in favour of team-based management, with the team accepting responsibility collectively for all aspects of the clinical and managerial activity. As discussed in Chapter 2, in practice, most assertive outreach teams have a modified version of the team-based approach, which includes elements of key-working responsibility, but it is evident that conflicting policy directives can potentially result in confusion, and lead to uncertainty in clinicians, mangers and commissioners of services. There is also an increasing awareness of differences in the assertive outreach model reported in the literature (Billings et al., 2003; Priebe et al., 2003; Wright et al., 2003; Burns et al., 2007).

Reflection point

In the UK, standard systems of care coordination advocate key working by one individual; 'the case manager'. Assertive outreach recommends providing care, via a shared team responsibility. Teams in the UK are required to marry the two concepts and provide care within the dynamic of individual care coordination and shared responsibility. How does your team reconcile these approaches and what are the resulting challenges?

A challenge faced by assertive outreach teams working in the UK is that of how to merge a model based on shared governance and the team approach, with designated statutory procedures around the CPA. The CPA has at its core the concept of a single, named individual leading the management and delivery of care and treatment in the community. However, research evidence from the US has indicated that the most successful outcomes for assertive outreach are predicated on close fidelity to the assertive outreach model, including the use of a whole team approach. These findings were of course from the US healthcare system, in the context of patchy and sometimes under-resourced community care and treatment, which contrasts with the UK's experience of well established and resourced generic care and treatment pathways in community mental health.

Assertive outreach in the UK operates alongside a number of other functional teams and within a set of centrally defined policies and procedures for community-based care and treatment. The question that arises is one of balance: how far in the direction of either pure team working or pure key working does each individual team travel? It appears at present that there is no definitive answer to this question and individual teams operate at each end of the spectrum of team-based or key worker-based responsibility, some providing an eclectic mix of both approaches.

Case study 3.4   'Flexibility' Manchester assertive outreach service

Three teams work with a total of 308 service users, in a largely inner city environment.

When our service was established in 2001, we adopted the teamwork approach. Care co-ordinators carried nominal caseloads, but the service was delivered by the team as a whole, with activity planned via a daily handover and weekly planning meeting. As the service expanded in size, it became increasingly difficult to maintain the team approach effectively. Two of the Manchester teams have over 100 service users each, which meant that handover and planning meetings became increasingly unwieldy. Team members struggled to balance care co-ordination responsibilities with contributing to the team approach. Larger caseloads also meant more communication failures and increased difficulties effectively managing risk.

In 2009 the service abandoned the whole team approach in favour of intensive case management with zoning. The weekly planning meeting was scrapped and the daily handover meeting became a daily zoning meeting. Care co-ordinators carry their own caseloads of twelve service users and professional roles notwithstanding, take responsibility for delivering all aspects of care. At the zoning meeting, all service users who are in crisis or who may be going into crisis are discussed and a plan for that day is formulated. This is where the team approach is still applied – if the care co-ordinator is absent or if the level of input required to meet a service user's needs is too high for one care co-ordinator to manage, other members of the team step in to participate in delivery of the service.

It's not assertive outreach in the traditional sense of the word: some of the flexibility and responsiveness has been lost and the culture of peer support and shared responsibility is weaker. However, care co-ordinators have welcomed the opportunity to manage their own workload and service users generally seem to prefer consistent support from a single individual to the whole team approach. Zoning certainly appears an effective tool for targeting the finite resources of the team. Whether, in the longer term, it will make any difference in terms of outcomes remains to be seen.

Nigel Spencer
Team Manager
Manchester Assertive Outreach Service (Central)

As outlined above, the provision of assertive outreach in England has been mandated by central government in the National Service Framework for Mental Health (NSF-MH) (Department of Health, 1999) and guidance on implementation was provided within the Mental Health Policy Implementation Guide (Department of Health, 2001). As discussed, this guidance provided clinicians with a blueprint of how teams in the UK should be established. The Health Secretary at the time of the publication of the NSF-MH, Frank Dobson MP, stated the following in the introduction to the NSF- MH:

> our programme of National Service Frameworks …. will lay down models of treatment and care which people will be entitled to expect in every part of the country. (Department of Health, 1999: 1)

Essentially, this reflected the assertion by the government at the time that everyone will receive the same healthcare despite their geographical location. However, variations in local budgets and local need have resulted in variations to models of community mental health, including assertive outreach.

In a review by Chisholm & Ford (2004) in England, it was found assertive outreach teams were not homogenous and that variations in some cases could be seen as a positive adaptation to the local community (e.g. teams addressing the needs of the BME community or homelessness populations). Within this review, Chisholm & Ford (2004) reviewed ten sites across England. They mapped service provision against the MH-PIG blueprint/model. There were stark contrasts between teams and teams applied different elements of the eligibility criteria suggested by the Department of Health. It was acknowledged that rural teams modified assertive outreach criteria, such as multi-disciplinary team components, 24 hour/7 days a week working patterns, caseloads of 1 to 10–1 to 12, a range of interventions and in vivo treatment. Chisholm & Ford (2004) found that teams in rural areas were usually staffed by a couple of practitioners, did not offer 24 hour/7 day a week support and usually had caseloads of 1 to 12–1 to 20; a range of interventions could only be available if the resources were there to support this and although in vivo treatment was possible, there were some barriers. Chisholm & Ford (2004) also found that the majority of clinical staff in English based assertive outreach teams was mental health nurses. Teams generally conducted the type of work expected from assertive outreach teams, such as social support, attention to physical and mental health, engagement with people with dual diagnosis (substance misuse) and general creative engagement strategies. However, it was clear from this review that the model of provision varied across England.

Alternative models of assertive outreach in the UK: assertive outreach for people with learning disability

Assertive outreach services work in a climate of ever-changing policy framework. Over the last 15 years, since the Disability Discrimination Act (1995), there have been a series of reports which have focused on access to the NHS and the importance of people who are disadvantaged and in minority groups such as people with LDs and the elderly, being able to access specialist services in the same way that other members of the community can. In 2005 MENCAP produced a report called 'Death by Indifference', which highlighted the plight of people with LDs who needed to use the NHS and the struggle their families had to try to get to the bottom of the poor care they felt their children had received. The resultant inquiry was entitled 'Healthcare For All' (Department of Health, 2008) and this highlighted the challenge of working with people with LDs, who are often 'not visible' to health services. The needs of this group and the elderly have arguably been overlooked and have not represented a priority for the NHS. At this time there is effectively no legislative framework covering disability discrimination and mental capacity in UK health services. Healthcare For All (Department of Health, 2008) recommended that there should be an explicit requirement to make 'reasonable adjustments to the provision and delivery of services for vulnerable groups, in accordance with disability equality legislation.' (Department of Health, 2008: 10). Healthcare organisations are expected to collect data and information necessary to allow people with LDs to be identified within all pathways of care provided. Trust boards should deliver effective, 'reasonably adjusted' health services for people who happen to have LDs.

It is estimated that people with LDs are three times more likely to develop schizophrenia (Turner, 1989). Mental health services for this population are patchy (Hassiotis et al., 2000), but it has been argued that assertive outreach may benefit clients (Burns et al., 1999; Hassiotis et al., 2001). However, a number of studies have found no difference between assertive outreach and standard care for people with LDs (Hassiotis et al., 2003; Martin et al., 2005). Presently, there remain only a few teams in the UK exclusively providing assertive outreach services to people with LDs. A published evaluation of an assertive outreach team for people with LDs in Oxfordshire demonstrated positive outcomes (Prakash et al., 2007). Prakash et al. (2007) describe this team as providing the usual level of support provided by an assertive outreach team, across a range of bio-psychosocial needs. They stated that referrals were accepted from the local community learning disability teams (CLDT), rather than the usual route via mental health teams. The eligibility criteria described was modified to the typical assertive outreach eligibility criteria as described by Stein & Test (1980) and the UK government (Department of Health, 2001):

- Evidence of severe and enduring mental illness.
- High frequency and intensity of challenging behaviour.
- Frequent planned/unplanned admissions to/referrals to inpatient units in the last two years.
- Currently receiving less than 24 hour/7 days a week paid support.

It is reported that the assertive outreach team was comprised of two qualified staff and two behavioural support workers. The psychiatrist from the referring CLDT remained the responsible medical officer (RMO). It is reported that the team operated a small caseload of 20 patients, with a care coordinator. Input from the assertive outreach team was not time unlimited and input from the team is reported to have been between two and five years. Prakash et al. (2007) described ways in which services can be innovative, and although they needed to modify and adapt the assertive outreach model, the assertive outreach spirit appears active in adopting an outreach approach meeting the needs of local users which had a positive effect on engagement. It seems that although variations of an assertive outreach model are seen as good practice in meeting the needs of people with LDs, there is little evidence to support investment in such a distinct model. However, there are case examples of assertive outreach teams that are providing a focussed approach for people with LDs.

Exemplar models of assertive outreach in Europe: the FACT model, the Netherlands

Alternative and evolutionary models of assertive outreach should not be condemned and, in fact, in some cases we can learn lessons from adapting a North American model to meet the diverse needs of local communities in other countries. In the Netherlands, doubts about the affordability and fit of the orthodox model in more rural populations resulted in the widespread implementation of the FACT or 'Function – Assertive Community Treatment' model (Bak et al., 2007; van Veldhuizen, 2007). There are now some 80 FACT teams in the Netherlands and a further 30 orthodox ACT teams in urban centres. In FACT the whole severely ill population is managed by one team and one staff group. Between 80 and 90% get recovery oriented ICM in a multi-disciplinary sectorised team covering a population of 50,000 typically receiving two to four home visits a month. A flexible 10–20% receive ACT level of service according to need from the same team using ACT principles of shared caseload, daily planning and review and frequent visits. Service users move between the two groups according to need with a simple team based decision drawing upon a manualised programme standard description. They may receive ACT level of care for a few weeks, a few months or longer. In this way the notion of ACT as a time unlimited service is comprehensively rejected.

> We also questioned whether there really was an absolute distinction between the 20% and the 80% group. Are they separate groups, or do patients sometimes belong to one group and sometimes to the other, depending on the thresholds of the system? We suspected that there was a great deal of exchange between the groups. We concluded that the difference between the two groups pertained only to the intensity of care and treatment at a particular point in time and did not have consequences for the composition and attitude of the teams. (van Veldhuizen, 2007: 425)

Indeed two respected US ACT proponents acknowledge that the FACT model has appeal, is correct to question the established thinking, and that the notion of time unlimited service appears increasingly impractical due to cost and is unnecessary given the long-term evidence of recovery (Bond & Drake, 2007). They go on to say that FACT is also correct to consider what services should be available for individuals who don't need ACT most of the time. At the time of writing the Dutch FACT model has five years of experience and has been evaluated positively within the Dutch context regarding cost and outcomes (Bak et al., 2007; Drukker et al., 2008).

Conclusion

Healthcare environments are ever changing and socio-political factors alongside clinical innovations can alter the face of service delivery. Assertive outreach teams are now operating in a twenty-first century health economy, a world apart from the challenges that existed for assertive outreach pioneers. Therefore, should assertive outreach stay static as 'retro-chic' or should it recognise the ever changing environment in which it operates and develop further, reaching new horizons and building on the work of the original pioneers. It seems that the UK and mainland European healthcare systems have distinct challenges and assertive outreach model fidelity is not a panacea to address all these issues; other factors can influence the outcomes of teams (Burns et al., 2001a; 2002; 2007), therefore, creativity, imagination, an ability to work across service boundaries and above all a critical lens may be required for the effective future implementation of assertive outreach services.

Assertive outreach teams, it seems, are evolutionary and there are many teams in the UK and the rest of Europe that have modified the model to meet local needs. However, Bond and colleagues stated: 'Adaptations may be intuitively appealing, but they require careful research before they can be recommended' (Bond et al., 2001: 151). As an assertive outreach community, we can learn a lot from our colleagues in the Netherlands and the FACT model has been carefully evaluated, providing an evidence base and a good rationale for modifying assertive outreach teams within a European context. The FACT model seems to fit within mental health service configuration in the UK. However, anecdotal evidence suggests teams operating a high level of assertive outreach model fidelity report good 'on the ground' outcomes for their service users.

Assertive outreach needs to adapt to a changing world and the model may seem 'out of kilter' with the notions of recovery and service user independence from mental health services – a no drop out policy may seem draconian when developing a recovery focus within assertive outreach teams. Only time will tell, however, this is an exciting time for assertive outreach and an exciting time for assertive outreach practitioners and service users to be creative and be part of the evolution!

References

Audini, B., Marks, I.M., Lawrence, R.E., Connolly, J. & Watts, V. (1994) Home based versus out patient/in patient care for people with serious mental illness. phase II of a controlled study. *British Journal of Psychiatry*, **165**, 204–210.

Bak, M., van Os, J., Delespaul, P., de Bie, A., Campo, J. & Poddighe, G., et al. (2007) An observational 'real life' trial of the introduction of assertive community treatment in a geographically defined area using clinical rather than service use outcome data. *Social Psychiatry Psychiatric Epidemiology*, **42**(2), 125–130.

Billings, J., Johnson, S., Bebbington, P., Greaves, A., Priebe, S. & Muijen, M., et al. (2003) Assertive outreach teams in London: staff experiences and perceptions. *British Journal of Psychiatry*, **183**, 139–147.

Bond, G.R. (1991) Variations in an assertive outreach model. *New Directions for Mental Health Services*, **52**, 65–80.

Bond, G.R., Drake, R.E., Mueser, K.T. & Latimer, E. (2001) Assertive community treatment for people with severe mental illness. Critical ingredients and impact on patients' disease management and health outcomes. *Disease Management and Health Outcomes*, **9**(3), 141–159.

Bond, G.R. & Drake, R.E. (2007) Should we adopt the Dutch version of ACT? Commentary on 'FACT: a Dutch version of ACT.' *Community Mental Health Journal*, **43**(4), 435–438.

Brooker, C. & Repper, J. (1998) Serious Mental Health Problems in the Community. The Significance of Policy, Practice & Research. In: *Serious Mental Health Problems in the Community. Policy, Practice & Research,* (eds. C. Brooker & J. Repper). pp. 4–13. Balliere Tindall, Edinburgh.

Burns, T., Creed, F., Fahy, T., Thompson, S., Tyrer, P. & White, I. (1999) Intensive versus standard case management for severe psychotic illness: a randomised trial. *Lancet*, **353**, 2185–2189.

Burns, T., Fioritti, A., Holloway, F., Malm, U. & Rössler, W. (2001) Case management and assertive community treatment in Europe. *Psychiatric Services*, **52**(5), 631–636.

Burns, T., Knapp, M., Catty, J., Healey, A., Henderson, J., Watt, H. & Wright, C. (2001) Home treatment for mental health problems: a systematic review. *Health Technology Assessment*, **5**(15), 1–139.

Burns, T., Catty, J., Watt, H., & Wright, C., Knapp, M. & Henderson, J. (2002) International differences in home treatment for mental health problems. Results of a systematic review. *British Journal of Psychiatry*, **181**, 375–382.

Burns, T. & Firn, M. (2002) *Assertive Outreach: A Manual for Practitioners.* Oxford University Press, Oxford.

Burns, T., Catty, J., Dash, M., Roberts, C., Lockwood, A. & Marshall, M. (2007) Use of intensive case management to reduce time in hospital in people with severe mental illness: systematic review and meta-regression. *British Medical Journal*, **335**(7615), 336–340.

Chisholm, A. & Ford, R. (2004) *Transforming Mental Health Care: Assertive outreach and crisis resolution in practice.* The Sainsbury Centre for Mental Health, London.

Department of Health (1990) *NHS and CommunityCommunity Care Act.* Department of Health, London.

Department of Health (1999) *Modern Standards and Service Models - National Service Frameworks.* Department of Health, London.

Department of Health (2001) *The Mental Health Policy Implementation Guide.* Department of Health, London.

Department of Health (2006) *Reviewing the Care Programme Approach.* Department of Health, London.

Department of Health (2008) *Health Care for all.* Department of Health, London.

Dincin, J., Wasmer, D., Witheridge, T.F., Sobeck, L., Cook, J. & Razzano, L. (1993) Impact of assertive community treatment on the user of state hopsital inpatient bed-days. *Hospital and Community Psychiatry*, **44**(9), 833–838.

Disability Discrimination Act (1995). Public Sector Informatrion. TSO.

Drake, R.E.,Goldman, H.H., Leff, H.S., Lehman, A.F., Dixon, L. & Mueser, K.T., et al. (2001) Implementing evidence-based practices in routine mental health service settings. *Psychiatric Services*, **52**(2), 179–182.

Drukker, M., Maarschalkerweerd, M., Bak, M., Driessen, G., Campo, J. & De Bie, A., et al. (2008) A real life observational study of the effectiveness of FACT in a Dutch mental health region. *BMC Psychiatry* **8**(93), 1–10.

Firn, M. (2007) Assertive Outreach: has the tide turned against the approach? *Mental Health Practice*, **10**(7), 24–27.

Ford, R., Barnes, A., Davies, R., Chalmers, C., Hardy, P. & Muijen, M. (2001) Maintaining contact with people with severe mental illness: 5 year follow up of assertive outreach. *Social Psychiatry and Psychiatric Epidemiology*, **36**, 444–447.

Gibson, J. & Leggett, C. (2000) *Assertive community treatment: Florence Nightengale travel scholarship reports.* Florence Nightengale Travel Scholarship, unpublished.

Hassiotis, A., Barron, P., & O'Hara, J. (2000) Editorial: mental health services for people with learning disabilities. *British Medical Journal,* **321**, 583–584.

Hassiotis, A., Ukoumunne, O., Byford, S., Tyrer, P., Harvey, K. & Piachaud, J., et al. (2001) Intellectual functioning and outcome of patients with severe psychotic illness randomised to intensive case management: report from the UK700 trial. *British Journal of Psychiatry,* **178**, 166–171.

Hassiotis, A., Tyrer, P., & Oliver, P. (2003) Psychiatric assertive outreach & learning. *Disability Services Advances in Psychiatric Treatment,* **9**, 368–373.

Hemming, M., Morgan, S. & O'Halloran, P. (1999) Assertive outreach: implications for the development of the model in the United Kingdom. *Journal of Mental Health,* **8**(2), 141–147.

Killaspy, H., Bebbington, P., Blizard, R., Johnson, S., Nolan, F. & Pilling, S., et al. (2006) The REACT study: randomized evaluation of assertive community treatment in north London. *British Medical Journal: Online Published,* 16 Mar., 1–6.

Lachance, K.R. & Santos, A.B. (1995) Modifying the PACT model: preserving critical elements. *Psychiatric Services,* **46**(6), 601–604.

Marks, I.M., Connolly, J., Muijen, M., Audini, B., Mcnamee, G. & Lawrence, R.E. (1994) Home-based versus hospital-based care for people with serious mental illness. *British Journal of Psychiatry,* **165**, 179–194.

Marshall, M. & Lockwood A. (1998) Assertive community treatment for people with severe mental disorders. *Cochrane database of systematic reviews.* Issue 2.

Martin, G., Costello, H., Leese, M., Slade, M., Bouras, N. & Higgins, S. (2005) An exploratory study of assertive community treatment for people with intellectual disability and psychiatric disorders: conceptual, clinical, and service issues. *Journal of Intellectual Disability Research,* **49**(7), 516–524.

McGrew, J.H., Bond, G.R., Dietzen, L. & Salyers, M. (1994) Measuring the fidelity of implementation of a mental health program model. *Journal of Consulting and Clinical Psychology,* **62**(4), 670–678.

McGrew, J.H., Wilson, R.G. & Bond, G.R. (1996) Client perspectives on helpful ingredients of assertive community treatment. *Psychiatric Rehabilitation Journal,* **19**(3), 13–21.

MENCAP (2007) *Death by indifference Report.* Mencap.

Minghella, E., Gauntlett, N., & Ford, R. (2002) Assertive outreach: does it reach expectations? *Journal of Mental Health,* **11**(1), 27–42.

Morago, P. (2006) Assertive community treatment: practice, ethical considerations and the role of social workers. *Cuadernos de Trabajo Social,* **19**, 7–23.

Mueser, K.T., Torrey, W.C., Lynde, D., Singer, P. & Drake, R.E. (2003) Implementing evidence-based practices for people with severe mental illness. *Behavior Modification,* **27**(3), 387–411.

Muijen, M., Cooney, M., Strathdee, G., Bell, R. & Hudson, A. (1994) Community psychiatric nursing teams: intensive support versus generic care. *British Journal of Psychiatry,* **165**, 211–217.

Muijen, M. (2006) Challenges for psychiatry: delivering the Mental Health Declaration for Europe. *World Psychiatry,* **5**(2), 113–117.

NICE (2009) *Schizophrenia: Core Interventions in the Treatment and Management of Schizophrenia in Primary and Secondary Care (Update).* National Institute for Health and Clinical Excellence, London.

Prakash, J., Andrews, T. & Porter, I. (2007) Service Innovation: assertive outreach teams for adults with learning disability. *Psychiatric Bulletin,* **31**, 138–141.

Priebe, S., Fakhoury, W., Watts, J., Bebbington, P., Burns, T. & Johnson, S., et al. (2003) Assertive outreach teams in London: patient characteristics and outcomes. Pan London assertive outreach study, Part 3. *British Journal of Psychiatry,* **183**, 148–154.

Priebe, S., Watts, J., Chase, M. & Matanov, A. (2005) Processes of disengagement and engagement in assertive outreach patients: qualitative study. *British Journal of Psychiatry,* **187**, 438–443.

Repper, J. & Brooker, C. (1998) 1. Serious Mental Health Problems in the Community. The Significance of Policy, Practice & Research. In: Brooker, C. & Repper, J. (Eds) (1998) *Serious Mental Health Problems in the Community London,* Bailliere, Tindall, pp. 3–13.

Ritchie, J.H., Dick, D. & Lingham, R. (1994) *The Report of the Inquiry into the Care and Treatment of Christopher Clunis.* HMSO, London.

Rowlands, P. (2004) The NICE schizophrenia guidelines: the challenge of implementation. *Advances in Psychiatric Treatment,* **10**, 403–412.

Ryan, T., Pearsall, A., Hatfield, B., Poole, R. & Ryan, T. (2004) Long term care for serious mental illness outside the NHS. A study of out of area placements. *Journal of Mental Health,* **13**, 425–429

Shaw, J., Appleby, L., Amos, T., McDonnell, R., Harris, C. & McCann, C., et al. (1999) Mental disorder and clinical care in people convicted of homicide: national clinical survey. *British Medical Journal,* **318**(7193), 1240–1244.

Stein, L.I. & Test, M.A. (1980) Alternative to mental hospital treatment. I. Conceptual model, treatment program and clinical evaluation. *Archives of General Psychiatry,* **37**, 392–397.

Tasker, J. (1998) *Locality Services in Mental Health. Developing Home Treatment and Assertive Outreach.* The North Birmingham Experience Booklet 4, Hove, England, Sainsbury Centre for Mental Health / North Birmingham MHT.

Teague, G.B., Bond, G.R. & Drake, R.E. (1998) Program fidelity in Assertive Community Treatment: development and use of a measure. *American Journal of Orthopsychiatry,* **68**(2), 216–232.

Turner, T.H. (1989) Schizophrenia and mental handicap: an historical review, with implications for further research. *Psychological Medicine,* **19**, 301–314.

Tyrer, P., Balod, A., Germanavicius, A., McDonald, A., Varadan, M., & Thomas, J. (2007) Perceptions of assertive community treatment in the UK and Lithuania. *International Journal of Social Psychiatry,* **53**(6), 498–506.

van Veldhuizen, J.R. (2007) FACT: a Dutch version of ACT. *Community Mental Health Journal,* **43**(4), 421–433.

Wane, J., Owen, A., Sood, L., Bradley, S.H.L. & Jones, C. (2007) The effectiveness of rural assertive outreach: a prospective cohort study in an English region. *Journal of Mental Health,* **16**(4), 471–482.

Williams C. (2006) *Assertive outreach team implementation within the United Kingdom: a critique and methodological analysis of the literature.* Unpublished MSc Thesis. The University of Manchester.

Witheridge, T.F. (1990) Assertive community treatment as a supported housing approach. *Psychosocial Rehabilitation Journal,* **13**(4), 69–75.

Witheridge, T.F., Dincin, J. & Appleby, L. (1982) Working with the most frequent recidivists: a total team approach to assertive resource management. *Psychosocial Rehabilitation Journal,* **5**(1), 9–11.

Wright, C., Burns, T., James, P., Billings, J., Johnson, S. & Muijen, M., et al. (2003) Assertive outreach teams in London: models of operation. Pan-London assertive outreach study, Part 1. *British Journal of Psychiatry,* **183**, 132–138.

Chapter 4

Cognitive behaviour therapy for assertive outreach service users

Robert Griffiths, Caroline Williams and Neil Harris

Introduction

There are striking parallels between the philosophies underpinning assertive outreach and Cognitive Behaviour Therapy (CBT) (Williams, 2008). Both approaches are collaborative, are designed to reduce dependency on services, improve autonomy and pro-social behaviours, encourage personal growth and promote adaptive behaviours.

The term familiar to many clinicians when describing cognitive behavioural interventions in psychosis services is Psychosocial Interventions (PSI). PSI is an umbrella term that encapsulates interventions designed to improve the well being of service users with severe mental health problems. The term PSI has become synonymous with cognitive behavioural interventions for psychosis and the practice of psychological therapies. Psychological therapies for psychosis, such as cognitive behaviour therapy for psychosis (CBTp), are firmly placed within the psychosocial skills repertoire (Brooker, 2001; Jones et al., 2004; Turkington et al., 2004) and evidence based guidance has recommended the use of cognitive behavioural approaches for people with a diagnosis of schizophrenia (both individual and family based interventions) (NICE, 2002; 2009). There is a trend within the literature, however, to move away from the term PSI, possibly due to an increased specific evidence base for CBTp.

Despite an increasing evidence base for CBTp, there is a paucity of literature exploring its use specifically within assertive outreach teams, although the approach has been recommended as a treatment option within this setting (SCMH, 1998; Department of Health, 2001). CBT has mainly been evaluated in outpatient clinics or (in the case of some CBTp trials) inpatient settings (Cupitt, 2010). Its utility in outreach settings, and the inherent challenges involved in delivering CBTp and CBT within these settings, has not been sufficiently explored, despite recommendations that assertive outreach is a perfect vehicle for delivering such interventions (Turkington et al., 2004).

This chapter explores the scope for using cognitive behavioural approaches within assertive outreach teams and examines related approaches in use, including interventions based on building hope and strengths and assisting in medication management.

Assertive Outreach in Mental Healthcare: Current Perspectives, First Edition. Edited by C. Williams, M. Firn, S. Wharne and R. Macpherson.
© 2011 Blackwell Publishing Ltd. Published 2011 by Blackwell Publishing Ltd.

The chapter will also explore the real world challenges in delivering CBT and CBTp within assertive outreach teams and will suggest solutions to some of these challenges. Due to the differing clinical approaches involved in 'standard' CBT (e.g. CBT for anxiety, anger, depression, etc.) and CBTp (e.g. CBT for voices, delusions, etc.), we have separated the term 'CBTp', when referring to CBT approaches specifically for psychosis, from the term 'CBT' when describing standard CBT approaches. We have avoided the use of the term PSI due the lack of clarity with the term when describing specific CBT interventions.

Cognitive behaviour therapy (CBT)

Cognitive behaviour therapy (CBT) is a psychological therapy based on Beck's (1964) cognitive model of emotional disorders. The central tenet of this model is that a person's emotional reactions are a consequence of their perceptions of a situation, rather than a consequence of the situation itself. An individual's perception of any given situation is thought to be governed by their beliefs about themselves and the world, which, in turn, have been learned through life experiences. These beliefs fall into two categories: unconditional beliefs, known as schemas or core beliefs (e.g. 'I'm a failure'), and conditional beliefs (e.g. 'If I'm always successful, people won't reject me'). When an individual experiences an event that either matches or clashes with their underlying conditional or unconditional beliefs, this generates 'negative automatic thoughts', fleeting thoughts that just seem to 'pop into our heads' without warning, often with themes relating to the person ('I'm useless'), the world ('This is a dangerous area') or the future ('I'll never succeed at anything'). If these thoughts are accepted uncritically, they can have a negative influence on the individual's emotions, physiology and behaviour – often leading to further cognitive distortions and patterns of behaviour that can, unintentionally, contribute to the maintenance of the person's difficulties.

CBT is a structured, time limited therapy that is primarily focussed on the problems a person is experiencing in the 'here and now'. The aim of CBT is to reduce the service user's level of emotional distress by focussing on misinterpretations, self defeating behaviour, and underlying attitudes and beliefs (Morrison et al., 2004). Therapy is guided by the principal of 'collaborative empiricism'. In other words, the therapist and service user working together to identify and evaluate the evidence for a particular belief, and giving consideration to alternative beliefs. This is achieved through the use of a questioning style known as 'guided discovery'. Here, rather than giving the service user direct answers to questions or using a didactic approach, the therapist guides the service user to reach their own conclusions by asking a series of questions that allow the person to explore the different facets of their experiences. One of the aims of therapy is for the person to learn the skills needed to autonomously evaluate their own thoughts, feelings and behaviours.

Although initially developed as a treatment for depression, CBT has since been applied to the treatment of a variety of disorders, including psychosis. Although not unequivocal, there is a relatively good evidence base to support the use of CBT for psychosis (CBTp). The most recent Cochrane Review of CBTp found it to be a promising but under evaluated intervention (Cormac et al., 2004). A more recent review of studies of CBTp conducted by Steel (2008) concluded that the evidence supported its use as an intervention for people with 'treatment resistant' psychosis – in other words, ongoing active positive or negative symptoms, despite adequate treatment – as is commonly seen in assertive outreach caseloads. The National Institute for Health and Clinical Excellence (NICE, 2006, 2009) deemed that the evidence base to support the use of CBTp was sufficiently strong that it should be part of the treatment for all service users with diagnoses of schizophrenia and bipolar affective disorder. Given that assertive outreach teams are specifically designed to work with people who have been given these diagnoses, teams should ideally be in a position to offer CBTp as part of the range of treatments available to service users.

Creating a team environment that is conducive to the delivery of CBT

Although there has been a large investment in training mental health staff in the delivery of psychological therapies, including CBTp (Brooker, 2001), this has not always translated into increased access to these interventions for service users. Common impediments to the implementation of CBTp in routine mental health practice are insufficient time, poor access to appropriate supervision, planned sessions being disrupted to carry out crisis work, difficulty identifying 'suitable' clients, a lack of appropriate knowledge and skills amongst staff, and psychological therapies being viewed as a low service priority by managers (Farhell & Cotton, 2002; Brooker et al., 2003). These barriers have been found to exist in a variety of clinical settings, including assertive outreach (Griffiths & Harris, 2008; Williams, 2008).

As well as needing appropriately trained staff, conditions within assertive outreach teams need to be right for staff to be able to transfer CBTp training into clinical practice. Factors which help with the implementation of CBTp in assertive outreach are staff having protected time specifically set aside for this work, reducing the care coordination responsibilities of therapists to allow them to concentrate on delivering CBTp, having the active support of senior clinicians and managers to keep the delivery of CBTp high on the assertive outreach team's list of priorities, and ensuring that therapists have access to appropriate supervision and ongoing training. It is also useful to develop a policy or protocol that outlines exactly how the team will deliver CBTp. This should provide details about how service users will be identified and recruited for therapy, who will deliver therapy and what provisions will be made to facilitate the delivery of CBTp (e.g. protected time or reduced caseload).

Reflection point

What problems can you identify when considering implementing CBT interventions within your assertive outreach team – are there are any barriers? How will you overcome these?

Who can deliver CBT to assertive outreach service users?

Assertive outreach teams are made up of practitioners from different professional backgrounds with varying levels of training and experience in the delivery of CBT. Generally, some members of the team will not have a core professional qualification. For this reason, team members will not all be offering the same levels or types of cognitive behavioural interventions. Clinical psychologists, because of the nature of their core professional training, are usually well placed to deliver CBT/CBTp. Practitioners from other professional backgrounds – such as nursing, social work and occupational therapy – may also have completed post-qualifying training in CBT and CBTp, and this staff resource should not be overlooked within assertive outreach teams. The British Association of Behavioural and Cognitive Psychotherapists (BABCP, 2008) guidelines on standards for the practice of CBT recommend that, in addition to a core professional qualification, practitioners are expected to have had at least two years post-qualification training and experience to provide CBT.

However, if only staff that have undertaken post-qualifying training in CBT are involved in delivering this intervention, it is likely to be perceived as a specialist intervention, separate from the routine functioning of the team. Potentially, this could lead to CBT being viewed as a low service priority, which may act as an impediment to its delivery. Assertive outreach service users are likely to derive more benefit from working with a team that has a culture where clinical practice is informed by CBT principles than a team where this work is seen as the sole responsibility of one or two 'experts'.

The illustration in Figure 4.1 is a model of how CBT practice can be disseminated throughout the whole team so that, to a greater or lesser extent, all staff are involved in its delivery and all service users derive some benefit from having CBT-trained staff working in the team. The principal of this model is that all service users who are ready, willing and able to engage in psychological therapy should be able to have access to CBT that is delivered by appropriately trained staff. However, at any one time, this is only likely to account for a small proportion of the team's overall caseload. It is likely that many more service users will be able to engage in short-term, structured CBT interventions, such as anxiety management, activity scheduling or relapse prevention. These can often be delivered by experienced members of the team, who may not have received post-qualifying training in CBT, under the supervision of CBT-trained staff. Finally, with appropriate training, all team members could incorporate elements of CBT into routine practice, such as working collaboratively with service users, setting SMART (specific, measurable, achievable, realistic, and time-limited) goals and understanding the links between thoughts, feelings and behaviour. CBT-trained staff can take a lead in developing this culture of CBT-informed practice through the delivery of training and supervision. It can also be useful to establish a regular meeting, facilitated by CBT-trained staff, to formulate a psychological understanding of service users' difficulties and to consider potentially beneficial psychological interventions. This serves several functions: promoting a psychologically informed approach to case management, making it easier to identify those service users who would benefit from individual therapy, and providing support and supervision for the team.

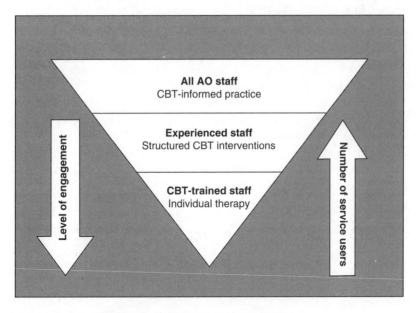

Figure 4.1 A model of CBT implementation in assertive outreach.

Overcoming difficulties in finding appropriate intervention environments

One of the fundamental principles of the assertive outreach model is that care is delivered in vivo. In other words, in the service users own environment, rather than, for example, hospital outpatient departments or other clinical settings. However, finding a suitable environment for psychological therapy can present challenges in assertive outreach. Service users' home environments are often chaotic and unsuitable for this kind of work. In some cases, service users may be homeless or in poor quality temporary accommodation. Consequently, finding a private, safe, and relaxed environment that is conducive to psychological therapy is a perennial problem for practitioners working in assertive outreach teams.

There is no simple solution to this problem. Although visiting service users at home fits most closely to the assertive outreach model, it may be difficult to find somewhere private to talk and there is always the possibility that other people living at the property will interrupt sessions. General Practice surgeries or voluntary sector organisations often have rooms available that therapists are able to access. However, service users are often less inclined to attend a service setting than they are to see mental health staff in their own home. Unconventional settings, such as fast food restaurants at quiet times, have been suggested as appropriate venues to undertake CBT interventions in vivo whilst sharing a social activity (Cupitt, 2010). Issues such as preserving client confidentiality and staff safety need to be taken into account when meeting in public places, but using creative solutions when selecting a venue can maximise the chances that a person will engage in psychological therapy. Public venues can also make good settings to conduct behavioural experiments, which enhance the quality of the therapy. Resolving dilemmas about where to meet requires the therapist to have some knowledge of, amongst other things, the service user's preferences about where they meet with assertive outreach staff, their general attitude to mental health services, their level of social functioning, and how motivated they are to attend therapy. Drawing on the rest of the multi-disciplinary team's knowledge of the service user is invaluable when making these decisions, as is working collaboratively with the service user, providing them with as many options as possible.

So far, this chapter has focused on the preconditions that are required before teams are in a position to deliver CBT interventions to service users, such as appropriately trained staff who have dedicated time to deliver CBT based interventions, and the practical arrangements that need to be made before sessions can take place, such as finding suitable venues to meet. Once these barriers to implementation have been dealt with, challenges still exist for therapists working with this often complex client group.

Attention to medication as a precursor to effective CBT

Service users receiving treatment through an assertive outreach team are likely to be prescribed psychotropic medication and response to treatment with medication can influence the choice and appropriateness of psychological interventions. In addition, a variety of CBT based interventions can improve the likelihood of increased efficacy of medicines and enhance service user's involvement in treatment.

At one end of the spectrum – perhaps as a result of treatment resistance, dangerous behaviour or symptoms that present a risk – service users may require high doses of medication such as antipsychotics or mood stabilisers and this has been identified by assertive outreach staff as a barrier to the effective use of psychosocial interventions (Williams, 2008). Medication side effects are mostly dose related and these can include cognitive impairment, for example, poor concentration, sedation, akinesia (impaired body movement) and akathisia (feelings of inner restlessness). These symptoms can interfere with the person's ability to engage with and benefit from CBT. Other side effects, such as sexual dysfunction or movement disorder, may result in the person prioritising this kind of difficulty. It is important that an assessment of side effects experience is made at an early stage in the process of prioritising CBT work with service users and before beginning therapy. This may be undertaken by the therapist or included as a criterion in a referral process. The use of rating scales can be used to assess these effects. The LUNSERS[*] (Day et al., 1995), for example, is a quick and easy method of assessing antipsychotic side effects.

At the other end of the spectrum is non-adherence with prescribed medication, either intentional or non-intentional. Non-adherence rates are estimated to be around 50% for people with a diagnosis of schizophrenia (Dolder et al., 2002) and between 20–66% for those with a diagnosis of bipolar disorder (Lingham & Scott, 2002). This figure is likely to be substantially higher in assertive outreach service users, as non-adherence is a common criterion for referral to outreach services. Engagement with assertive outreach services is enhanced when service users' concerns about medication are addressed and CBT principles and interventions can be used to explore medication related experiences. Providing information can enable the person to understand how medication can help and

---

[*] Liverpool University Neuroleptic Side Effects Rating Scale.

using role-play and rehearsal to develop negotiation skills increases the likelihood of achieving concordance or shared decision making (Harris, 2009). Other exercises, based on CBT techniques, can aid this process of examination and discovery; looking back to see how medicines have helped or hindered, tying medication decisions to periods of illness or wellness, examining the pros and cons of medication and looking forward, identifying goals and the part medication will play in their achievement. Working with the person's beliefs about medication, such as their subjective effects, the person's ideas about self-sufficiency and self-reliance and their perceptions about illness are areas that affect medication taking. The principles of working with delusions are appropriate here; developing clarity, rating conviction and finding evidence.

Attention to a service user's pharmacological treatment is an important facet in developing effective CBT formulations, not only in establishing the optimum conditions from which to begin treatment but as a possible target for CBT itself. The use of medication within assertive outreach services is explored further in Chapter 6.

Reflection point

What is the therapeutic alliance?
How can this be used in relationship building and engaging clients?

The importance of the therapeutic relationship in CBT for assertive outreach service users

One of the strongest predictors of a successful outcome in CBT – as with many other treatment approaches – is the therapeutic relationship that exists between therapist and service user (Katzow & Safran, 2007). As Newman points out,

> Though cognitive therapy has developed a positive reputation as being conceptually sophisticated and technically rich, it does in fact pay close attention to the therapeutic relationship. (Newman, 2007: 165)

People are often referred to assertive outreach teams because they have had difficult experiences with mental health services, which can result in service users actively avoiding contact with services or, in some cases, hostility towards staff. Although the assertive outreach teamwork approach provides the opportunity for people to develop multiple attachments with the team, very often service users will find it difficult to develop secure attachments, and working with this can be a challenge (see Cupitt et al. (2010) for more on this subject). Assertive outreach service users are also likely to have experienced problems with unemployment, social exclusion, and may have a history of difficult or traumatic personal relationships – factors which are all associated with poorer outcomes in therapy (Beutler, 2002). Therefore, the quality of the therapeutic relationship is likely to be especially important when working with this client group. There is evidence that a good therapeutic relationship between assertive outreach staff and users that are new to the service is predictive of improved treatment adherence and reduced levels of hospitalisation (Fakhoury et al., 2007).

The main components of the therapeutic relationship, according to Hardy et al. (2007), are the affective bond and partnership, the cognitive consensus on tasks and goals, and the relationship history of both participants. They propose a three-stage model that seeks to explain how the therapeutic relationship evolves in therapy. According to this model, the initial focus of therapy should be on establishing a relationship and engaging the service user in the process of therapy. As well as predicting a better outcome, establishing a good therapeutic relationship early on has been shown to increase the chances of people remaining in therapy (Martin et al., 2000). The objectives of initial meetings, therefore, should be to get a sense of the service user's expectations about therapy, to instil a sense of hopefulness about the potential benefits of therapy, and to develop their motivation to engage in therapy (the influence of hope on therapy is looked at in more detail later in this chapter). At this stage of therapy it is important to focus on the humanistic conditions of empathy, warmth and genuineness (Rogers, 1957), negotiating shared goals and establishing a collaborative framework.

Once the therapeutic relationship has started to become established – where the service user is motivated to attend therapy and has a degree of hope about therapy's potential benefits – the aim is to begin to develop this relationship further. The objectives for the second stage of therapy, therefore, are for the service user to trust the therapist, to be open during therapy, and to have a degree of commitment to working with the therapist. To achieve this Hardy et al. (2007) emphasise the importance of exploring the relationship between the service user and therapist, looking specifically for what Leahy (2008) refers to as 'schematic mismatch' (roughly equivalent to the concept of counter transference in psychodynamic therapy). Schemas are specific learned rules that govern our behaviour and help us to make sense of the world (Beck, 1964). To illustrate the sorts of difficulties that schematic mismatch can cause in therapy, Leahy gives the example of a therapist with high standards becoming impatient with a service user whose progress is slower than expected. The therapist's unintentional expressions of frustration confirm the service user's belief that it is unsafe to trust the therapist, damaging the therapeutic relationship as a consequence. Another example would be a therapist who has schemas about being abandoned or rejected and is concerned that service users will end therapy if they are given tasks that are too demanding. The unintended consequence of this may be to activate a service user's schemas about being incapable of completing difficult tasks.

Like everyone, therapists will have a range of personal and interpersonal schemas that influence their relationships with other people. It is useful for therapists to try to reflect on this and to use supervision to explore this further, with the aim of reducing the chances of schematic mismatch negatively impacting on the therapeutic relationship (see Leahy (2007) for more on this topic). Exploring the therapeutic relationship in supervision is particularly important when working with assertive outreach service users, who are likely to have lots of interrelated, complex problems, such as anxiety, depression, psychotic symptoms and substance misuse. Progress in therapy is likely to be relatively slow and, in many cases, service users will end therapy prematurely. Therapists can sometimes feel overwhelmed by the complexity and severity of service users' problems and, without appropriate supervision, they can be left feeling frustrated, which can lead to demoralisation and de-motivation.

Maintaining the therapeutic relationship is the third and final stage of Hardy et al.'s (2007) model. The objectives are to maintain the service user's satisfaction with therapy, to strengthen the working alliance and for the service users to be able to express their emotions openly, while starting to explore their view of themselves. This can be achieved by strengthening the collaborative nature of the relationship, identifying and repairing possible ruptures to the therapeutic relationship, and dealing with any dissatisfaction the service user may have with therapy or the relationship.

Assertive outreach service users are likely to have been in contact with mental health services for a significant amount of time prior to being referred for CBT and may have previous experience of therapy. If this is the case, it is useful to ask about how helpful they found this and what they liked and disliked about therapy; as well as which problems they would like to focus on now and what they would like to get out of therapy on this occasion. This can facilitate the development of the therapeutic relationship by anticipating potential problems that could arise in therapy, emphasising the collaborative nature of therapy and demonstrating to the service user that the therapist is taking their problems seriously and is committed to helping them.

Therapists should expect to work with service users for longer time periods than usual in order to allow adequate time for the therapeutic relationship to be established. In our experience, it is often useful to first establish a trusting relationship with service users in a non-therapy context (for example, by assisting with practical difficulties that are causing the service user high levels of stress) and, once this has been established, move to a more traditional model of CBT if this is thought to be appropriate for the service user.

In our experience, it is often the case that assertive outreach service users drop out in the early stages of CBT, prior to the establishment of a therapeutic relationship. One of the strengths of the assertive outreach model is that service users will often work with several members of the team (Goodwin, 2003). Efforts should be made to ensure that these attachments are maintained during therapy, so that if the relationship with the therapist does break down, the service user still has a good relationship with other team members. In this way, if a service user disengages from therapy, they have not necessarily disengaged from the team as a whole.

Recovery style and CBT for assertive outreach service users

There is evidence that a person's psychological adjustment to psychosis influences the extent to which they will engage with mental health services and psychological therapy. McGlashan et al. (1975) identify two broad categories of 'recovery style' in people who have experienced psychosis: 'integrative' and 'sealing over'. It is thought that people with a sealing over recovery style cope with psychosis by minimising the importance of the experience. They also have a tendency to be less curious about the episode than people who attempt to integrate the experience of psychosis into the narrative of their lives. Tait et al. (2003) found that the process of sealing over begins as soon as a person ceases to experience the symptoms of psychosis and that a sealing over recovery style is negatively associated with engagement with mental health services.

This has implications for the timing of offers of psychological therapy for assertive outreach service users. Tait et al. (2003) recommend that service users should be offered psychological interventions before they experience a full remission of psychotic symptoms. Assertive outreach service users are likely to experience frequent episodes of psychosis and numerous admissions to hospital. Although these experiences are often traumatic and disruptive for the person, these episodes can be an opportunity to engage them in therapy, before the process of sealing over has started.

There is some evidence that people with a sealed over recovery style are more likely to drop out of CBTp than those with an integrative style because they are less curious about their experience of psychosis and because they minimise the impact of the psychotic episode (Startup et al., 2006). However, therapists should be cautious about promoting an integrative recovery style in people for whom sealing over is their usual recovery style because, in some cases, they may be removing a useful defensive process (McGlashan et al., 1987). It is generally more useful to try to work with the person's existing recovery style. It is also worth noting that people tend to have better therapeutic outcomes when they are autonomously motivated to engage in psychological therapy (Ryan & Deci, 2008). Service users should not be pressurised to enter therapy.

The influence of hope on assertive outreach service users' attitude to CBT

Although CBT has a relatively good evidence base to support its use, and even though many assertive outreach teams have skilled, enthusiastic members of staff who are keen to offer CBTp, the uptake of structured therapy by service users is often very low. The consequence of this is that service users miss out on a potentially beneficial intervention and, without the opportunity to practice and maintain CBT skills, staff can start to feel dispirited and deskilled. So why is it that, despite the best efforts of assertive outreach teams, service users are often reluctant to engage in therapy?

One factor that may play a role in determining whether or not service users accept offers of therapy is their sense of hope. Snyder et al. (1991) define hope as 'a positive motivational state that is based on an interactively derived sense of successful (a) agency (goal-directed energy) and (b) pathways (planning to meet goals)'. In order to achieve our goals, according to hope theory, we must have a sense of how we are going to move from the present to an imagined future. This is achieved by planning potential routes that will enable us to reach our goals – known as 'pathways'. In addition, we also require a perception of ourselves as capable of using these pathways to achieve our goals – this is the motivational component of hope theory and is referred to as 'agency thinking'. In order for an individual to be hopeful about achieving their goals, both pathways and agency thought are needed.

Whether we have high or low levels of hope in connection to particular domains of our life is determined by the outcome of our previous goal pursuits and is thought to be

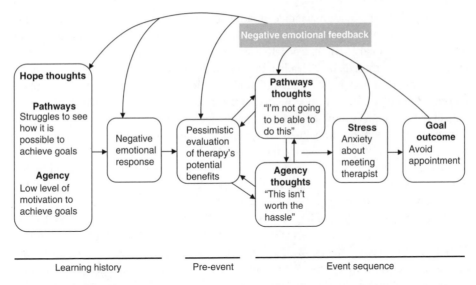

Figure 4.2 A hypothetical negative response to an offer of psychological therapy in someone with low hope. (Adapted from Snyder, 2002). Reproduced by permission from Taylor & Francis Ltd. http://www.informaworld.com

learned over the course of our lives. Individuals who have been repeatedly thwarted in their attempts to achieve goals, or who have suffered high levels of trauma, are more likely to have low levels of hope (Snyder, 2002). This is especially significant when work-ing with assertive outreach service users because it is well documented that individuals with psychosis have experienced higher levels of traumatic life events than the general population (Mueser et al., 1998). In addition to having experienced trauma, assertive outreach service users are also more likely to be unemployed, single and socially isolated. It is reasonable to surmise, therefore, that assertive outreach service users will have lower levels of hope than the general population.

In comparison to individuals with high levels of hope, people with low levels of hope are less able to develop clearly articulated pathways, will experience negative emotions in relation to the pursuit of goals, and are more easily diverted from task relevant thoughts by self-critical rumination about how badly they are performing. The consequence of this is that low hope individuals are less able to achieve their goals compared to those indi-viduals with high levels of hope. This is compounded by the fact that each incident of goal nonattainment further reduces an individual's level of hope for the future (Snyder, 2002). Developing service user's level of hope improves the chances of them continuing with therapy and is associated with positive outcomes (Hardy et al., 2007).

Based on Snyder's (2002) cognitive model of hope, Figure 4.2 is a hypothetical illus-tration of why someone with low levels of hope might struggle to attend an appointment for psychological therapy. Moving from left to right, when the person with low hope is offered an appointment for therapy, their learning history means that they find it difficult to identify possible pathways and lack the necessary motivation to help them achieve this goal. They also experience a negative emotional response to the offer, a consequence of previous occasions where the person has not achieved their goals. At this point, the person with low hope is likely to make a negative appraisal of how worthwhile achieving the goal of attending therapy actually is, leading to negative pathways and agency thoughts. Added to this, stressful events increase the probability of hopeful thoughts of goal-attainment becoming derailed. Within hope theory, stress is defined as anything that acts as an impediment to hopeful thinking. In our example – as a consequence of the negative emotions associated with pursuing goals, a pessimistic evaluation of therapy's potential benefits, negative pathways and agency thoughts, and the impact of stress caused by feeling anxious about meeting the therapist – the person avoids the therapy appointment, which in turn leads to negative emotional feedback, such as feelings of shame, that will influence the pursuit of future goals.

Because Snyder's theory of hope is based on a feed-forward and feedback model, every incident of goal non-attainment will reduce the likelihood of future goal achievement. Therefore, offering therapy before the person is ready can have a doubly negative effect because, not only will they fail to attend that appointment, but it also means that they are less likely to attend future therapy appointments.

Implications of hope theory for assertive outreach service users

Given that assertive outreach teams are likely to be working with people who are low in hope, what can we do to maximise the chances that service users will engage in psychological therapy? The timing of offers of therapy is crucial in determining whether the offer is accepted. For many service users, it may not be appropriate to offer psychological therapy before efforts have first been made to raise their overall level of hope. This might be achieved by helping the person to attain more easily achievable goals. Not only will this have the effect of increasing the person's degree of hope to a level where they may consider accepting offers of therapy, it is also likely to have other positive benefits, such as improving the person's engagement and relationship with the team.

When offering CBT to a service user, it is important to identify any potential stressors or barriers to therapy that could derail the person's goal of attending therapy at the outset. For example, practical considerations such as the venue for therapy, the time of the appointment and whether the person is able to get to the appointment unassisted should all be taken into account. In addition, people may hold preconceptions about what therapy will entail that makes the process feel threatening, making them less inclined to attend. It is important to check out people's expectations of therapy. Any specific anxieties or worries that the service user has about therapy should be explored to see what changes can be made to make the experience feel safer. See Box 4.1 for some key points on building hope.

In spite of our best efforts, very often people will still struggle to attend structured therapy sessions. When this happens it is vital that the service user is not made to feel blamed or as if they have let anybody down. The likelihood is that people will already be experiencing negative emotional feedback – guilt or shame, for example – as a

---

Box 4.1 Building Hope: Key Points

Hope is the ability to plan how we can achieve our goals, combined with the necessary energy to put the plan into action.

- People who are low in hope will struggle to achieve their goals compared to those with high levels of hope.
- Each incident of goal non-attainment reduces a person's level of hope still further.
- Helping the person to achieve smaller, more manageable goals will increase their level of hope.
- If a person's level of hope increases, they may be more inclined to accept offers of therapy.

---

consequence of failing to attain the goal of attending therapy. Additional external negative feedback will only serve to diminish the individual's level of hope still further, reducing the person's ability to work towards future goals. It is more useful to re-evaluate what assistance the person actually needs, before exploring alternative ways of helping them. It may be that they are not ready to engage in therapy at this time. As has already been discussed, assertive outreach service users who do not engage in structured psychological therapy can still benefit from a psychologically-informed approach to case management.

Reflection point

What benefits can CBT interventions bring to your team?

Seeking strengths

Ryan & Morgan (2004) advocate a strengths based approach to the delivery of assertive outreach. Building hope is challenging and difficult in clients who feel hope has abandoned them or that they do not have the skills or strengths to rebuild their lives and manage their symptoms. As discussed previously in this chapter, CBT classically challenges negative thinking, with a focus on the 'problem' (Leahy, 2001). Service users are aware they have a 'problem' and may have discussed this at length over many years with practitioners and, therefore, could feel they have become their label or 'problem'. This is a difficult environment in which to instil hope. The client may possess depressive schema, such as 'I am worthless', 'I am useless' and unhelpful assumptions such as 'What's the point in trying, I'll never succeed'. Therefore, instilling hope and optimism at the beginning of therapy is key to successful CBT intervention.

Taking a strengths based approach as described by Kuyken et al. (2009) is arguably a key intervention when working with assertive outreach service users. Kuyken et al. (2009) argue that engaging with service users through a strengths focus helps clients to seek ways of solving problems in more creative and imaginative ways. Clients may find

---

Box 4.2   A strengths approach in CBT: the case of 'Phil'

(key – C = Clinician / P = Phil)

C: I noticed that last week you said you felt hopeless and that you were not as good as others.

P: Yes, nothing works out for me and I can't seem to get better or manage my paranoia, you know?

C: You worry nothing works out for you and nothing gets better? ... well I wonder if we could shift the focus and look at your strengths today, so we can import some of your strengths to help you solve your current problem?

P: Strengths ... I haven't got any!

C: Ok, that is a common reaction, but can I ask if you remember a time you overcame something, despite all the odds?

P: Yes, when I was in detox – I haven't touched a drink for 15 years.

C: You remember how you coped when you were in detox?

P: Yeah, I had to be strong, my Mam said she didn't want to see me again.

C: What did you do to remain, as you say in your own words, 'strong'?

P: I attended the AA meetings and also attended the self help groups, I was organised and I put into practice what we discussed in the groups. I got irritable once or twice with the staff, but I had to manage it, which I did, because I was so violent, but I did it – I had to though as I didn't want to go back on the booze.

C: That must have been hard, but you sounded motivated, was that the case?

P: Yes I had to be – It was difficult, I struggled at first, but I managed it.

C: So, having a goal, something to help motivate you, helped?

P: Yeah.

C: Ok, Looking back, would you say you had strengths at the time in combating that problem?

P: (smiling) Yes, I never looked at it like that before.

C: Tell me why you have never seen it like that before?

P: I have never felt good about myself, which is why I drank in the first place, so I don't recognise myself as strong.

C: What gets in the way of tapping into those strengths today?

P: The paranoia is so strong and it takes over, you know?

C: You mentioned detoxing was difficult, but you managed to get through – you remained resilient to the problems and have done so since. Is the paranoia as difficult to manage as the urge to drink was?

P: No, nothing is as bad as that.

C: So, if nothing is as bad, do you think we could try and develop a plan to build the strengths you have into helping solve today's problem? The qualities you mentioned that make you resilient – being organised, undertaking self help and putting things into practice.

P: Yes, I could give that a go (smiling).

---

identifying strengths difficult and assisting the client in identifying their strengths by engaging in discussing an area of their life they enjoy or are good at, is the first step in the identification of strengths (Padesky & Mooney, 2009). This enables the therapist to build a personal model of resilience (PMR™) (http://www.padesky.com) with their client. The PMR™ is a collaborative document which resembles a management plan for strengths and allows the service user to build and implement a strengths based paradigm in achieving recovery. See Kuyken et al. (2009) for a more detailed account of a CBT strengths based approach (also see Box 4.2, above).

Conclusions

It has been suggested that assertive outreach teams create an ideal environment in which to provide CBT/CBTp for people with severe and enduring mental health problems who live in the community (Turkington et al., 2004). However, implementing CBTp and CBT approaches within assertive outreach teams is challenging. As described above, success-ful implementation requires a focus on a strategic, team based approach rather than the employment of a lone practitioner trained in CBT. Ideally, the aim of CBT implementa-tion should be to train all staff in CBT-informed interventions (Cupitt, 2010) – rather than solely focus on the recruitment of one or two psychological therapists – to create a culture where CBT principles permeate the routine clinical practice of the team.

Solutions exist to many of the clinical, practical and systemic challenges inherent in delivering CBT within an assertive outreach setting. However, barriers remain, par-ticularly when delivering interventions to those who are reluctant to engage with men-tal health services. Instilling hope, maximising the benefits of medication, adapting to an individual's recovery style and taking a strengths based approach can assist in improving engagement, reducing resistance and allow for successful clinical imple-mentation. However, we should recognise that CBT does not suit everybody. Choice is not only an important aspect of engendering a recovery paradigm (CSIP Choice & Access Programme, 2006), but service user choice has also been recommended when offering psychological interventions (NICE, 2002; 2009). CBT should, therefore, be part of a range of treatments and interventions that assertive outreach teams are able to provide.

CBTp has a promising evidence base and is a recommended psychological treatment for people with psychosis. It can also help assertive outreach service users with a dual diagnosis (Haddock et al., 2003). Assertive outreach teams need to ensure that they have local policies that promote a culture which supports the implementation of CBT and other psychological therapies for all service users, including those considered 'treatment resist-ant'. More AO teams can then start to offer this beneficial, evidence based treatment routinely to their service users.

References

BABCP (2008) *Criteria for Provisional Accreditation as a Cognitive and/or Behavioural Psychotherapist*. British Association for Behavioural and Cognitive Psychotherapies.

Beck, A.T. (1964) Thinking and depression. II: theory and therapy. *Archives of General Psychiatry*, **10**, 561–571.

Beutler, L.E., Harwood, T.M., Alimohamed, S. & Malik, M. (2002) Functional Impairment and Coping Style. In: *Psychotherapy Relationships That Work: Therapist Contributions and Responsiveness to Patients*, (ed. J. Norcross). pp. 145–174. Oxford University Press, Oxford.

Brooker, C. (2001) A decade of evidence based training for work with people with serious mental health problems: progress in the development of psychosocial interventions. *Journal of Mental Health*, **10**, 17–31.

Brooker, C., Saul, C., Robinson, J., King, J. & Dudley, M. (2003) Is training in psychosocial interventions worthwhile? Report of a psychosocial intervention trainee follow-up study. *International Journal of Nursing Studies*, **40**, 731–747.

Cormac, I., Jones, C. & Campbell, C. (2004) Cognitive behaviour therapy for psychosis. *Database of Systematic Reviews*, **2**, 1–46.

CSIP Choice & Access Programme (2006) *Our Choices in Mental Health – A Framework for Improving Choice for People Who Use Mental Health Services and their Carers.* Community Services Improvement Partnership, London.

Cupitt, C. (2010) Cognitive Behaviour Therapy. In: Cupitt, C. (ed.) (2010) *Reaching Out: The Psychology of Assertive Outreach Hove*, Routledge, pp. 186–206.

Day, J.C., Wood, G., Dewey, M. & Bentall, R. (1995) A self-rating scale for measuring neuroleptic side-effects. Validation in a group of schizophrenic patients. *British Journal of Psychiatry*, **166**, 650–653.

Department of Health (2001) *The Mental Health Policy Implementation Guide.* Department of Health, London.

Dolder, C.R., Lacro, J.P., Dunn, L.B. & Jeste, D.V. (2002) Antipsychotic medication adherence: is there a difference between typical and atypical agents? *American Journal of Psychiatry*, **159**, 103–108.

Fakhoury, W.K.H., White, I. & Priebe, S. (2007) Be good to your patient: how the therapeutic relationship in the treatment of patients admitted to assertive outreach affects rehospitalisation. *The Journal of Nervous and Mental Disease*, **195**, 789–791.

Farhell, J. & Cotton, S. (2002) Implementing psychological treatments in an area mental health service: the response of patients, therapists and managers. *Journal of Mental Health*, **11**, 511–522.

Goodwin, A.M. (2003) Dilemmas in providing psychological therapy as an integral component of mental healthcare. *Psychoanalytic Psychotherapy*, **17**(2), 150–162.

Griffiths, R. & Harris, N. (2008) The compatibility of psychosocial interventions (PSI) and assertive outreach: a survey of managers and PSI-trained staff working in UK assertive outreach teams. *Journal of Psychiatric and Mental Health Nursing*, **15**, 479–483.

Haddock, G., Barrowclough, C., Tarrier, N., Moring, J., O'Brien, R. & Schofield, N., et al. (2003) Cognitive-behavioural therapy and motivational intervention for schizophrenia and substance misuse: 18-month outcomes of a randomised controlled trial. *British Journal of Psychiatry*, **183**(5), 418–426.

Hardy, G., Cahill, J. & Barkham, M. (2007) Active Ingredients of the Therapeutic Relationship that Promote Client Change: A Research Perspective. In: *The Therapeutic Relationship in the Cognitive Behavioural Psychotherapies*, (eds. P. Gilbert & R.L. Leahy). pp. 24–42. Routledge, Hove.

Harris, N. (2009) Exploring Medication Issues with Service Users: Achieving Concordance. In: *Medicines Management in Mental Health*, (eds. N. Harris, J. Baker & R. Gray). pp. 189–207. Care Wiley - Blackwell, Chichester.

Jones, C., Cormac, I., Silveira da Mota Neto, J.I. & Campbell, C. (2004) Cognitive behaviour therapy for schizophrenia (Cochrane Review). *The Cochrane Library*, Issue 4.

Katzow, A.W. & Safran, J.D. (2007) Recognizing and Resolving Ruptures in the Therapeutic Alliance. In: *The Therapeutic Relationship in the Cognitive Behavioural Psychotherapies*, (eds. P. Gilbert & R.L. Leahy). pp. 90–105. Routledge, Hove.

Kuyken, W., Padesky, C.A. & Dudley, R. (2009) *Collaborative Case Conceptualization. Working Effectively with Clients in Cognitive Behavioral Therapy.* Guilford Press, New York.

Leahy, R.L. (2001) *Overcoming Resistance in Cognitive Therapy.* Guilford Press, New York.

Leahy, R.L. (2007) Schematic Mismatch in the Therapeutic Relationship: A Social-Cognitive Model. In: *The Therapeutic Relationship in the Cognitive Behavioural Psychotherapies*, (eds. P. Gilbert & R.L. Leahy). pp. 229–254. Routledge, Hove.

Leahy, R.L. (2008) The therapeutic relationship in cognitive-behavioural therapy. *Behavioural and Cognitive Psychotherapy*, **36**, 769–778.

Lingham R. & Scott J. (2002) Treatment non-adherence in affective disorders. *Acta Psychiatrica Scandinavica*, **150**, 164–172.

Martin, D.J., Garske, J.P. & Davis, M.K. (2000) Relation of therapeutic alliance with outcome and other variables: a meta-analytic review. *Journal of Consulting and Clinical Psychology*, **68**, 438–450.

McGlashen, T.H., Levy, S.T. & Carpenter, W.T. (1975) Integration and sealing over: clinically distinct recovery styles from schizophrenia. *Archives of General Psychiatry*, **32**, 1269–1272.

McGlashen, T.H. (1987) Recovery style from mental illness and long term outcome. *Journal of Nervous and Mental Disease*, **175**, 681–685.

Morrison, A.P., Renton, J.C., Dunn, H., Williams, S. & Bentall, R.P. (2004) *Cognitive Therapy for Psychosis: A Formulation Based Approach*. Brunner-Routledge, Hove.

Mueser, K.T., Trumbetta, S., Rosenberg, S.D., Vidaver, R., Goodman, L.A., & Osher, F., et al. (1998) Trauma and PTSD in severe mental illness. *Journal of Consulting and Clinical Psychology*, **66**, 493–499.

Newman, C.F. (2007) The Therapeutic Relationship in Cognitive Therapy with Difficult-to-Engage Clients. In: *The Therapeutic Relationship in the Cognitive Behavioural Psychotherapies*, (eds. P. Gilbert & R.L. Leahy). pp. 165–184. Routledge, Hove.

NICE (2002) *Schizophrenia: Core Interventions in the Treatment and Management of Schizophrenia in Primary and Secondary Care*. National Institute for Health and Clinical Excellence, London.

NICE (2006) *Bipolar Disorder: The Management of Bipolar Disorder in Adults, Children and Adolescents, in Primary and Secondary Care*. National Institute for Health and Clinical Excellence, London.

NICE (2009) *Schizophrenia: Core Interventions in the Treatment and Management of Schizophrenia in Adults in Primary and Secondary Care (up date)*. National Institute for Health and Clinical Excellence, London.

Padesky, C.A. & Mooney, K.A. (2009) Uncover Strengths and Build Resilience with CBT: A Four Step Model. Interactive workshop seminar, Manchester, UK June 18th 2009, User Friendly Psychiatry Ltd.

Rogers, C.R. (1957) The necessary and sufficient conditions of therapeutic personality change. *Journal of Consulting Psychology*, **21**, 95–103.

Ryan, P. & Morgan, S. (2004) *Assertive Outreach: A Strengths Approach to Policy and Practice*. Churchill Livingstone, Edinburgh.

Ryan, R.M. & Deci, E.L. (2008) A self-determination theory approach top psychotherapy: the motivational basis for effective change. *Canadian Psychology*, **49**, 186–193.

SCMH (1998) *Keys to Engagement. A Review of Care for People with Severe Mental Illness who are Hard to Engage with Services*. Sainsbury Centre for Mental Health, London.

Snyder, C.R., Irving, L.M. & Anderson, J.R. (1991) Hope and Health: Measuring the Will and the Ways. In: *Handbook of Social and Clinical Psychology: The Health Perspective*, (eds. C.R. Snyder & D.R. Forsyth). pp. 285–305. Pergamon, New York.

Snyder, C.R. (2002) Hope theory: rainbows in the mind. *Psychological Inquiry*, **13**, 249–275.

Startup, M., Wilding, N. & Startup, S. (2006) Patient treatment adherence in cognitive behaviour therapy for acute psychosis: the role of recovery style and working alliance. *Behavioural and Cognitive Psychotherapy*, **34**, 191–199.

Steel, C. (2008) Cognitive therapy for psychosis: current evidence and future directions. *Behavioural and Cognitive Psychotherapy*, **36**, 705–712.

Tait, L., Birchwood, M. & Trower, P. (2003) Predicting engagement with services for psychosis: insight, symptoms and recovery style. *British Journal of Psychiatry*, **182**, 123–128.

Turkington, D., Dudley, R., Warman, D. & Beck, A.T. (2004) Cognitive behaviour therapy for schizophrenia: a review. *Journal of Psychiatric Practice*, **10**, 5–16.

Williams, C.H.J. (2008) Cognitive behaviour therapy within assertive outreach teams: barriers to implementation: a qualitative peer audit. *Journal of Psychiatric and Mental Health Nursing*, **15**, 850–856.

Chapter 5

Dual diagnosis: putting policy into practice

Rory Allott, Ian Wilson and Mike Firn

Introduction: the context

Definition

Dual diagnosis refers to people concurrently receiving a mental health and substance misuse diagnosis. In the United States (US) the common term is dual disorder and the literature also uses the term comorbidity. As a group, they are far from homogenous. The nature and degree of people's mental health problems *and* substance misuse varies widely. At one end of the spectrum, assertive outreach teams work with people who have received a diagnosis of bipolar disorder, are asymptomatic, smoke small amounts of cannabis and show few negative consequences of their substance misuse. At the other end, assertive outreach teams work with people who have been diagnosed with schizophrenia, use crack cocaine daily, present with multiple psychotic symptoms and show many social and health consequences of the substance misuse. The treatment approach necessarily varies according to where along this spectrum people with a dual diagnosis lie.

Prevalence

Estimates of the prevalence of dual diagnosis in assertive outreach caseloads vary widely owing to methodological and geographical differences. The Pan-London Survey of assertive outreach teams found that 29% of service users met criteria for a dual diagnosis (Priebe et al., 2003). The study's authors have suggested this figure is surprisingly low (Fakhoury & Priebe, 2006). Our experience in the Manchester Assertive Outreach team (MAO) has been that substance misuse is the rule rather than the exception, with around 70% of service users reporting problematic substance use (Schulte & Holland, 2008). These prevalence rates are much higher than would be expected in the general population (Regier et al., 1990).

Assertive Outreach in Mental Healthcare: Current Perspectives, First Edition. Edited by C. Williams, M. Firn, S. Wharne and R. Macpherson.
© 2011 Blackwell Publishing Ltd. Published 2011 by Blackwell Publishing Ltd.

The challenges of a dual diagnosis

As has been reported elsewhere, the majority of people meeting diagnostic criteria for a dual diagnosis are dependent on alcohol (Barrowclough et al., 2001). Around a third report cannabis use and fewer are dependent on crack cocaine (10%), amphetamines (7%) and opiates (4%) (Barrowclough, 2007).

The consequences of substance misuse appear to be significant and reach across multiple domains (see Maslin (2003) for a review). Many of our clients prioritise substance use over food and bills and consequently become malnourished and in severe financial debt. Substance misuse can exacerbate psychotic symptoms and lead to increasingly bizarre behaviours (e.g. chasing snakes around the room, running naked in the street) that can be perceived by others as threatening, leading to homelessness and social exclusion. The likelihood of self-harm and homicide is increased and there are high rates of physical health problems related to both the mode of use (e.g. injecting and blood borne viruses) and the direct consequence of substance misuse itself (e.g. overdose or liver function problems). The challenge for assertive outreach teams is clear: dual diagnosis is associated with poorer clinical and social outcomes.

Meeting the challenge of a dual diagnosis

Drug and alcohol services have traditionally offered interventions focussed on medical treatments for opiate and alcohol dependencies. Opiate users form the smallest group of substance users in assertive outreach. In one team in MAO, there are only two opiate users from an entire caseload of 86 clients. Some medical treatments offered for substance dependency (e.g. disulfiram; dexamphetamine) can exacerbate psychosis and are rarely used in assertive outreach services. Compounding this situation, many people using assertive outreach services find it difficult to engage with traditional services (Hussein-Rassool, 2006) and at least half report finding pharmacological treatments unacceptable and consequently show poor adherence (Patel & David, 2004).

The poor fit between traditional drug and alcohol services and the complex needs of people with a dual diagnosis has been recognised over the last 15 years, both in the United Kingdom (UK) and in the US. In response to these needs, the so-called 'integrated dual diagnosis model' emerged (Drake et al., 2004). Policy has concluded that integrated care by a single team delivers better outcomes than serial care (sequential referrals to different services) or parallel care (more than one service engaging with a patient at the same time) Abou-Saleh (2004).

Assertive outreach and a long-term approach form the core of the integrated dual diagnosis model aiming to respond to the chaos and disengagement that can ensue when some people with mental health problems use substances. In addition, interventions for both substance misuse and mental health problems are provided in an integrated way such that they 'appear seamless, with a consistent approach, philosophy, and set of recommendations. The need [for the individual with a dual diagnosis] to negotiate with separate clinical teams, programs, or systems disappears' (Drake et al., 2004: 470).

A Cochrane Review (Cleary et al., 2007) comparing integrated models of care versus treatment as usual, did not demonstrate that providing dual diagnosis interventions from one assertive outreach team rather than standard case management was more effective. The two major studies in this review were the New Hampshire Dual Diagnosis Study (Drake et al., 1998) and the study by Essock et al. (2006) in Connecticut. An interesting US study of homeless clients with dual diagnosis had a three arm design comparing integrated assertive community treatment (ACT) versus non integrated ACT versus standard care (Morse et al., 2006). No significant differences were found between the three models of care. Despite these limited findings from a small number of methodologically rigorous studies, it is interesting that many commentators and policy makers appear to accept the validity of the integrated approach and the suggestion that integrated treatment programmes improve outcomes (Mueser, 2004).

Best Practice

The Department of Health (2002) issued guidance recommending that mainstream mental health services take responsibility for addressing the needs of people with a dual diagnosis, drawing on support from substance misuse services. The guidance highlights the key role that assertive outreach teams must play in working with people with a dual diagnosis and recommended that all staff in assertive outreach should be trained and equipped to work with this population. It recommended that services match their interventions to service users' readiness to change and identify the following core interventions that staff should be skilled in:

1   Motivational Interviewing (MI) to establish engagement and build motivation to change.
2   Increasing social support, vocational activity and establishing good interagency links with drug services to support active efforts at abstinence or reduction.
3   Relapse prevention to prevent the frequent occurrence of slips back into substance use.

This chapter outlines the approach of the MAO team in working with service users receiving a dual diagnosis. In keeping with the Department of Health (2002) guidance and the explicit strategy within the team of working within a staged approach, it is organised into the four stages of intervention: engagement, building motivation, active interventions and relapse prevention. Case examples are provided to show how the mainstreaming model described above is provided in MAO. The chapter will highlight the role of training and supervision in supporting this model of working and the need to overcome specific barriers to ensure its implementation.

Engagement

Managing the chaos

Initial contacts with service users who have a dual diagnosis start by meeting their basic needs to ensure that the service user experiences quick, tangible progress toward engagement. The focus of these early contacts draws on the team's expertise and skill mix to meet the challenges of unmet basic needs such as housing, finance and welfare interventions to

Table 5.1 Item S9 DACTS

Criterion	Score 1	2	3	4	5
DUAL DISORDERS (DD) MODEL: team uses a stage-wise treatment model that is non-confrontational, follows behavioural principles, considers interactions of mental illness and substance abuse, and has gradual expectations of abstinence	Team fully based on traditional model: confrontation; mandated abstinence; higher power etc.	Team uses primarily traditional model: e.g. refers to AA; uses inpatient detox & rehabilitation; recognises need for persuasion of clients in denial or who don't fit AA	Team uses mixed model: e.g. DD principles in treatment plans; refers clients to persuasion groups; uses hospitalisation for rehab; refers to AA, NA	Team uses primarily DD model: e.g. DD principles in treatment plans; persuasion and active treatment groups; no hospitalisation for rehab, nor detox. except for medical necessity; refers out some s/a treatment	Team fully based in DD treatment principles, with treatment provided by team staff

(Teague et al., 1998)

prevent eviction and combat homelessness, and to ensure that people access benefit entitlements to secure food and utilities. The behaviour, culture, attitudes and values of the team are important and the approach is neatly summarised in item S9 of the Dartmouth Assertive Community Treatment Scale (see Table 5.1; DACTS Teague et al., 1998). This scale for evaluating assertive outreach services uses a 1–5 rating scale for best practice where 5 is highest fidelity.

Case study 5.1

Jim is a 35 year old single man who injects amphetamines, heroin and uses prescribed methadone. In addition to substance misuse, Jim persistently hears voices abusing him and goading him to fight. Jim fluctuates in his belief that the voices were real or part of a mental health problem. Believing they were real, he locked himself in his house, barricading the doors and stayed awake for long periods using amphetamines, holding a hammer to protect himself. Following reports that he might harm a stranger or possibly take a lethal injection of amphetamines, his Community Mental Health Team admitted him to a psychiatric ward. During this inpatient stay, Jim was referred and accepted to MAO. Before the team had engaged with Jim on the ward, the inpatient team discharged him, viewing his repeated intravenous amphetamine use on the ward as the primary precipitant of his psychosis and therefore seeing the admission as futile (see later for a discussion around the role of attitudes in dual diagnosis).

Jim was given a lift to his house, where the assertive outreach team discovered a gas meter with a debt of over £200, a rewired electricity supply, little furniture, several crack pipes and syringes lying around and no food. Jim had spent all his benefits on substances and therefore the team purchased food for him. During this contact and subsequent contacts in the first week, a housing and welfare officer from the team reinstated Jim's gas supply, organised the safe wiring of his electrics, conducted a benefits review and secured a community care grant for carpeting and furniture.

Building motivation

Resolving housing issues and meeting service user's basic needs is only the beginning of an intervention and should not become an end in itself. So often, assertive outreach teams get no further. Stopping here though creates a dangerous situation whereby the assertive outreach team may inadvertently reinforce substance misuse by removing its consequences and, with that, some of the service user's motivation to change. Whilst harm minimisation strategies are part of the staged approach to dual diagnosis (and often the only approach while the individual remains firmly pre-contemplative) the team aim to help the service user move up the stages towards recovery. For these initial engagement and stabilising strategies to work, they need to be conducted as part of larger assessment and intervention plan.

Assessment and intervention

The process of working with someone with a dual diagnosis is no different from working with other clients in assertive outreach. A thorough assessment of risk and need is undertaken before planning appropriate interventions. Although much of the content of this

---

Box 5.1   Dual Diagnosis: Areas for assessment

Patterns of substance misuse and degree of dependence/withdrawal problems.
Assessment of physical, social and mental health problems.
Consideration of the relationship between substance misuse and mental health
  Problems.
Consideration of any likely interaction between medication and other substances.
Assessment of carer involvement and need.
Assessment of knowledge of harm minimisation in relation to substance misuse.
Assessment of treatment history.
Determination of individual's expectation of treatment and their degree of motivation for
  change.
Need for pharmacotherapy for substance misuse. (Department of Health, 2002)

---

assessment is the same as with service users who are not misusing substances there are
additional specific areas to consider for service users with a dual diagnosis (see Box 5.1).

The conduct of this assessment, and how the information from it is used, is important in
working with people who have a dual diagnosis. As mentioned previously, people experiencing mental health problems and using substances feel stigmatised and are often marginalised from both health services and society. It is, therefore, essential that opportunities for
building motivation to change and engaging the service user are maximised throughout any
assessment or intervention.

Facilitating assessment and intervention: motivational interviewing

Motivational interviewing (MI) is an evidence-based counselling style that has become
the core interviewing style recommended for use with people with a dual diagnosis, both
here and in the US (Department of Health, 2002; CSAT, 2005). MI has been demonstrated to improve engagement with psychiatric services, reduce substance misuse and
increase adherence to psychiatric medication (Kemp et al., 1998; Swanson et al., 1999;
Barrowclough et al., 2001). MI is a collaborative, person-centred form of guiding that
elicits and strengthens motivation for change in a range of health related behaviours
(Miller & Rollnick, 2009). Its application has been developed in three separate ways:

- As a stand-alone method that both builds motivation for change and helps a client plan
  for change once a commitment has been made.
- As a prelude to a subsequent intervention (e.g. prescribing medication, delivering cognitive behavioural therapy, engaging in a work placement).
- As a style that permeates routine practice, which is called upon especially where issues
  of motivation become central.

The use of MI in dual diagnosis integrates all three of these applications. All contacts
with service users employ the core skills of MI to guide conversations, such that they are

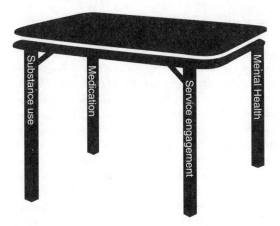

Figure 5.1   Four legged table.

more likely to talk about the possibilities of changing their behaviour in four key areas: substance misuse, medication adherence, service engagement and problematic behaviours linked to their mental health problem. Extending Martino and colleague's (2002) three-legged stool analogy, we have construed these areas as the four legs of a table for ease of memory (see Figure 5.1).

Using core communication skills (open questions, affirmations, reflective listening and summaries) the client is helped to explore their core values and goals and articulate the ways that they think taking medication, reducing substance use and staying engaged with the service can help them to achieve these. At the same time, MI attempts to reduce conflict with the service user and the likelihood of them arguing for the status quo (substance use, avoiding staff, missing their depot injection).

One key area of change, which deserves special mention, is behaviour tied to people's mental health problems. Just as people may be ambivalent about taking medication or reducing substance use, so too will they be ambivalent about altering behaviours, which they believe, keep them safe from harm and further distress. An example of this is where the service user believes they are being pursued by the secret service and consequently remain at home all day with their curtains shut. Rather than offering change-focused interventions aimed at eliminating this avoidance (e.g. cognitive behaviour therapy, support work), MI acknowledges that there are benefits for the client in maintaining the status quo and staying at home. In this case, by avoiding the secret service, the service user also manages to stay away from other people who he fears might find out he has mental health problems. Starting from a position of acceptance reduces resistance, increases engagement and facilitates the client to explore how their behaviour is coming between them and their expressed goals. Only when a client has articulated why they might like to change and, crucially, heard their own reasons for why their current behaviour cannot continue, might the conversation move toward a commitment to change and staff discussing interventions that might support that.

Case study 5.2   Jim and amphetamine use

MI was used early on in the assessment process with Jim. Firstly, the Clinical Psychologist in the team explored with Jim his reasons for substance use. He was already committed to abstaining from heroin and was consequently being prescribed methadone by the Community Drug Team to support this. His amphetamine use, on the other hand, alleviated his depressed mood, which he mostly attributed to the denigrating voices he heard, and reportedly was the only thing that helped him to get out of bed in the morning. Exploration of his key values and goals showed that Jim had previously worked and wanted to return to employment. Moreover, Jim valued his family's view of him, which, at the time, was extremely negative because of his amphetamine use. He wanted to show them that he could succeed in his life. Finally, Jim ultimately wanted to have a girlfriend. All of these goals, to some extent or other, were being prevented by Jim's continued amphetamine use. The excerpt below illustrates how the worker strategically uses reflective listening to both communicate empathy and selectively reinforce Jim's talk about the problems of amphetamine use and the benefits and possibility of change.

> *Jim: The speed's the only thing that gets me up in the morning without it I'm a mong and wouldn't get anything done.*
> *Worker: You can't imagine being able to do anything without the speed.*
> *Jim: Well, that's the thing – I can't get up without it because I'm depressed, but I know I'll never get anything done while I'm still a drug addict.*
> *Worker: The speed's a bit of a short term fix for the depression, but in the long term it's getting in the way of what you want.*
> *Jim: Yeah. Who's going to employ a smack head who's using 3 grams of speed every day.*
> *Worker: And that's something you really want; full time employment … But taking speed everyday is somehow stopping you do that.*

Case study 5.3   Jim and mediation adherence

MI was also used to explore Jim's attitudes toward medication. The excerpt below illustrates how the worker commenced discussions around medication from a 'no change' stance to reduce resistance. The excerpt also illustrates how the four target behaviours (see Table 5.1) appear in most conversations and there is a need for the therapist to remain focussed on these.

> *Jim: They're just goading me to fight. I dunno, I think they just want to do my nut in. Every time I go outside there's no one there. I'm not scared. I'm ready for them. I shout out my door 'c'mon just show yourself, come and have it'.*
> *Worker: It sounds awful, and you're not sure whether they're voices in your head or they're real.* (Reflecting implicit ambivalence around the reality of voices).
> *Jim: I'm convinced they're real, but then I never ever see them.*
> *Worker: And I guess the medication has no impact on them at all.* (Strategically overstating medication's ineffectiveness)
> *Jim: Well, I wouldn't say 'at all'. If I take a stack load at night the voices do stop and I get some sleep.*
> *Worker: The meds do eventually stop the voices and when that happens you think; 'maybe it is in my head'* (Reflecting talk about the benefits of medication and also ambivalence about the reality of voices).
> *Jim: Yeah, I read somewhere that speed can make people psychotic and my dad reckons that's what's happened to me.*
> *Worker: But you're not convinced.*

Jim: Well they're just so real when they're shouting and they're there whether I use speed or not.

Worker: It sounds like they really do your head in and sometimes you end up shouting at them or going outside to see if they're there. You're confused as to whether they're real because you can hear them so clearly, but reflecting on it now you're thinking that; a. you've never seen them, b. you've read something about speed causing people to hear voices and c. they seem to disappear when you take meds. (Summary reflecting positives of medication and ambivalence about the reality of voices).

The excerpt also shows how an MI style can elicit valuable information for assessment and risk management. Here, instead of instantly assessing risk of overdose or providing education regarding the appropriate use of Olanzapine, the team member took the opportunity to build commitment to taking medication and develop ambivalence regarding the reality of voices. The information elicited in this session led to a risk management plan that involved Jim collecting daily prescriptions of Olanzapine alongside his methadone to prevent its misuse. MAO took a lead in establishing this plan in close collaboration between the General Practitioner (who provided the daily prescriptions), the Community Drug Team (who regularly monitored substance use), the pharmacy (who would alert us to non adherence) and a non-statutory drug project that supported Jim to collect his medication every day. The importance of multi-agency working is returned to later.

Adapting MI for psychosis

Some authors have suggested the need to adapt MI for working with people with psychosis (Martino et al., 2002). We have found that we have needed to slow the pace of MI for some people and make slight changes to the way we reflected and summarised; offering less complex reflections and detouring emotional material that led to distressing psychotic symptoms (e.g. thought disorder, voice hearing). As noted above, the trained individuals in the team use MI throughout their routine practice and, therefore, the approach extends beyond the usual one or two sessions, as it was originally conceived (Miller & Rollnick, 2009). This ensures that MI responds to the ongoing, changing needs and challenges presented by people with a dual diagnosis.

We have discovered that accurate reflective listening and empathy can sometimes generate paranoia, the service user believing the therapist was reading their mind. To counteract this risk, we sometimes make use of a greater proportion of simple reflections over complex ones, thereby avoiding reflecting emotion, heightening distress and exacerbating psychosis:

CLIENT: I'm tormented, the only way I can keep going is by knocking myself out on alcohol.

SIMPLE REF: The alcohol knocks you out. (A simple reflection aiming to direct the client toward an exploration of the effects of alcohol without reflecting distress.)

COMPLEX REF: You're desperate to find a way out of the torment. (A complex reflection using emotion to direct the client's exploration of ways to cope with voice hearing that may or may not include alcohol.)

Like others working with this group (Carey et al., 2001; Martino et al., 2002), we have used written materials to help people with memory problems, made sure that sessions were brief, and met people wherever they preferred (e.g. at home, a café, in the park, etc.). We have avoided reflecting on traumatic life events, which this group has experienced more than any other, as this too can exacerbate psychosis and feelings of hopelessness. Instead, we have placed more emphasis on affirming the client and ensuring that there is a strong relationship. Whilst all of these 'adaptations' show some difference in emphasis, none of them are fundamentally different from the spirit of MI or its principles. Moreover, the adaptations are suggested whilst acknowledging the risk of casting a diagnostic shadow over everyone attracting a dual diagnosis, who in reality comprise a group of varied individuals with varying problems and a multitude of resources.

Training

Many mental health staff report feeling ill-equipped when working with clients with a dual diagnosis (Ryrie & McGowan, 1998). Some report hopelessness regarding treatment outcome and make moralistic judgements regarding substance use (Seigfried et al., 1999; Richmond & Foster, 2003). Having a capable workforce is vital to achieving the mainstreaming of dual diagnosis interventions in mental health services. *Closing the Gap* (Hughes, 2006) attempts to address these gaps in knowledge and skill. It is a framework that outlines the capabilities required for working with people receiving a dual diagnosis and provides a blueprint for training and service development (see Box 5.2). It is divided into three sections: values and attitudes; knowledge and skills; and practice development, with each capability given three levels: core, generalist and specialist.

Given what we have learned so far of the concentration of dual diagnosis in assertive outreach services, teams should include staff with skills at levels 2 and 3.

Healthcare workers tend to psychologically distance themselves from people with a dual diagnosis in comparison to friends they know who misuse substances and other non-using clients (Ralley et al., 2008). A consequence of this is that workers may avoid contact with people with a dual diagnosis and this may contribute to poorer outcomes.

Box 5.2   Capabilities framework for dual diagnosis

Level 1 Core
Aimed at all workers in contact with this service user group e.g. primary care workers, A & E staff, non-statutory agency workers.

Level 2 Generalist
Generic post-qualification workers in non-specialist roles (secondary and tertiary care) e.g. community mental health workers, substance misuse workers.

Level 3 Specialist
Those people in senior roles that have specific experience or qualifications, a special interest or specific role in dual diagnosis, and who have a practice development, and/or training remit related to dual diagnosis.

The training programme within MAO has therefore included training both in the interventions recommended for dual diagnosis (e.g. MI) as well as a clear focus in supervision on the attitudes that staff hold. In the case example of Jim, he was discharged primarily because of his substance use, and negative attitudes can be expressed explicitly or covertly throughout the healthcare system which can lead to shortfalls in care. As well as supporting staff within MAO to develop the necessary skills and attitudes for working with people with a dual diagnosis, it has been necessary to offer training to other healthcare providers, such as supported accommodation and inpatient services.

The impact of training in dual diagnosis – the evidence base

The COMO study (Hughes et al., 2008) was a randomised controlled trial in which community mental health team case managers were randomly allocated to receive dual diagnosis training and follow-up supervision, or no training. Training had only a modest impact on attitudes towards working with people with a dual diagnosis. Significant gains were made in knowledge and self evaluated skills in the training group. The COMPASS study (Graham et al., 2006) found gains in knowledge and confidence in five UK assertive outreach teams who received six half days of dual diagnosis training. Assertive outreach teams had access to the training manual and an integrated dual diagnosis specialist. However, there was no significant difference when the teams that had received the training were compared to those who had not had the training. Given the significant need for training, there clearly needs to be a further research on what works in training to produce measurable differences in attitude change, skill acquisition and, ultimately, client outcomes. These studies show that achieving changes in knowledge, skills and attitudes in teams is not straightforward and in our view can only come through team-based training, development and supervision.

Active interventions

Medical interventions for drug and alcohol misuse

The medical management of substance misuse primarily falls into the following broad categories: the physical management of acute detoxification; the treatment of overdose; the pharmacological management of detoxification; withdrawal from alcohol; substitute prescribing (mainly for opiates); the use of medications that reduce cravings (e.g. acamprosate to reduce cravings in alcohol); and the use of opiate antagonists (e.g. naltrexone). Most of these medical interventions are provided within specialist drug and alcohol services and organised according to the guidelines set out in the national framework of substance misuse services (NTA, 2002; 2006a; 2006b).

Models of Care (NTA, 2002; 2006a) set out the national framework for commissioning the treatment of adult drug misuse in England, describing best practice in drug treatment. A sister document outlined a similar framework for alcohol misuse (NTA, 2006b). Both provide a stepped care model of service provision organised around a four-tier system. Tiers one and two provide low level screening, assessment and intervention (e.g. education, brief interventions), whereas levels three and four provide more specialist assessment and interventions (e.g. inpatient detoxification, structured day programmes) aimed at people with more complex needs.

Achieving integration between mental health services and the four tiers of substance misuse services can be challenging when presented with the range of difficulties associated with dual diagnosis. Most clients with a dual diagnosis would expect to access tiers' three and four services, though the reality is often not so clear-cut. As previously mentioned, this client group have a tendency not to engage with treatment agencies, to disengage from treatment and are typically poor at attending appointments (Hussein-Rassoul, 2006). Sometimes when the chaos becomes too difficult, interventions usually delivered by tiers' three and four substance misuse services must be organised and delivered 'in-house', which takes considerable expertise, professional commitment and tenacity. The team must have the knowledge, skills and interagency links to ensure the effective delivery of these interventions. This is largely achieved in MAO through a dual diagnosis network, a network of over 200 service users, substance misuse and mental health workers from both statutory and non-statutory organisations. It meets quarterly and offers opportunities for networking and, in partnership with the local university, offers intensive training to mainstream mental health staff (including MAO) such that they can deliver the core interventions for substance misuse.

Relapse prevention

Relapse is a common part of both substance misuse and severe and enduring mental health problems (Carey, 1995). Interventions aimed at the prevention and management of relapse are therefore vital. The dual diagnosis team provide an outpatient clinic that focuses on supporting clients who are actively making changes in their substance misuse. This has the advantage of providing a setting where the events surrounding relapse can be viewed in a more dispassionate, neutral and analytical fashion than might be the case by services more actively engaged in other areas of a client's care (especially where a relapse into substance misuse has resulted in an inpatient admission).

At one time the issue of relapse was not discussed in treatment programmes (Dennison, 2003). It was as though therapists believed that talking about the subject would make it happen. Avoiding this discussion means losing an opportunity to be prepared in advance for the situation if it occurs – and how to move from relapse to recovery. A method of learning to avoid relapse in the future is to view previous patterns of relapse as a 'learning experience' instead of a catastrophic failure. A detailed 'analysis' of previous relapse cycles can be undertaken to identify triggers and high-risk situations.

Triggers and high-risk situations

Relapse prevention helps the client to identify triggers and high risk situations that leave them vulnerable to using substances and support them to find alternative ways of coping with these. Triggers and high-risk situations mostly fall into three main areas: people (e.g. a drug using boyfriend), places (e.g. the pub) and things (e.g. a glass previously used for smoking crack). Feeling depressed, interpersonal conflict and direct or indirect social pressures have been associated with 75% of reported relapses (Dennison, 2003). Coping strategies for high risk situations can be separated into two categories:

- Specific – planning for a particular event, skills training, cognitive reframing.
- Global – making wider lifestyle changes in order to anticipate or avoid them.

The general principle behind relapse prevention is to help the client to move from a resourceless to a resourceful state, to review previously successful strategies and to encourage their use in the future, whilst avoiding those behaviours that have been less successful. As with relapse prevention for psychosis, there is an emphasis placed on recognising early warning signs and to use periods of relapse as opportunities for learning that can be useful in the future.

Cravings

Another significant factor in a high number of relapses is a craving for substances. They can vary in intensity and, importantly, are time-limited. Enabling clients to learn to cope with cravings is an important component of relapse prevention work. Workers can help clients to learn to recognise triggers and reduce exposure to them. Sometimes, new behaviours can be introduced that can help clients to find ways of distracting themselves through alternative activities (e.g. reading, exercise, talking to someone about the cravings, etc.). Most people never learn that cravings are time-limited, because they assuage them by using the substance before they begin to slowly subside. Keeping a cravings diary can bring greater awareness of when and how they occur and this can enable people to gain enough confidence to wait until they begin to subside.

If the management of lapses fail, the task for the assertive outreach team involves returning to a motivational interviewing style to engage the client, re-motivate them and revisit previous substance reduction goals. The challenge for the team is to sustain therapeutic optimism at a time when the client and those around them may be finding it difficult to do so. Clinical supervision is the primary mechanism through which we achieve this in our service.

Conclusions: turning policy into practice

Co-morbid substance misuse and mental health problems are common in assertive outreach teams. Using substances in the context of a mental health problem can multiply its associated problems and generate a huge number of challenges for both substance misuse *and* mental health services. Multiple problems require multiple interventions and this can mean involving other agencies. The challenge is to ensure that the many health and social care workers that surround the client with a dual diagnosis develop the appropriate knowledge, skills and attitudes that, the evidence now shows, can contribute to their recovery. A further challenge is to find ways of overcoming cultural and organisational differences to provide seamless care across agencies. Assertive outreach teams are ideally placed to go one step further and provide a one-stop-shop for service users when appropriate. Our experience in MAO shows that although it is not always possible to provide every intervention from within a single team, the team can promote positive, hopeful attitudes to working with clients with a dual diagnosis and provide the skills and interventions to help even those with the most complex needs.

References

Abou-Saleh, M.T. (2004) Dual diagnosis: management within a psychosocial context. *Advances in Psychiatric Treatment*, **10**, 352–360.

Barrowclough, C., Haddock, G., Tarrier, N., Lewis, S., Moring, J. & O'Brien, R., et al. (2001) Randomised controlled trial of cognitive behavioural therapy plus motivational intervention for schizophrenia and substance use. *American Journal of Psychiatry*, **158**, 1706–13.

Barrowclough, C. (2007) The development and evaluation of therapy for psychosis and substance misuse. Paper presented at 'Handling og håb for mennesker med dobbeltdiagnose' 27–29. August 2007 Aarhus, Danmark.

Carey, K. (1995) Treatment of substance use disorders and schizophrenia. In: *Double Jeopardy: Chronic mental illness & substance use disorders*, (eds. A. Lehman & L. Dixon). pp. 85–108. Harwood Academic, Chur, Switzerland.

Carey, K., Purnine, D.M., Maisto, S.A. & Carey, M.P. (2001) Enhancing Readiness-to-Change Substance Abuse in Persons with Schizophrenia: A Four-Session Motivation-Based Intervention. *Behavior Modification*, **25**, 331–384.

Center for Substance Abuse Treatment (2005) *Substance Abuse Treatment for Persons With Co-Occurring Disorders*. Treatment Improvement Protocol (TIP) Series 42. Substance Abuse and Mental Health Services Administration, Rockville, U.S.

Cleary, M., Hunt, G.E., Matheson, S.L., Siegfried, N. & Walter, G. (2007) Psychosocial interventions for people with both severe mental illness and substance misuse. *Cochrane Database of Systematic Reviews* 2007, Issue 4.

Dennison, S. (2003) *Handbook of the dually diagnosed patient*. Lippincott, Philadelphia.

Department of Health (2002) *Mental Health Policy Implementation Guide: Dual Diagnosis Good Practice Guide*. Department of Health, London.

Drake, R.E., McHugo, G.J., Clark, R.E., Teague, G.B., Xie, H. & Miles, K. (1998) Assertive community treatment for patients with co-occurring severe mental illness and substance use disorder: a clinical trial. *American Journal of Orthopsychiatry*, **68**(2), 201–215.

Drake R.E., Essock, S.M., Shaner A., Carey K.B., Minkoff, K. & Kola, L., et al. (2004) Implementing dual diagnosis services for clients with severe mental illness. *Journal of Lifelong Learning in Psychiatry*, **II**(1), 102–110.

Essock, S.M., Mueser, K.T., Drake, R.E., Covell, N.H., McHugo, G.J. & Frisman, L.K. (2006) Comparison of ACT and standard case management for delivering integrated treatment for co-occurring disorders. *Psychiatric Services*, **57**(2), 185–196.

Fakhoury, W.K. & Priebe, S. (2006) An unholy alliance: substance abuse and social exclusion among assertive outreach patients. *Acta Psychiatrica Scandinavica*, **114**(2), 124–131.

Graham, H., Copello, A., Birchwood, M., Orford, J., McGovern, D. & Mueser, K. (2006) A preliminary evaluation of integrated treatment for co-existing substance use and severe mental health problems: impact on teams and service users. *Journal of Mental Health*, **15**, 577–591.

Hughes, E. (2006) *Closing the Gap: A capability framework for effectively working with people with combined mental health and substance use problems (dual diagnosis)*. University of Lincoln, Mansfield.

Hughes, E., Wanigaratne, S., Gournay, K., Johnson, S., Thornicroft, G. & Finch, E., et al. (2008) Training in dual diagnosis interventions (the COMO Study): randomised controlled trial. *BMC Psychiatry*, **8**, 12.

Hussein-Rassool, G. (2006) Understanding dual diagnosis: An overview. In: *Dual Diagnosis Nursing*, (ed. G. Hussein-Rassool). pp. 3–15. Blackwell, Oxford.

Kemp, R., Kirov, G., Everitt, B., Hayward, P. & David, A. (1998) Randomised controlled trial of compliance therapy. 18-month follow-up. *British Journal of Psychiatry*, **172**, 413–419.

Martino, S., Carroll, K., Kostas, D., Perkins J., & Rounsaville, B. (2002) Dual diagnosis motivational interviewing: a modification of motivational interviewing for substance-abusing patients with psychotic disorders. *Journal of Substance Abuse Treatment*, **23**(4), 297–308.

Maslin, J. (2003) Substance Misuse in Psychosis: Contextual Issues. In: *Substance Misuse in Psychosis: Approaches to Treatment and Service Delivery*, (eds. H.L. Graham, A. Copello, M.J. Birchwood & K.T. Mueser). pp. 3–23. John Wiley & Sons, Chichester.

Miller, W.R. & Rollnick, S. (2009) Ten things that motivational interviewing is not. *Behavioural & Cognitive Psychotherapy*, **37**, 129–140.

Morse, G.A., Calsyn, R.J., Klinkenberg, W.D., Helminiak, T.W., Wolff, N. & Drake, R., et al. (2006) Treating homeless clients with severe mental illness and substance use disorders: costs and outcomes. *Community Mental Health Journal*, **42**(4), 377–404.

Mueser, K.T. (2004) Clinical Interventions for severe mental illness and co-occurring substance use disorder. *Acta Neuropsychiatrica*, **16**, 26–35.

NTA (2002) *Models of Care for Treatment of Adult Drug Misusers Parts One & Two*. National Treatment Agency, Publications, London.

NTA (2006a) *Models of Care for Treatment of Adult Drug Misusers: Updated*. National Treatment Agency, Publications, London.

NTA (2006b) *Models of Care for Adult Alcohol Misusers*. National Treatment Agency, Publications, London.

Patel, M.X. and David, A. (2004) Predictive factors and enhancement strategies. *Community Psychiatry*, **6**(9), 357–361.

Priebe, S., Fakhoury, W., Watts, J., Bebbington, P., Burns, T. & Johnson, S., et al. (2003) Assertive outreach teams in London: patient characteristics and outcomes. Pan London assertive outreach study, Part 3. *British Journal of Psychiatry*, **183**, 148–154.

Ralley, C., Allott, R., Hare, D.J., & Witowski, A. (2009) The use of the repertory grid technique to examine staff beliefs about clients with dual diagnosis. *Clinical Psychology and Psychotherapy*, **16**(2), 148–158.

Regier, D.A., Farmer, M.E., Rae, D.S., Locke, B.Z., Keith, S.J. & Judd, L.L., et al.(1990) Comorbidity of mental disorders with alcohol and other drug abuse. Results from the Epidemiologic Catchment Area (ECA) Study. *Journal of American Medical Association*, **264**(19), 2511–2518.

Richmond, I.C. & Foster, J.H. (2003) Negative attitudes towards people with co-morbid mental health and substance misuse problems: an investigation of mental health professionals. *Journal of Mental Health*, **12**, 393–403.

Ryrie, I. & McGowan, J. (1998) Staff perceptions of substance use among acute psychiatric inpatient. *Journal of Psychiatric and Mental Health Nursing*, **5**, 137–148.

Seigfried, N., Ferguson, J., Cleary, M., Walter, G. & Rey, J.M. (1999) Experience, knowledge and attitudes of mental health staff regarding patients' problematic drug and alcohol use. *Australian and New Zealand Journal of Psychiatry*, **33**, 267–263.

Schulte, S. & Holland, M. (2008) Dual diagnosis in Manchester, UK: practitioners' estimates of prevalence rates in mental health and substance misuse services. *Mental Health and Substance*

Use: dual diagnosis, **1**(2) 118–124. http://www.informaworld.com/smpp/title~db=all~content=t
777186830~tab=issueslist~branches=1 - v11

Swanson, A.J., Pantalon, M.V. & Cohen, K.R. (1999) Motivational interviewing and treatment
adherence among psychiatric and dually diagnosed patients. *Journal of Nervous and Mental
Disease*, **187**, 630–635.

Teague, G.B., Bond, G.R. & Drake, R.E. (1998) Program fidelity in assertive community treatment:
development and use of a measure. *American Journal of Orthopsychiatry*, **68**(2), 216–232.

Chapter 6

Use of medication in assertive outreach

Rob Macpherson and Tom Edwards

Case study contributors: Vinnie Farrell and Mike McKenzie

Introduction

Assertive outreach involves working with service users whose illness has been difficult to treat, for a variety of reasons. Although there are many ways to help these individuals, optimising medical treatment is an essential aspect and can on occasions help people on their path to dramatic, life changing recovery. The two major challenges in using medication in assertive outreach teams are treatment resistance and non-compliance, and these, not uncommonly, occur together. This chapter will focus on the challenge of working in community based settings with people who continue to have a high level of symptoms, who may have a framework for understanding their difficulties which differs greatly from the medical view and who may openly oppose attempts to persuade them to take treatment.

> I've had hospital admissions for the last 12 years and been treated under the assertive outreach team for the last 4. I was diagnosed first with depression but then that changed to schizoaffective disorder. At first, my symptoms would improve, but that never seemed to last. (Comments of a service user)

Treatment of psychosis: 'the state of the art'

> The great tragedy of science- the slaying of a beautiful hypothesis by an ugly fact. T.H. Huxley (1825–1895)

There is extensive evidence that use of antipsychotic medication is effective in the treatment of schizophrenia and schizoaffective disorder, both as an acute treatment of illness episodes and in the prevention of relapse (NICE, 2009). A problem with the research evidence has been that randomised controlled trials have tended not to look beyond short term treatment (three to six months) and generally exclude people with substance misuse or compliance problems, so it is difficult to extrapolate research findings to the people who receive treatment in assertive outreach teams.

Assertive Outreach in Mental Healthcare: Current Perspectives, First Edition. Edited by C. Williams, M. Firn, S. Wharne and R. Macpherson.
© 2011 Blackwell Publishing Ltd. Published 2011 by Blackwell Publishing Ltd.

'Typical' antipsychotics such as Chlorpromazine and Haloperidol have been used widely in the treatment of severe mental illness since the 1960s. The so called 'second generation', or 'atypical' antipsychotic drugs (with a reported reduced risk of neurological side effects) have been developed over the last two decades. These drugs, which include Olanzapine, Risperidone, Quetiapine and Aripiprazole, were reputed to have superior efficacy for positive and negative symptoms and favourable effects on cognitive functioning. However, Heres et al. (2006) concluded that much of the evidence for these claims was based on short-term studies, with selected patient groups, high dropout rates and outcomes focussing on symptom ratings selected to demonstrate certain findings, in the context of pharmaceutical industry funding. Despite initial hopes and claims, systematic reviews and meta-analyses have shown only partial, or sometimes no superiority of the second generation antipsychotics (Geddes et al., 2000; Leucht et al., 2009).

These findings have contributed to a widespread debate in the academic literature regarding the use of randomised controlled trials (RCTs) as the 'gold standard' method for establishing treatment efficacy, due to concerns about lack of real-world considerations and clinical relevance of RCTs. It has been argued that some sources of bias, such as exclusion criteria (for example impaired capacity due to illness related factors, arbitrary age cut-offs, excluding women due to concerns about conception while in the trial), are an inherent part of RCT protocols and make generalisation of results impossible (Hodgson. et al, 2007). Use of rating scales to define change may have limited relation to clinicians' views of improvement and reporting of side effects has often been highly selective.

There is a renewed interest in *observational studies*, in which treatment outcomes are compared in natural settings over prolonged periods, with clinically meaningful outcomes, such as drug discontinuation or hospitalisation. The main weaknesses of this form of research are the lack of true randomisation and possible ratings bias, which limit interpretation of findings. However, the risk of over-estimating the treatment effect has been challenged by studies demonstrating similar outcomes from both types of study (Concato et al., 2000) and these researchers argued that observational studies are more likely to produce consistent and meaningful outcomes as they relate to a broad spectrum of the population at risk. Hodgson et al. (2007) suggested that in examining treatment efficacy in the clinical setting, evidence from RCTs, observational studies and pragmatic trials in real life settings should be triangulated.

Recent trials evidence

In response to the dilemma about the efficacy of first versus second generation antipsychotics, the National Health Service (NHS) Health Technology Assessment R&D Office in the United Kingdom (UK) and National Institute of Mental Health in the United States (US) developed large clinical trials, with wide inclusion criteria and extended follow up periods. The UK Cost of Utility of the Latest Antipsychotic Drugs in Schizophrenia Study (CUtLASS) (Jones et al., 2005) was an open, randomised trial comparing typical and atypical antipsychotics excluding Clozapine. This study found no advantage of second generation antipsychotic drugs in relation to symptoms or quality of life after one year; in fact, those receiving first generation antipsychotic drugs were reported to have done rather better. The patients reported no preference for either drug class and there was no significant difference in rates of major side effects, including extra-pyramidal problems such as stiffness and tremor, which have been generally seen as a problem of the first generation drugs. The study found no difference in efficacy for negative symptoms or cognitive deficits.

The US Clinical Antipsychotic Trials of Intervention Effectiveness (CATIE) (Lieberman et al., 2005) was a double blind, multi-centre trial. Patients with chronic schizophrenia were randomly allocated to groups taking the atypical drugs Risperidone, Quetiapine, Olanzapine, Ziprasidone, or the medium potency typical antipsychotic Perphenazine. The main outcome was discontinuation of medication for any reason, including side effects, lack of efficacy or service user preference. Clinicians started trial medication within double blind conditions (i.e. they did not know which drug was being given). Olanzapine was found to have the lowest discontinuation rate, but it also had the highest side effect profile. However, there was no significant difference between the other atypical drugs or Perphenazine in terms of effectiveness or side effects. In total, 74% of patients were discontinued from the initial, randomised treatment within 18 months. Questions have been raised as to whether Perphenazine was the best choice as a typical antipsychotic, as it is little used in some countries (including the UK) and may have some 'atypical' characteristics, rather like Sulpiride.

The Schizophrenia Outpatient Health Outcomes (SOHO) study (Haro et al., 2007) was a large scale, open, pan-European observational study, which examined outpatient treatment over up to three years, of over 10,000 cases of schizophrenia. The results gave many insights into social functioning, patterns of treatment and factors associated with relapse and remission. In general high rates of antipsychotic switching/discontinuation were found (up to 66% for Quetiapine); Olanzapine and Clozapine were found to have the lowest discontinuation rates. Some 65% of patients achieved remission, in keeping with findings from other long-term studies (Hodgson et al., 2007).

These observational and pragmatic trials have taken a new approach to studying treatment in schizophrenia, going beyond short-term efficacy comparisons and instead comparing the outcome of drug treatments in real-world settings, allowing more meaningful comparisons with clinical practice. The results imply that with careful prescribing (use of lower doses and avoiding high potency drugs), first generation antipsychotics may be as effective as second generation antipsychotics in schizophrenia. These findings have important implications for assertive outreach clinicians, where service user choice and attempts to maximise treatment effectiveness and tolerability over the longer term are of particular importance.

Side effects of antipsychotics

The most troublesome side effects reported by people taking antipsychotics are sedation, weight gain, extra-pyramidal affects (commonly akathisia, stiffness or tremor) and sexual dysfunction which can be linked to hyper-prolactinaemia (NICE, 2009). Autonomic effects including blurred vision, constipation and dry mouth are also common, particularly with first generation drugs. Several antipsychotics have been shown to affect ventricular repolarisation in the heart, leading to a risk of ventricular arrhythmias. Tardive dyskinesia (involuntary oro-facial and trunk movements) is a late onset side effect which may be less common with second generation drugs.

Table 6.1   Treatment options to address antipsychotic side effect problems

Antipsychotic adverse effect	Suggested antipsychotic treatment
Sedation	Sulpiride, Risperidone, Aripiprazole, Haloperidol
Weight gain	Amisulpiride, Aripiprazole, Haloperidol
Extra-pyramidal side effects	Quetiapine, Aripiprazole, Olanzapine, Clozapine
Increased cholesterol, glucose intolerance	Amisulpiride, Aripiprazole, Ziprasidone
Postural hypotension	Sulpiride, Aripiprazole, Risperidone, Amisulpiride
ECG changes, QT prolongation	Aripiprazole, Olanzapine
Sexual side effects (may be related to hyper-prolactinaemia)	Quetiapine, Aripiprazole, Ziprasidone

(from The Maudsley Prescribing Guidelines, 9th edition, Taylor et al., 2007)

Of particular concern has been the association between the metabolic syndrome (hypertension, obesity, insulin resistance and dyslipidaemias, a possible precursor to type II diabetes) and second generation antipsychotics (American Diabetes Association, 2004). Awareness of the high prevalence of other high risk lifestyle factors in people with psychosis such as smoking, poor diet and exercise (Department of Health, 2006a), has led to a consensus that people taking these drugs longer term should receive regular physical health screening. Antipsychotic side effects cannot always be overcome, but Table 6.1 suggests treatment changes to address these.

Assessment when treatment is not working

A thinker sees his own actions as experiments and questions – as he attempts to find out something. Success and failure are for him answers above all. Friedrich Nietzsche (1844–1900)

There are many possible reasons for poor response to treatment. The starting point to address these is to take a full history, assess the mental state and make both a psychiatric diagnosis and a formulation about why treatment is not working. Pharmacists, nurse prescribing colleagues and psychiatric trainees may undertake the assessment, but the use of a team based reflective session may create the space to fully explore the situation. The aim is to reach a formulation explaining why treatment problems occurred and what can be done to address these. Box 6.1 shows areas to assess.

Treatment resistance

Your treatment does not make any difference to the voices at all, the only useful thing it does is give me a good night's sleep. (Quote from a service user after 12 years treatment with antipsychotics)

Box 6.1   Assessment when treatment is not working

- The service user's view – what treatment worked, which caused side effects, which was the best/worst treatment so far. Attitudes to Clozapine and intramuscular treatment.
- Treatment history – all medications used, response, side effects, as recorded in the case notes.
- Has there been an attempt to use a cognitive behaviour therapy (CBT) approach and if so what was the outcome? Has family work been undertaken, if the person lives with family/carers?
- Complicating factors – use of substances including alcohol, cannabis, stimulants. Lifestyle issues, stress due to homelessness or other major social difficulties.
- Attitudes to illness – does the person see paranoid ideas, voices as due to psychosis, does he or she see him- or herself as ill and needing treatment?
- Present and past side effects – particularly weight gain, sedation, other serious problems.
- Views of other key people – include current and past team members, inpatient team, views of family/carers (with consent of the service user).
- Careful physical assessment to exclude possible physical causes of mental illness, co morbid physical illness. Consider drug interactions affecting antipsychotic treatment.

Table 6.2   Service users' and professionals ranking of factors in medication compliance

Factors influencing compliance	Service user	Professional
Efficacy of medication	1	5
Side effect self management	2	7
Positive medication attitudes	4	10
Side effects	6	2

Ranking: 1 – most important, 10 – least important

Treatment resistance refers to a poor response to treatment in terms of ongoing psychosis or poor social functioning, difficulties generally accumulating over a number of illness episodes. The standard definition is failure to respond to sequential use of two antipsychotic drugs given at optimal dose for four to six weeks, one of which must be second generation. Treatment resistance can refer to resistant positive or negative symptoms of psychotic illness.

Assessment follows the principles set out above. Assessing attitudes to treatment, acceptance of illness and side effects are all of particular importance as understanding the service user's perspective may unlock barriers to treatment: Table 6.2 (from Kikkert et al. (2006)) compares service user and professional attitudes regarding compliance.

Professionals in assertive outreach teams are likely to be able to build up a detailed picture of attitudes to treatment and side effects of different medication, over a prolonged period. This can be achieved through repeated discussions with service users and others and it is possible that using rating scales as listed in Box 6.2 may help to assess how these factors change over time.

Box 6.2   Rating scales of use in assertive outreach

Brief Psychiatric Rating scale (BPRS); (Overall & Gorham, 1962). A scale measuring severity of psychopathology.
Engagement Measure (EM); (Hall et al., 2001). Measures staff rated engagement including
attention to compliance with treatment.
KGV scale (KGV); (Kravieka, Goldberg & Vaughn, 1977). A scale rating psychopathology
which can be useful in assessing symptoms accurately and planning treatment.
Knowledge about Schizophrenia Inventory (KASI); (Barrowclough et al., 1987). Assesses
the knowledge about illness and treatment, can be used with service users and carers.
Liverpool University Neuroleptic Side Effect Rating Scale (LUNSERS); (Day et al., 1995)
Positive and Negative Syndrome Scale (PANSS); (Kay et al., 1987). Rates psychopathology including scales for positive, negative symptoms and general psychopathology. Often
used in pharmaceutical trials.
Social functioning scale (SFS); (Birchwood et al., 1990). Assesses social functioning across
a range of domains.

Formally assessing compliance with treatment may be important when this is in doubt
and may include trial supervised administration of medication, as well as serum testing of
medication levels (although this is not available for all antipsychotics).

Case study 6.1   Supporting use of medication in the Liverpool assertive outreach team

*Liverpool assertive outreach team is part of Mersey Care NHS Trust, covering a population of 220,000
in Central and South Liverpool. The area has high levels of poverty, deprivation and a sizable ethnic
minority population, with Mini scores in the range of 111–132. The current caseload is 135.*

*We supply oral medication for approximately 35% of our service users in our team. About half
are on Clozapine, which is dispensed from the hospital pharmacy to our office each week. Some
prescriptions are ordered from the hospital pharmacy, the rest are collected from local pharmacies.
Clearly it is not a strategy to be used with all service users and teams need to guard against
fostering dependence, seeing this support as a time-limited intervention and passing back the
responsibility for dealing with medication as the service user becomes more stable, as part of the
recovery plan.*

*Supporting service users to obtain and sometimes administering medication in the home involves
some challenges:*

– remembering to order prescriptions on time throughout the week.
– ensuring appropriate storage is available.
– travelling to different pharmacies and waiting for medication to be dispensed.
*– this work is often the focus for any conflict over treatment and will directly expose negative
attitudes about taking medication.*

*As well as creating a very untidy work space, it can be a time consuming process with obvious
cost implications!*

*However we continue to do this as the benefits far outweigh the problems we may encounter.
Many assertive outreach service users are hard to engage and have poor social functioning and
difficulty maintaining contact with services. They may have difficulty accessing primary care
services, perhaps due to previous negative experiences. Building trusting, collaborative relationships*

with service users and carers is a key component of engagement and needs a high level of consistent, face to face contact. Helping with medication can be a positive engagement strategy for the team, demonstrating how the team is different from more traditional services and willing to engage in helpful, practical everyday activities. The task of medication management is often seen as beneficial by service users and carers and can reduce stress and anxiety.

Medication management must be more than simply picking up and delivering medication. It promotes dialogue around efficacy, concordance, side effects and co morbidity and may facilitate collaborative working with service users and their carers in a way that more formal approaches may fail to achieve. This can be valuable when assessing symptoms, managing risk and identifying early warning signs of relapse.

Treatments of use in resistant psychosis

Much depends on the assessment of the cause of treatment resistance and the resulting formulation of a management plan to address this. Occasionally taking pills can be a problem for some individuals and preparations available in syrup form or tablets which melt rapidly on the tongue may be preferred.

Intramuscular antipsychotics

The NICE guidelines on the treatment of schizophrenia (2009) advise that depot antipsychotic medication should be considered in patients who have a history of non-compliance with oral medication. Long acting injections are given in the UK to between a quarter and a third of people being treated for schizophrenia at the time of writing (Barnes et al., 2009). Certainty of treatment administration is probably the key advantage of this form of treatment, but it is important to recognise that intramuscular treatment is not helpful or acceptable to all. Some individuals are nervous of injections and others reject the idea of accepting treatment passively, or due to embarrassment. Problems of pain and lumps at the injection site can be distressing. There is evidence that a significant number of people started on intramuscular preparations default from these (Young et al., 1999). However, there is some evidence of improved outcomes with first generation antipsychotic long-acting injections, rather than oral preparations (Haddad et al., 2009). A number of service users prefer depot medication, perhaps due to the greater convenience and the certainty of this form of treatment in those leading a chaotic lifestyle.

Using Clozapine in the assertive outreach team

Although it was first discovered and used as long ago as 1958, Clozapine remains the only antipsychotic which has shown efficacy in treatment resistant schizophrenia. After its launch in the 1970s, reports of the serious side effect agranulocytosis led to a partial international withdrawal of its use. The paper by Kane et al. (1988) showed that Clozapine had greater efficacy in treatment resistant schizophrenia than conventional antipsychotic treatment. Clozapine was subsequently reintroduced in the UK with special licensing arrangements, which restrict use to treatment resistant illness and require regular blood testing. NICE guidelines for the treatment of schizophrenia (2009) state that service users whose psychosis has not responded to the sequential use of at least two antipsychotics at adequate dosage, of which at least one should be a second generation antipsychotic, should be given a trial of Clozapine. Use of Clozapine is a standard part of most assertive outreach teams' work.

Starting Clozapine and monitoring treatment

Starting Clozapine is complex and needs to be explained to the service user as a major intervention, which if helpful will continue for a number of years. Informing service users involves discussing benefits and side effects (including agranulocytosis, metabolic syndrome and cardiac problems), and will establish whether the individual has capacity and agrees with the treatment plan. Where possible the involvement of carers in planning treatment is also important. In practice, issues of capacity are complex as people with treatment resistant illness may have cognitive impairment and thought disorder. Assessment of capacity should be made following guidance in the Mental Capacity Act (2005), unless the patient is detained under the Mental Health Act (1983). If the clinical team believes that it is right to start Clozapine and the patient lacks capacity, then consultation with the service user, carers and if appropriate an Independent Mental Capacity Advocate (IMCA) will establish whether treatment is in the individual's best interests. Seeking a second opinion from another experienced clinician is advisable in this scenario.

Concern over the possibility of major haematological side effects in the early stages of treatment has led to a cautious approach to initiation of Clozapine in the community. It has been demonstrated that the resources and intensity of care provided by assertive outreach teams make this possible (O'Brien & Firn, 2002) and many teams now adopt this approach as standard. Exceptions include individuals with physical health concerns related to possible side effects. Community initiation of treatment fits with assertive outreach principles of home based care and also patient preference. Avoiding admission and providing proactive support around adherence and the blood testing arrangements for Clozapine markedly increases access to this effective treatment.

Baseline physical checks are required before initiation and the service user should have a physical examination and be weighed. During the first month of treatment, the dose is gradually titrated upwards and two or three daily physical health checks ensure that problems such as pyrexia and tachycardia are detected and addressed at an early stage. Standard regimes for dose titration and physical health monitoring during initiation can be found in the Maudsley Prescribing Guidelines (Taylor et al., 2007).

The measurement of serum Clozapine levels has become standard practice in recent years. Where service users respond poorly to Clozapine, the dose should be adjusted in order to achieve serum levels of 0.35–0.5 mg/L. There is evidence that serum Clozapine levels relate to side effects and to some extent predict EEG changes (Khan et al., 2005); serum levels greater than 1.0 mg/L are associated with a higher frequency of seizures. Prophylactic use of Sodium Valproate to reduce the risk of seizures may be considered

Table 6.3 Clozapine side effects

Common side effects (%)	Serious side effects (less than 1%)
Drowsiness (39%)	Agranulocytosis (low white blood cell count)
Hypersalivation (30%)	Myocarditis (inflammation of heart muscle)
Fast heart rate (25%)	Seizures
Dizziness (19%)	Orthostatic hypotension (low blood pressure)
Constipation (14%)	Thromboembolism (blood clots)

Data from http://www.drugs.com/sfx/clozaril-side-effects.html

when at a standard therapeutic dose of Clozapine, serum Clozapine levels are found to be above the therapeutic range.

Smoking increases metabolism of Clozapine by inducing liver enzymes. Plasma concentrations of clozapine vary considerably at a given dosage and this variation may be greater in heavy smokers receiving lower doses of Clozapine, increasing the risk of subtherapeutic concentrations (Diaz et al., 2005). Adjustment of Clozapine dose in patients who stop smoking during treatment is important, to avoid elevated serum Clozapine levels and risk of toxicity.

Monitoring Clozapine treatment and managing side effects

There are a range of common and potentially serious Clozapine side effects, as seen in Table 6.3. Special concerns have been raised about the risks of the metabolic syndrome, as Clozapine appears to have a higher risk of weight gain, compared with other antipsychotics.

Service users take Clozapine for prolonged periods and need help to manage these problems. Hypersalivation reduces over time and is often treated with Hyoscine or Pirenzepine, although the evidence for either is limited. Close working with cardiology colleagues is needed to address the range of cardiac problems. Constipation should be addressed early with high fibre diet, bulk-forming and stimulant laxatives. Dietary advice is advised before initiation and weight gain can be so severe as to require cessation. Nocturnal enuresis may be missed if not actively assessed and may respond to dose timing changes and evening fluid restriction.

Using Clozapine in the assertive outreach team

Working with service users who comply inconsistently and disengage from services, results in some particular challenges using Clozapine and licensing arrangements further complicate the picture. Where a break in treatment (often due to intermittent non-compliance) goes beyond 48 hours, the Clozapine monitoring services will recommend stopping treatment and dose retitration, as from treatment initiation. This can create a clinical crisis as there is a risk of rebound psychosis upon abrupt withdrawal of Clozapine (Moncrieff, 2006). The lead clinician needs to discuss with the respective Clozapine monitoring service agency team whether the balance of risks is best addressed by Clozapine cessation and full retitration (risking relapse), by restarting the previous dose (risking side effects), or the usual solution of rapidly retitrating, over three to six days, to the former dose. When service users miss blood tests, the monitoring service agency will generally agree to continuation of treatment for a period (one week in service users having monthly tests), but the team will need to rapidly obtain the necessary blood result, to ensure no break in treatment.

The intensity of assertive outreach service provision over seven days and the team approach mitigates the barriers to maintaining individuals on Clozapine. The team has the ability to support medication adherence at home and ensure blood samples are obtained, with many teams having staff trained to take blood. This is labour intensive in the early, more chaotic stages of treatment but where long-term benefits occur this activity is very often seen as a beneficial investment.

Augmentation of Clozapine

The treatment effect of Clozapine may take a number of months to become apparent. The classic study by Kane et al. (1988) showed that Clozapine was probably helpful to some extent in 30–50% of patients with treatment resistant schizophrenia and these results were fairly typical of subsequent research (Iqbal et al., 2003), using optimal doses of Clozapine. In contrast to other antipsychotic treatments, peak response occurs in the 12–24 week period, but in an open trial by Conley et al. (1997), there was found to be little clinical advantage in extending treatment with Clozapine beyond eight weeks, if no response was observed.

So how can clinicians best help those who do not respond well to Clozapine? Research on augmentation of Clozapine with other antipsychotics has been limited. There is developing evidence (although as yet no randomised trial) for the use of Amisulpiride (Munro et al., 2004), which may be effective and allow Clozapine dose reduction. A favourable randomised controlled trial of Clozapine augmentation with Sulpiride (Shiloh et al., 1997) supports its use. There is most evidence regarding Risperidone, including a number of randomised controlled trials, with mixed results which do not really support its use in Clozapine augmentation beyond empirical trial. A randomised trial of augmentation with Aripiprazole (Chang et al., 2008) suggested limited benefits, restricted to mildly alleviating negative symptoms. It seems logical to avoid augmentation with typical antipsychotics and drugs with marked effect on electrical activity in the heart, such as Olanzapine and Quetiapine.

Other forms of Clozapine augmentation depend on the service user's symptom pro-file: there is limited evidence to support the use of mood stabilisers including Sodium Valproate, Lamotrigine and Lithium, but these treatments may cause problematic drug interactions and caution is advised. Carbamazepine is not generally seen as a good choice for Clozapine augmentation due to its risk of agranulocytosis. Fish oils have often been used clinically and are sometimes sought out by interested service users or carers looking for more 'natural' forms of treatment. There have been supportive ran-domised trials (Puri et al., 1998) and this may be worth trying, although gastrointesti-nal side effects and weight gain can occur. In her review, Sweeting (2006) noted that whenever considering use of multiple medications it is important to consider the possibility of additional side effects, pharmacological interactions, compliance problems and cost effectiveness.

Antipsychotic polypharmacy and use of high dose antipsychotics

The practice of combining two (or more) antipsychotic drugs, sometimes called 'polypharmacy' was criticised in the first and second NICE Guidelines for schizophrenia (2002 and 2009). Concerns about excess total antipsychotic dosages, multiplication of side effects and lack of demonstrated efficacy are generally accepted in the psychiatric profession (Kreyenbuhl et al., 2007). However, some results from observational studies have challenged the perceived lack of efficacy (Haro et al., 2007) and an extensive audit of UK prescribing (Harrington et al., 2002) found that nearly half of antipsychotic prescriptions were for more than one drug.

The use of high dose antipsychotics, that is, at doses (including all medication given) greater than recommended in the British National Formulary, is seen in up to a quarter of inpatients (Harrington et al., 2002) and is used mostly to manage aggression among inpatients and resistant psychosis. The practice has caused concern particularly in relation to possible cardiac side effects and sudden death, which was found to be 2.4 times more likely in people taking antipsychotics (Ray et al., 2001). A report by the Royal College of Psychiatrists (2006) advised against use of high dose antipsychotics unless evidence-based strategies have failed, and then only as a carefully monitored therapeutic trial, led by a fully trained psychiatrist, with ECG monitoring. However, the report concluded that most clinicians have experience of a small number of service users who do well on combination and higher dose treatment and that some individuals may have genetically determined differences in response profiles, that 'may justify a degree of dose finding in clinical practice'.

Reflection point

Use of medication 'off licence'
It is common for patients who are on an effective dose of an antipsychotic medication, to continue to have active problems with psychosis or negative symptoms and the team will often be faced with the dilemma of treating a patient where there is limited evidence (at least, evidence from randomised, controlled trials) from which to draw, to plan treatment.

Think through how you could research this problem and what resources inside and outside your team could be of use.

It seems likely that the reason clinicians use antipsychotic polypharmacy or high dose antipsychotic treatment is not due to lack of awareness of potential problems or a lack of concern for the service user. The dilemma is whether, faced by a service user with significant morbidity, we do nothing, or to bring about a clinical improvement offer a trial of a treatment 'off licence'.

Faced with these difficult issues, there is little research to help us plan treatment when standard antipsychotic approaches have failed. The use of high dose Olanzapine may have a place and there are studies to support its use (Dursun et al., 1999), but at high doses Olanzapine starts to show many problems of first generation antipsychotics and can be poorly tolerated (Kelly et al., 2003). Given the current evidence, combining antipsychotics (other than Clozapine) cannot be advocated unless other options have been exhausted. However it is interesting to note that NICE guidelines (2009) include a discussion about 'the problem of attribution of benefits', following treatment with a second drug, a problem which 'leaves uncertain the optimal treatment in the longer term'. Sweeting (2006) noted that combined treatment is common and advised that if a decision is made to combine treatment, drug choice might logically be made on the basis of differing receptor profiles. There were also recommendations on the basis of current evidence for the use of: Olanzapine, with either Amisupiride or Risperidone: or Quetiapine with Risperidone.

Another approach which has little evidence in its support but is common, is the use of treatments targeting secondary disorders which complicate psychotic illness, such as mood disorders. Antidepressant or mood stabilising medication may be used alongside antipsychotic medication to treat specific symptoms. The lack of research evidence means that each treatment has to be seen as an empirical trial in each case, and the continuation of treatment should be decided on the basis of individual response.

Medication management

The effective use of medication is best seen as a collaborative process, aiming to achieve a good understanding of the aims of treatment and realistically a balance of wanted and unwanted effects. These outcomes are best achieved in a positive therapeutic relationship and this can take time and commitment for all involved. In Box 6.3 there are some useful resources which can help to provide information to staff, service users and carers about medication used in assertive outreach.

Box 6.3   UK Resources to support the use of medication in assertive outreach teams

NICE, the National Institute for Health and Clinical Excellence Guidelines for the treatment of schizophrenia (2009), bipolar disorder (2006): http://www.guidance.nice.org.uk
The British association of Psychopharmacology Guidelines on the treatment of bipolar disorder, depression and substance abuse disorders: http://www.bap.org.uk
The British National Formulary (updated 6 monthly, contains a complete list of all medicines which can be prescribed (and proprietary medicines) in the United Kingdom.
The Maudsley Prescribing Guidelines (Taylor et al., 2007) contains advice on prescribing all psychotropic medication, including treatment in special circumstances such as differing medical conditions and treatment resistance.
http://www.nwmhp.nhs.uk/pharmacy; a useful website which contains information about treatment and printable information leaflets.
The National Psychosis Service: based at the Bethlem Royal Hospital, provides a multidisciplinary second opinion service and potentially inpatient treatment for treatment resistant psychosis: http://www:Psychosis Outpatient Service Maudsley

---

Non-medical prescribing

Non-medical prescribing was introduced in the UK in 2003 (Department of Health, 2006b). Although from 2006 non-medical prescribers have been able to prescribe independently for any condition within their competence, practitioners mostly use supplementary prescribing, within parameters set out in a clinical management plan agreed with the service user and supervising psychiatrist. This fits with the assertive outreach team approach – medication is often delivered as part of an assertive outreach treatment package and non-medical prescribing allows adjustments to be made in a timely manner for those who find it hard to access services.

Some international literature on nurse prescribing has been positive: Mundinger et al., (2000) reporting similar outcomes for nurse and doctor prescribing and high service user satisfaction for nurse prescribing. The development has not been universally welcomed in the UK and there have been concerns about the adequacy of training and possible risks to service users' safety (Avery & James, 2007). A survey of mental health staff in a UK Trust (Tomar et al., 2008) found that most psychiatrists did not feel confident to act as supervisors and both nurses and psychiatrists expressed concerns. This was undertaken before widespread use of non-medical prescribing and it will be interesting to follow professional views as practice becomes more widespread.

Case study 6.2   Nurse prescribing in assertive outreach – Mike McKenzie, Cheltenham assertive outreach team manager

I have been a nurse prescriber for over a year, working in an assertive outreach team. During my 26 day training I studied pharmacology, anatomy and physiology and prescribing principles, including legal aspects. I wrote case studies and considered ethical issues, including pharmaceutical company influence and the challenge of working with clients who lack capacity. I found it reassuring to learn that nurse prescribers should not prescribe beyond their limits of competence and experience.

I have mainly prescribed antidepressant and antipsychotic medications within clinical management plans, agreed with the client and consultant. I can give repeat prescriptions, change the dose and stop treatment if needed. I cannot prescribe benzodiazepines independently, due to current legislation. This type of medication is commonly used to alleviate stress-related anxiety, and I have wide experience of using short term benzodiazepine treatment to help service users through crisis. It is at times frustrating that non-medical prescribing of this treatment is restricted, but I have prescribed benzodiazepines through supplementary prescribing, supervised by a medical practitioner.

A recent case highlighted the value of non-medical prescribing: a client on Clozapine repeatedly missed doses and was at risk of relapse and problems related to special licensing arrangements. I was able to discuss the case with the psychiatrist and staff in the supported accommodation involved. We agreed that if the client missed his evening medication there was an 'as required' prescription available to nursing staff to give in the morning, which the client was encouraged to take. I provided the prescription, explained the plan to all involved and wrote a detailed care plan. Over a period of time the client learned more about the importance of regular compliance and I supported the accommodation team, who were anxious about possible relapse and the risks of stopping and starting treatment. His condition gradually stabilised and he started to take medication regularly.

Psychoeducation

People receiving assertive outreach services often have limited knowledge about their treatment, even after many years of taking it. Psychoeducation aims to improve understanding and knowledge of illness, treatment options – including coping strategies and medication – and leads to more effective coping. It often involves family carers and can be an important part of a family intervention. Sometimes staff worry that knowledge about mental illness and medication side effects may destabilise the mental health of a service user and reduce concordance. However, this is not in practice likely to occur. In a systematic review of psychoeducation versus standard levels of knowledge provision in schizophrenia, Pekkala & Merinder (2007) concluded that psychoeducation was associated with a significant reduction in both risk of relapse and readmission rates when followed up at 9–18 months. For the large part the implementation of psychoeducation by members of an assertive outreach team should be reasonably achievable within the standard engagement and initial treatment approach – many of the interventions are inexpensive and time efficient and can be delivered by all team members.

Compliance therapy

Medication compliance is often thought of as a particular problem in psychiatric conditions, but it features to some degree in all medical treatments. Optimising compliance in assertive outreach services has particular challenges because psychotic illness often affects cognition and attitudes to treatment. The importance of the issue is emphasised by the fact that in schizophrenia relapse rates over two to three years increase from 20% to 80% when medication is stopped (Jones & Marder, 2008).

Compliance therapy is an intervention spanning a number of techniques, including psychoeducational, motivational interviewing and cognitive approaches, as summarised in Box 6.4 (after Kemp et al. (1998)).

A Cochrane Review of formal compliance therapy versus non specific counselling (McIntosh et al., 2006) showed no clear benefit for the more formal approach and NICE Schizophrenia Guidance (2009) does not recommend compliance therapy to be offered routinely. This leaves assertive outreach clinicians with a dilemma, as the problem of non compliance is often a major focus of clinical work. In practice, eclectic approaches which incorporate elements of compliance therapy alongside strengths-based and recovery focused work are likely to be necessary and over time, helpful. Dolder et al. (2003) found that combined educational, behavioural and affective (e.g. discussing emotional responses to the issues) strategies were most effective in improving concordance and reducing relapse and readmission to hospital.

Incentives, leverage and coercion

In the new 2007 amendments to the Mental Health Act (1983), Community Treatment Orders (CTO) were introduced for England and Wales. The CTO is an enabling power (at the discretion of the clinical team) which allows enforced community treatment of service

---

Box 6.4   The principles of compliance therapy

Indirect benefits of medication are addressed – e.g. 'getting on better with other people'.

- Differences between symptoms and illness side effects are openly addressed.
- Highlight the risk that stopping treatment may affect individual goals such as getting a job.
- Challenge common misnomers – e.g. medication is addictive, or medication leads to loss of personality.
- Symptoms/problems used as targets for treatment.
- Meanings attached to medication are explored.
- Discussion of the protective nature of medication concordance – e.g. reduced risk of hospitalisation or losing work.
- Discussion of the natural wish to stop medication if well.

---

users who must see members of the community team, and can be recalled to hospital if they refuse medication. The CTO is an explicitly coercive means to try to address patterns of non-compliance and relapse, the 'revolving door' cycle. UK assertive outreach teams have a central role in implementing CTOs, as in Canada, United States, Australia and New Zealand where CTOs have been available for some time. In practice, CTOs are likely to be used primarily to allow longer-term treatment of people with relapsing psychosis, with long acting intramuscular antipsychotics (Mullen et al., 2006).

Case study 6.3   Financial incentives

Five non-adherent patients of an assertive outreach team in East London were offered a financial incentive of between £5 and £15 to take long acting intra muscular antipsychotic medication. Four patients accepted the proposal. Three did not have an admission to hospital once on the scheme despite having 539 combined hospital days in the 2 years before receiving money for medication. A survey of assertive outreach team managers in England was conducted by the service alongside the incentives to seek opinion on the acceptability of the practice. 70 responses were elicited, attitudes to the practice were mainly negative and no others teams had used this approach and a range of ethical objections and concerns for therapeutic relationship were raised. (Claassen et al., 2007)

The question of whether financial incentives are acceptable has been further explored by focus groups of stakeholders and the efficacy of the practice clinically is currently subject to a cluster randomised controlled trial. (Priebe et al., 2009) (see also Ford & Priebe (2007))

A broader discussion about issues relating to leverage, coercion and personal autonomy in assertive outreach practice is found in Chapter 12.

Conclusions and future considerations

Assertive outreach teams work at the most complex end of the spectrum of severe mental illness, with service users who have co-morbid illness, of multi-factorial aetiology, which is difficult to treat. However, it is the challenge of working with people who have these difficulties which often attracts mental health professionals to work in assertive outreach. An ability to accept uncertainty and to adopt a realistic framework for what can be achieved and how long this will take, is a necessary aspect of this type of work.

We have available a range of effective medications to help people with standard and treatment resistant psychotic illness. We need to use all members of the team appropriately and employ interventions targeted at improving symptoms and treatment compliance, in order to achieve the best outcomes for service users. As a specialist team working with small, defined caseloads of service users, assertive outreach teams should be expected to offer accurate and detailed assessments of their service users and should provide up to date, evidence based approaches to treatment. A challenge for the future, for all those working in specialist teams like this, will be whether in an NHS which focuses increasingly on measuring outcomes, and commissioning services on this basis, we can continue to demonstrate the value of this form of community psychiatry, which targets one of the most disadvantaged, disenfranchised groups in society.

References

American Diabetes Association (2004) Consensus development conference on antipsychotic drugs and obesity and diabetes. *Diabetes Care*, **27**, 596–601.

Avery, A.J. & James, V. (2007) Developing nurse prescribing in the UK. *British Medical Journal*, **335**, 316.

Barnes, T.R.E., Shingleton-Smith, A. & Paton, C. (2009) Antipsychotic long-acting injections: prescribing practice in the UK. *British Journal of Psychiatry*, **195**, 37–42.

Barrowclough, C., Tarrier, N., Watts, S., Vaugh, C., Bamrah, J.S. & Freeman, H.L. (1987) Assessing the functional value of relatives' knowledge about schizophrenia: a preliminary report. *British Journal of Psychiatry*, **151**, 1–8.

Birchwood, M., Smith, J., Cochrane, R., Wetton, S. & Copestake, S. (1990) The Social Functioning Scale. *British Journal of Psychiatry*, **157**, 853–859.

Chang, J.S., Ahn, Y.S., Park, H.J., Lee, K.Y., Kim, S.H. & Kang, U.G., et al. (2008) Aripiprazole augmentation in Clozapine-treated patients with refractory Schizophrenia: an 8-week, randomized, double-blind, placebo-controlled trial. *Journal of Clinical Psychiatry*, **69**, 720–731.

Claassen, D. (2007) Financial incentives for antipsychotic medication: ethical issues. *Journal of Medical Ethics: Journal of the Institute of Medical Ethics*, **33**(4), 189–193.

Concato, J., Shah, N. & Horowitz, R.I. (2000) Randomised controlled trials and the hierarchy of research designs. *New England Journal of Medicine*, **342**, 1887–1892.

Conley, R.R. & Buchanan, R.W. (1997) Evaluation of treatment-resistant schizophrenia. *Schizophrenia Bulletin*, **23**, 663–674.

Day, J.C., Wood, G., Dewey, M. & Bentall, R. (1995) A self-rating scale for measuring neuroleptic side-effects. Validation in a group of schizophrenic patients. *British Journal of Psychiatry*, **166**, 650–653.

Department of Health (2005) *Mental Capacity Act*. Department of Health, London.

Department of Health (2006a) *Choosing Health: Supporting the Physical Health Needs of People with Severe Mental Illness*. Department of Health, London.

Department of Health (2006b) *Improving Patients Access to Medicines*. Department of Health, London. http://www.nwmhp.nhs.uk/pharmacy

Department of Health (2007) *Mental Health Act*. Department of Health, London.

Diaz F.J., de Leon, J., Josiassen, R.C., Copper, T.B. & Simpson, G.M. (2005) Plasma clozapine concentration coefficients of variation in a long-term study. *Schizophrenia Research*, **72**, 131–135.

Dolder, C.R., Lacro, J.P., Leckband, S. & Jeste, D.V. (2003) Interventions to improve antipsychotic medication adherence: a review of recent literature. *Journal of clinical Psychopharmacology*, **23**(4), 389–399.

Dursun, S.M., Gardner, D.M., Bird, D.C. & Flinn, J. (1999) Olanzapine for patients with treatment-resistant schizophrenia: a naturalistic case – series outcome study. *Canadian Journal of Psychiatry*, **44**, 701–704.

Ford, R. & Priebe, S. (2007) Money for medication: financial incentives to improve medication adherence in assertive outreach. *Psychiatric Bulletin Royal College Psychiatry*, **31**, 4–7.

Geddes, J., Freemantle, N., Harrison, P., Bebbington, P. & Geddes, J. (2000) Atypical antipsychotics in the treatment of schizophrenia: systematic overview and meta-regression analysis. *British Medical Journal*, **321**, 1371–1376.

Haddad, P.M., Taylor, M. & Niaz, O.S. (2009) First generation antipsychotic long acting injections v. oral antipsychotics in schizophrenia; systematic review of randomised controlled trials and observational studies. *British Journal of Psychiatry*, **195**, 20–28.

Hall, M., Meaden, A., Smith, J. & Jones, C. (2001) The development and psychometric properties of an observer-rated measure of engagement with mental health services. *Journal of Mental Health*, **10**(4), 457–465.

Haro, J.M., Suarez, D., Novick, D. Brown, J., Usall, J. & Naber, D. (2007) Three-year antipsychotic effectiveness in the outpatient care of schizophrenia: observational versus randomized studies results. *European Neuropsychopharmacology*, **17**(4), 235–244.

Harrington, M., Lelliot, P., Paton, C., Konsolaki, M., Sensky, T. & Okocha, C. (2002) Variation between services in polypharmacy and combined high dose of antipsychotic drugs prescribed for in-patients. *Psychiatric Bulletin*, **26**(11), 418–420.

Heres, S., Davis, J., Maino, K., Jetzinger, E., Kissling, W. & Leucht, S. (2006) Why Olanzapine beats risperidone, risperidone beats quetiapine, and quetiapine beats olanzapine: an exploratory study of head to head comparison studies of second generation antipsychotics. *American Journal of Psychiatry*, **163**, 185–194.

Hodgson, R., Bushe, C. & Hunter, R. (2007) Measurement of long-term outcomes in observational and randomized controlled trials. *British Journal of Psychiatry*, **1191**, 78–84.

Iqbal, M.M., Rahman, A., Husain, Z., Mahmud, S.Z., Ryan, W.G. & Feldman, J.M. (2003) Clozapine: a clinical review of adverse effects and management. *Annals of Clinical Psychiatry*, **15**, 33–48.

Jones, P.B., Barnes, T.R.E., Davies, L., Dunn, G., Lloyd, H. & Hayhurst, K.P., et al. (2006) Randomised controlled trial of the effect on quality of life of second vs first generation antipsychotic drugs in schizophrenia: cost utility of the latest antipsychotic drugs in schizophrenia study (Cutlass 1). *Archives of General Psychiatry*, **63**(10), 789–796.

Jones, P.B. & Marder, S.R. (2008) Psychosocial and Pharmacological Treatments for Schizophrenia. In: *Cambridge Textbook of Effective Treatments in Psychiatry*, (eds. P. Tyrer & K.R. Silk). pp. 469–480. Cambridge University Press, Cambridge.

Kane, J. M., Honigfeld, G., Singer, J. & Meltzer, H. (1988) Clozapine in treatment-resistant schizophrenics: a double-blind comparison with Chlorpromazine. *Psychopharmacology Bulletin*, **24**(9), 62–67.

Kay, S.R., Opler, L.A. & Lindenmayer, J.P. (1987) The Positive and Negative Syndrome Scale (PANSS): rationale and standardisation. *British Journal of Psychiatry*, **155**(suppl. 7), 59–67.

Kelly, D.L., Conley, R.R., Richardson, C.M., Tamminga, C.A. & Carpenter, W.T. (2003) Adverse effects and laboratory parameters of high dose Olanzapine versus Clozapine in treatment resistant schizophrenia. *Annals of Clinical Psychiatry*, **15**(3–4), 181–186.

Kemp, R., Kirov, G., Everitt, B., Hayward, P. & David, A. (1998) Randomised controlled trial of compliance therapy. *British Journal of Psychiatry*, **172**, 413–419.

Khan, A.Y. & Preskorn, S.H. (2005) Examining concentration-dependent toxicity of clozapine: role of therapeutic drug monitoring. *Journal of Psychiatric Practice*, **11**(5), 340–343.

Kikkert, M.J., Schene, A.H., Koeter, M.W.J., Robson, D., Born, A. & Helm, H., et al. (2006) Medication adherence in schizophrenia: exploring patients', carers', and professionals' views. *Schizophrenia Bulletin*, **32**(4), 786–794.

Kravieka, M., Goldberg, D. & Vaughan, M. (1977) A standardised psychiatric assessment scale for rating chronic psychotic patients. *Acta Psychiatrica Scandinavica*, **55**, 299–308.

Kreyenbuhl, J.A., Valensteen, M., McCarthy, J.F., Ganoczy, D. & Blow, F.C. (2007) Long-term antipsychotic polypharmacy in the VA health system: patient and treatment patterns. *Psychiatric Services*, **58**(4), 489–495.

Leucht, S., Corves, C., Arbter, D., Engel, R.R., Li, C. & Davos, J.M. (2009) Second-generation versus first generation antipsychotic drugs for schizophrenia: a meta-analysis. *Lancet*, **373**, 3–41.

Lieberman, J.A., Stroup, S., McEvoy, J.P., Swartz, M.S., Rosenheck, R.A. & Perkins, D.O., et al. (2005) Clinical Antipsychotic Trials of Intervention Effectiveness (CATIE) Investigators. Effectiveness of antipsychotic drugs in patients with chronic schizophrenia. *New England Journal of Medicine*, **353**(12), 1209–1223.

McIntosh, A., Conlon, L., Lawrie, S. & Stanfield, A.C. (2006) Compliance therapy for schizophrenia. *Cochrane Database of Systematic Reviews*. Issue 3.

Moncrieff, J. (2006) Does antipsychotic withdrawal provoke psychosis? Review of the literature on rapid onset psychosis (supersensitivity psychosis) and withdrawal-related relapse. *Acta Psychiatrica Scandinavica*, **114**(1), 3–13.

Mullen, R., Dawson, J. & Gibbs, A. (2006) Dilemmas for clinicians in use of Community Treatment Orders. *International Journal of Law and Psychiatry*, **29**, 535–550.

Mundinger, M.O., Kane, R.L., Lenz, E.R., Totten, A.M., Tasi, W. & Cleary, P.D., et al. (2000) Primary care outcomes in patients treated by nurse practitioners or physicians: a randomised trial. *Journal of American Medical Association*, **283**(1), 59–68.

Munro, J., Matthiason, P., Osborne, S., Travis, M., Purcell, S. & Cobb, A.M., et al. (2004) Amisulpride augmentation of Clozapine: an open non-randomised study in patients with schizophrenia partially responsive to Clozapine. *Acta Psychiatrica Scandinavica*, **110**(4), 292–298.

NICE (2002) *Schizophrenia: Core Interventions in the Treatment and Management of Schizophrenia in Primary and Secondary Care*. National Institute for Health and Clinical Excellence, London.

NICE (2006) *Bipolar Disorder: The Management of Bipolar Disorder in Adults, Children and Adolescents, in Primary and Secondary Care*. National Institute for Health and Clinical Excellence, London.

NICE (2009) *Schizophrenia: Core Interventions in the Treatment and Management of Schizophrenia in Primary and Secondary Care*. National Institute for Health and Clinical Excellence, London.

O'Brien, A. & Firn, M. (2002) Clozapine Initiation in the Community. *Psychiatric Bulletin*, **26**, 339–341.

Overall, J.E. & Gorham, D.R. (1962) The Brief Psychiatric Rating Scale. *Psychological Reports*, **10**, 799–812.

Pekkala, E. & Merinder, L. Psychoeducation for schizophrenia. In: *The Cochrane Library*, Issue 3, 2007. Chichester, John Wiley & Sons Ltd.

Priebe, S., Burton, A., Ashby, D., Ashcroft, R., Burns, T. & David, A., et al. (2009) Financial Incentives to improve adherence to anti-psychotic maintenance medication in non-adherent patients – a cluster randomized controlled trial (FIAT). *BMC Psychiatry*, **9,** 61.

Puri, B.V. & Richardson, A.J. (1998) Sustained remission of positive and negative symptoms of schizophrenia following treatment with eicosapentaenoic acid. *Archives of General Psychiatry*, **55**(2), 188–189.

Ray, W.A., Meredith, S., Thapa, P.B., Meador, K.G., Hall, K. & Murray, K.T. (2001) Antipsychotics and the risk of sudden cardiac death. *Archives of General Psychiatry*, **58**(12), 1161–1167.

Royal College of Psychiatrists (2006) Consensus statement on high-dose antipsychoticmedication (Council Report 138), Royal College of Psychiatrists.

Shiloh, R., Zemishlany, Z., Aizenberg, D., Radwan, M., Schwartz, B. & Dorfman-Etrog, P., et al. (1997) Sulpiride augmentation in people with schizophrenia partially responsive to Clozapine. A double blind placebo controlled study. *British Journal of Psychiatry*, **171**, 569–573.

Sweeting, M. (2006) Management of Medication When Treatment is Failing. In: *Enabling Recovery: The Principles adn Practice of Rehabilitation*, (eds. G. Roberts, S. Davenport, F. Holloway & T. Tattan). pp. 146–157. Gaskell, London.

Taylor, D., Paton, C. & Kerwin, R. (2007) *The Maudsley Prescribing Guidelines*, 9th Edition. Informa Heathcare, London.

Tomar, R., Jakovljevic, T., & Brimblecombe, (2008) Psychiatrists' and nurses' views of mental health nurse prescribing: a survey. *Psychiatric Bulletin*, **332**, 364–365.

Young, J.L., Spitz, R.T., Hillbrand, M. & Daneri, G. (1999) Medication adherence failure in schizophrenia: a forensic review of rates, reasons, treatments and prospects. *Journal of the American Academy of the Law*, **27**(3), 426–444.

Chapter 7

Relatives', friends' and carers' experiences: involvement and support

Simon Wharne, Sara Meddings, Tizzie Coleman
and Jo Coldwell

Introduction

According to evidence-based guidance for the treatment of people diagnosed as suffering from schizophrenia, it is expected that mental health teams in England and Wales should offer formal, cognitive behavioural family interventions in their daily work (NICE, 2009). Assertive outreach teams work with service users who are particularly isolated and distressed, so family interventions often need to be adapted. In forming a therapeutic alliance with their service users, workers will try to help re-engage them with families and friends. However, it is sometimes appropriate to think about current networks, such as neighbours, landlords or various workers, as a kind of family. Where 'informal carers' are providing substantial support, teams can struggle to promote recovery, particularly when they are under pressure to 'take the burden of care' from families and communities. Referrals are often taken when service interventions, over many years, have not adequately resolved problems or treated illness. Sometimes there are ongoing conflicts and, perhaps, many complaints because concerned people do not feel that needs are met or risks resolved, so assertive outreach teams must then find a mediating role within this complexity.

When workers spend time with family members or other carers they can gain understanding and offer practical help. This can enable families and other networks to recognise and support the positive contributions that those who are diagnosed with psychosis can make. This valuing is more likely to be achieved where workers have offered different ways of delivering interventions, from individual contacts, to family support meetings, to more formal family therapy. However, in this work, care is needed to maintain a confidential service for each individual. So, the use of formulation and team reflection are highlighted in this chapter as a means to foster understanding. The use of procedures, such as Safeguarding Vulnerable Adults (in England and Wales), are also highlighted as a means to give structure to risk management interventions. Meanwhile, the value of more informal unstructured engagement is discussed, while the need for strong team-based support is recognised in this challenging work.

Assertive Outreach in Mental Healthcare: Current Perspectives, First Edition. Edited by C. Williams, M. Firn, S. Wharne and R. Macpherson.

How do we think about families?

Working with families and other informal carers has been central to the assertive outreach approach since its first introduction. Working collaboratively through social networks and providing psycho-education became an established adaptation, particularly where community services were scarce. Family aided Assertive Community Treatment (FACT) placed the family at the centre of the team's approach (McFarlane, 1997). However, dilemmas have emerged. People using services often express views that are different from their relatives or friends and each of these people will have their own needs and concerns, so workers face conflicting demands. Families will have established patterns of interaction and shared understandings, so the introduction of psychological or psychiatric interpretations, with associated statutory powers, might be experienced as threatening and intrusive. Services may polarise descriptions of one person as a carer and another as the 'cared for person', losing the complexity of family relationships. For example, in East Sussex we have worked with a husband acting as a carer to his wife who uses assertive outreach services, but she is a carer to him, regarding his physical disability. Similarly, an audit of two assertive outreach teams (Meddings et al., 2007) found that whilst 95% of service users were single (or widowed, separated or divorced), 37% of these people had children and 6% identified themselves as carers.

We have found that even when our service users live independently, many of them would not achieve a stable existence without many hours of support provided by family members and other informal carers. So when our workers talk about these arrangements using terms such as 'community placement', in which a 'package of care' is provided, in what way are carers included and supported? Workers are often concerned with 'professional standards', while family members might ask if someone 'really cares'. So is caring an exercise of some kind of technical expertise, or an informal emotion-based activity, or both? With increasing economic migration in modern Western societies family support might be diluted, so should teams replace what has been lost, or, following recovery philosophies, should they promote social inclusion by supporting families and communities in developing their own capacities? Prior to community care in the UK, old Victorian institutions did in some ways attempt to replace family and community (Pilgrim & Rogers, 1993). Some commentators now claim a 'burden of caring', has been placed on families following the closure of long-term institutional care (Harvey et al., 2008; see also Box 7.1). Carers are thought of as facing a number of losses or compromises, but potentially benefiting from the knowledge that workers impart (McFarlane et al., 1996). Rather than only working with individuals or families, many assertive outreach teams use a 'Community Psychology' approach (Meddings et al., 2010) in which psychological understandings are employed to enhance social support networks. In contrast to this, in other cultures, professionalised community care is still limited or completely absent.

Warner (2000) discusses two studies which compare towns in Italy and America. Some 70% of people with psychosis in Italy were living with family, compared with 17% of the Anglo-American sample. In Italy they had greater social recovery and quality of life associated with their more frequent contact with their family, being less worried about money and security of housing, with more opportunity for employment. However, the relatives in

---

Box 7.1   Traditional extended family support

Seloilwe (2006) observes the phenomena of multiple or collective care giving. In this study of Botswana community care, it was found that most families had many dependants, including children and elderly relatives, along with people who suffered mental health problems. Those who provided care included both adults and children. However, adult men more often made decisions, provided money, food and clothing or other material goods. They delegated domestic care tasks. Persons who earned less could be asked to leave their employment to contribute to care giving activities.

Italy struggled more with the stresses of living with someone with psychosis. They neglected their pastimes, felt stressed and depressed, and felt more critical of their relative. This is concerning given that research in the UK shows that people are more likely to relapse when they are in contact with stressed and critical families for more than 35 hours per week (Vaughn & Leff, 1976; Barrowclough & Tarrier, 1998; Kavanagh, 1992). It is perhaps significant that the Italian families gained more limited supported from services. Warner (2000) advocates that the value of families should be recognised and that they should be supported financially, in a manner that is linked with education and coping support. Recovery rates from psychosis have been found to be higher in 'developing countries' than in the West and this is hypothesised to be because people are less stigmatised, more supported by extended families and more likely to be in employment (Warner, 1994). In Nigeria people who are diagnosed as suffering from an enduring mental health problem gain material, social and emotional support from around five family members: siblings, uncles and aunts, cousins and in-laws (Ohaeri, 1998). Some 96% of patients are accompanied for their first appointment at the psychiatric hospital by relatives (Franklin et al., 1996). In contrast, in Western societies, it is much less common for people to be accompanied by family members when attending appointments and if they are, questions might be raised about 'co-dependence'. More emphasis is placed on individuality in modern Western societies and this might hinder the social integration of people who develop psychotic illness. Families might be seen as exacerbating the condition, particularly when emotional distress is displayed. So we might be drawn into using the unhelpful notion of 'problem families', which use up our resources, rather than generally promoting the well-being and social inclusion of everyone we have contact with. This chapter will try to explore and understand these conflicting notions.

Reflection point

Research evidence suggests that in countries where mental health problems are not usually discussed within families, people with these problems are less stigmatised and more socially included. So, consider the complex professional understanding of mental health problems that you have developed; can you use this knowledge to build communities, or is it only useful for defining the manner in which an individual deviates from some kind of social norm?

A burden or a reward

The experience of being a relative of someone served by an assertive outreach team is multi-faceted, but the dominant narrative focuses on the 'burden' of care. A recent literature search found over 300 articles relating to the burden associated with schizophrenia and only six which attempted to include positive aspects (Coldwell et al., in press). Difficulties experienced by family members include financial hardship and practical demands; problems with roles and relationships within the family and outside; disruption of household activities and psychological distress (Hoenig & Hamilton, 1966; Fadden, 1998). Relatives caring for someone with mental health problems are more likely to experience mental and physical health problems themselves than people in the general population (Singleton et al., 2002).

Assertive outreach has often employed a 'strengths' philosophy (Rapp & Goscha, 2006) and we notice that 'burden' is affected by how people perceive their roles and responsibility, how they create meaning and their sense of reciprocity (Schwartz & Gidron, 2002). So, burden can be decreased through sharing information, emotional support, respite breaks and financial support (Askey et al., 2009). When we explore the rewarding aspects of relationships, families report that their relatives with serious mental health problems provide companionship, news about family and friends; they listen to problems and give advice (Greenberg et al., 1994). People with serious mental health problems contribute to the personal growth of families: to a familial sense of increased appreciation and closeness; self-value and purpose; and life satisfaction (Schwartz & Gidron, 2002). The opportunity for people to contribute to their families, when they have a diagnosis of psychosis, is mediated by the way family members conceptualise this illness (Coldwell et al., in press). There might be a belief that the person is not capable of contributing to meeting the needs of others, or that putting demands on them would lead to a relapse of their mental health problems. Taking back control, hope and opportunity are central to recovery (Repper & Perkins, 2003). Although opportunities to contribute to family life often arise spontaneously, support from assertive outreach teams may increase the likelihood that these opportunities will be taken up (see Box 7.2 for different family experiences).

Box 7.2   Different experiences in each family

Coldwell et al. (in press) found that for some people who developed severe psychotic illness, the experience drew the family closer together as members shared values and dealt with worry, fear and concern together. Other families found that living through the experience of acute illness created physical and emotional distance; through hospitalisation, homelessness or legal processes. Where families were able to stay together through emotional and physical separation, then opportunities for mutual support developed. People with a diagnosis of psychosis were able to give practical support to other family members, such as help with shopping, gardening and technology, as well as caring for elderly relatives, young children and family pets. They could also provide emotional support, in companionship, or being there for family members when others did not have the time.

'*I pick my nephew up from school every Monday.*' (service user, in Coldwell et al., in press)

Box 7.3   Feedback from siblings

Throughout their discussions, the respondents portrayed complex feelings of fear, anger, guilt, loss, and loneliness that they associated with the presence of an emerging and chronic mental illness in a brother or sister ... Yet, in spite of the negative and raw memories and emotions, all of the participants were willing to consider the positive effects of the illness for themselves and their family. Throughout, they wished for their sibling to be well. (Lukens et al., 2004: 496–497)

Within models of 'stress-vulnerability' (Zubin & Spring, 1977; Rosenfarb et al., 2006), the positive value given to the act of contributing suggests that this is experienced as a protective factor. Also, positive contribution might help foster individual resilience, enabling adjustment and adaptation, as well as strengthening intra-familial relations and the ability to adjust family roles, increasing the whole family's resilience (Enns et al., 1999; Greeff et al., 2006) (see Box 7.3). In Stern et al. (1999), it was found that when the carers of relatives with serious mental health problems are able to see positives in their situation, when they believe that mental health problems are an opportunity for learning and they utilise external resources in order to cope, then they are able to make sense of their experiences and manage difficulties proactively. So teams might support families to notice more contributions and reciprocity in their relationships. This is consistent with an integrated systemic and psycho-social approach which builds on individual and family competencies and strengths (Meddings et al., 2010).

From understanding to practical help

Recovery and social inclusion are the primary task of assertive outreach, but teams must first achieve a form of engagement. Understanding the complex negotiations that take place in family or friendship networks is essential in this work and the best way of understanding a particular family is to spend time with them, listening to them and appreciating what each member of the family says. People are experts concerning their own families, their strengths, difficulties and how they manage these and practical help has always been one of the most valued interventions in assertive outreach, see Box 7.4.

Box 7.4   Getting to the practical issues

At a family work session, Susan complained 'what's the point of all this talking, when will someone help me sort out my son's flat?' Susan explained that she had been visiting John every weekend and doing all his washing and cleaning. She then learned that the team had been trying to visit to help with these tasks but John had not been answering the door, as he worried the workers might be impostors. When the team did gain access, the flat had appeared clean and tidy and John had said that he could manage. During this session, John agreed to his mother having copies of appointment letters so that she could remind him to let the team in and so that she could let go of some of the practical input. The team were then able to assess and support John in exercising his daily living skills. Susan was able to spend more enjoyable time with him.

As professionals, we draw on our own experiences of life and family. As discussed in Chapters 10 and 11, it is important to distinguish behaviours that are normal within a culture from those that are not. For example, many of us as students may have initially lived in squalor, when we first left our parental homes, while clearly most of us would not have been incapacitated by symptoms of mental illness. Again, perhaps not everyone in a family shares tasks such as cleaning the toilet; often men leave this to women, and we have noticed some of our male clients also wanting to do this. Again, many of us will have experienced the normal competition with our siblings and from this experience we may appreciate and normalise the experience of siblings of our service users, who may have complex feelings of guilt or resentment, especially if their own needs were usurped by the needs of an older sibling developing psychosis. We must ensure that our formal assessments, such as observing 'mental capacity' or 'daily living skills', act to inform negotiations in families, rather than applying stigmatising labelling to particular family members.

Reflection point

Consider the understanding that you bring from your own experiences of family life. How do you use this understanding in your professional role?

Relatives' experiences; what do families want from assertive outreach?

It is crucial that teams work with service users and relatives to further their own recovery aims. Clinicians prioritise symptom-reduction more than service-users and their relatives (Repper & Perkins, 2003). In relation to mental health services generally, relatives want information, recognition, support, involvement in decision making, communication, and good coordinated services (Shepherd et al., 1995; Noble & Douglas, 2004). In 2003 the mental health charity Rethink conducted a survey asking 1450 carers about their experiences of accessing services and found that, although things were improving, quality and accessibility varied, leaving some carers without support or information. The most frustrating aspect was not being able to access help when they or their relative needed it. One in four carers had been turned away when they sought help from a professional. Other issues included lack of information, and not having regular contact with professionals.

Case study 7.1   A mother's experience

Owing to misdiagnosis, our daughter spent four years in different psychiatric units and was eventually referred to a rehabilitation unit where we (her parents and carers) first became aware of and had contact with the assertive outreach team. Our experiences with the local psychiatric units had left us exhausted, disillusioned, bitter and beaten. We had been treated with suspicion, the usual disdain for the carer's opinion and knowledge about their offspring and had generally been made to feel that we were the cause of her illness; that we were not wanted and did not matter. We were therefore very suspicious of any new services that were about to be offered.

We had, for the first three years of her detainment been told, that for reasons of confidentiality, we could not discuss matters relating to her mental health. During the last year, the staff had worked with us and our daughter to break down the barriers, gain her confidence and pursue the aim of working together as a team. The assertive outreach team worked alongside and very slowly we learnt that this service appeared to be 'onside'. It was a new experience for us to be asked about her likes, dislikes, her reaction to the surroundings, our opinion of her illness, how it affected her, how it affected us as a family etc. This different approach and new attitude began to allay the fears we had expected. Suddenly we were considered, we were included, our opinions mattered and it began to look as if we were all working towards the same goal: the mental and physical well-being of our daughter.

Our first impressions of the new team were reserved. Looking back, this was undoubtedly due to any new situation where staff appear to be in authority, where there appear to be 'sides', where the staff are comfortable amongst those with whom they work and where the carer is an unknown quantity. Gradually, as we began to know the various characters and they began to realise that we were reasonable, caring parents, the barriers started to break down. Information was flowing both ways and opinions were being sought and questions were asked and answered honestly. When our daughter was discharged, the assertive outreach team visited twice a week.

We have been asked to attend relatives and families evenings which give the carer an opportunity to meet with staff, to share experiences, to ask questions, to meet other relatives who share similar situations and to share some of the good and not-so-good experiences of working with the assertive outreach team. Carers of those with a psychotic illness have been dealt a very rough deal and therefore the opportunity to meet informally with staff to discuss general and personal issues in a 'safe' environment is of great benefit both to the carers and to assertive outreach team workers. As a consequence of these evenings, a fellow carer and I are setting up an advisory group aimed at working with the assertive outreach team to improve services.

*There is obviously a fine line to be drawn between us (carers) finding ourselves being and wanting to be dependent on the assertive outreach team. It is the first time we have met this way of working and it is reassuring to be sharing responsibilities. We have been and are being encouraged by them to try to become less engaged with our daughter in order to encourage her towards independence but, as resources are limited, (time, travel, area covered, lack of staff) we find that the pursuit of the so-called 'meaningful activities' falls back on us. Catch 22: the team looks for an activity, introduce our daughter to it, she will not willingly engage for some reason or other and **we** are left to pursue the goal. Unfortunately, I feel that if I keep drawing this to the attention of the team, they will interpret my concerns as over dependency on their services. The team is aware that when a carer has time on their own, it is a necessary opportunity for the carer to take 'time in the head' which translated means a clear head to think **for** oneself and **of** oneself without constant awareness of the person you care for.*

As our daughter does not have any friends or acquaintances of her own age and as we are relatively old parents, the younger female assertive outreach team workers provide some companionship for which she is so desperately in need. Ideally, in my opinion, an assertive outreach team service would provide workers who could befriend the user by accompanying them to the occasional evening's entertainment or class and remain with them for a few hours thus ensuring companionship and consistency and therefore, in time, promoting confidence in various and new situations. In our daughter's case, she is not very willing to engage in activities designed for those she terms 'mentally ill' and therefore provides an extra challenge to an under-resourced service. We are aware that our daughter needs encouragement to pursue any activity as, apart from her illness, the medication flattens responses, mood and enthusiasm and therefore any participation in an event needs long-term and consistent and persistent engagement by staff.

We are aware that we are supported by the assertive outreach team, that information is freely given and received, that our opinions are listened to, that we are equals in our ability to make our daughter's life easier. We have watched relationships develop between the staff and our daughter and seen more trust develop between personalities but we feel that the team must be consistent in their approach to helping her become more independent and building her confidence. Too often our daughter will be told of times to be met, places to be visited, hours to be spent on a certain day. The day will arrive and a telephone call will announce that the time has changed, that so-and-so cannot make it today, that they will only visit for an hour instead of the planned three hours or that they will ring back ... if they do. Our daughter has missed approximately eight vital years in which to experience all 'normal' ways of maturing and has therefore developed not only more dependency on us as parents but has also retained the childlike quality of 'expectation' which, when the services, for whatever reason, change an arrangement, upsets her mental well-being and causes anxiety. This anxiety in turn causes us to question the reliability of the team. We have had cause to complain about and highlight serious specific and significant concerns regarding CPA meetings, outcomes and appointments and occasions when errors have occurred. Although we have felt that these incidents might have altered our relationship with the services (and possibly with our daughter), we have always been encouraged to continue to raise issues and have not felt victimised for having done so.

The negative impact on a person's physical and mental health, when caring for some-one who suffers from severe mental health problems, is reduced when they feel valued and respected by professionals; when they have choice regarding their caring responsi-bilities and are given information on their role in relation to the diagnosis of the person they care for (Pinfold & Corry, 2003). In relation to assertive outreach specifically, McFarlane et al. (1996) found family members reported improvements in objective aspects of the care provided and in subjective experience of feeling burdened. In a qualita-tive study, Hayward et al. (2004) found that carers appreciated access to the assertive outreach team and considered the contact they had to be good quality. They valued the practical assistance given to service users who, they believed, had increased autonomy and involvement in new activities. However, some carers felt unsupported at times, found accessing the service difficult and wanted more help and information. Wane et al. (2009) found that with support from assertive outreach, parents felt reassured, valued and involved, where previously they experienced a distressing series of crises, feeling excluded from their caring role by services and by their child. The diverse and complex nature of each family was noted (see Box 7.5 for what families find valueable).

Hughes (2007) found that the relatives of people using assertive outreach services valued education and information; support and concern from the team especially at times

---

Box 7.5   What do families value?

Families value assertive outreach teams taking the time and effort to learn about and un-derstand them:

> *somehow they get to know the family better because they come visit and it's the whole idea of outreach so its reaching the patient rather than the patient reaching them ... don't have to explain so much to the professionals ... they have more of an understanding of stuff that goes on inside the house.* (Irena in Hughes, 2007)

> **Box 7.6**　Feedback from family carers in Hughes (2007)
>
> *... if they are involved there's more than one person ... I don't suppose I do any less with the AOT, it's just that you don't feel you're doing it all on your own.* (Ann)
>
> *If Cathy's going through a bad patch, they could maybe phone up and say, 'Well we know Cathy's going through a bad patch, we're doing x, y, z. How are you getting on?'.* (Maureen)
>
> *They've [assertive outreach workers] helped her to be independent. They have supported her and the system they put her through ... they've guided her through this path she had to go along to get her independence and teach her how to do things and how to manage a house and how to pay your bills and they've done all that for her.* (Maureen)
>
> *What the outreach worker has done is to have the family come back together type of thing, you know you live in a family sometimes but you don't know your family... the family therapy has been really helpful, learnt a lot from it but that's something I don't think we'd have got if we hadn't had the outreach worker.* (Irena)

of crises; workers taking time to understand the family; willingness to meet in their environment; flexibility; being included; sharing responsibility for monitoring their relative (see Box 7.6). Their main coping strategies were gaining information, accessing support and positively appraising the situation. Participants described how these coping strategies were particularly needed during times of crises. They reported that assertive outreach teams improved their lives, and family relations, and they felt less distressed. Some also gained support from carers groups, from other families and friends.

Learning from psychological/systemic theory

There is a vast literature which can give insights and frameworks for understanding the individuals and families with whom we work. Burbach et al. (2007) and Meddings et al. (2010) discuss how these can be utilised within assertive outreach, within a strengths based and recovery oriented framework. We recognise that many problems facing families arise from well-intended failed solutions as people try to deal with prior difficulties (Fisch et al., 1982). Families can be seen as facing problems rather than as problem families with high expressed emotion (EE): 'EE is an operational "thermometer" of stress in a *particular* relative-sibling (or spouse) relationship at a *particular* time' (Smith & Birchwood, 1990: 657). We can see interactional cycles whereby one person's thoughts and behaviour influence another's (Burbach et al., 2007).

Simple formulations can be used to help the team and family understand an interactional process. In Figure 7.1, one parent has tried their best for their son with psychosis by looking after him and doing everything for him, even leaving work to do so, but this has created new stresses for each of them and his son has lost more skills. In a second example, Janet is shouting at voices, her mother worries about her and confronts her, this

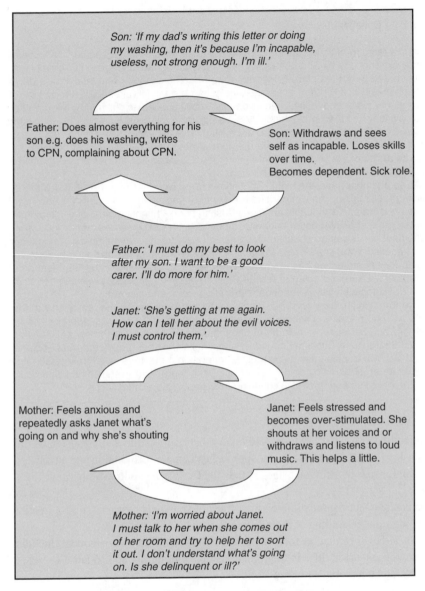

Figure 7.1   High EE interaction 'over-involved – over-concerned'.

leads to Janet becoming more stressed and trying harder to control them, but as we know, stress makes voices worse.

   The whole team approach is a key feature of assertive outreach and one of the strengths of this is that we can also formulate our understanding of families as a team. Everyone can contribute knowledge and experience, using their particular professional expertise. Multiple perspectives can generate debate, and move our understanding forward, inform-ing the care planning process. A formal structure is often used and these sessions are

---

Box 7.7   Case formulation

During a team formulation session, we drew a family tree which highlighted the losses and abuse experienced by Sharon's family. Her grandfather had spent time in a psychiatric institution and had killed himself. Her father had been diagnosed with bipolar disorder, and his father with schizophrenia, perhaps indicating a genetic vulnerability. We noticed how Sharon, her sister and mother had all been sexually abused as children by her grandfather and how they had then found themselves, as adults, in relationships which included domestic violence. Sharon had been in the care system from the age of seven, where she had also been abused. The family tree made us more aware of her niece, who, we realised, could also be at risk of abuse. It also helped us to have compassion for her family who had also been hurt by inter-generational difficulties.

As so often happens, the team had a sense of 'no wonder Sharon struggles with mental health problems' and 'no wonder she is wary of engaging with services'. We saw how her voices and 'paranoid' thoughts about not trusting people might be grounded in the reality of her life experience. We better understood how Sharon's experiences and difficulties in engagement had triggered troubling thoughts and feelings in team members. We understood how her sister's apparent over-involvement might be seen as her doing her best and making up for not protecting her when they were younger. We noticed how the team and her sister were drawn into trying to rescue Sharon, but also sometimes violated her boundaries, for example by giving her depot medication which she disliked.

The formulation influenced our practice. Our compassion for the family enabled us to support Sharon in strengthening those relationships which she found supportive by working with her and her sister to help them understand one another. At the same time we supported Sharon to maintain her boundary about not seeing her grandfather. Our understanding of our own transference helped us to moderate our pull to rescue her, instead respecting her as an adult who could make choices and learn from mistakes and who could be assertive with us and trusted in changing from depot to oral medication.

---

often facilitated by psychologists, although other team members may also take this role. Whomsley (2010) discusses several approaches to team formulation and advocates using different formats at different stages in the client's assertive outreach journey:

- An engagement formulation learning from the person's past and current relationships and their understanding of their difficulties.
- A resources formulation focusing on their power in their environment, including the strengths and difficulties in their relationships with family and friends.
- A risk and a moving-on formulation.

Within the teams where we work we have adapted Lake's (2008) approach to team formulation which draws on cognitive, behavioural, systemic and psychoanalytic ideas (see Box 7.7). The process promotes understanding, fosters empathy and enables us to use interventions more appropriately (Wane et al., 2009).

Systemic understandings are powerful and workers who use reflective practice might find themselves addressing issues within their own team. Teams can slip into patterns of interaction that are like a family, for example, where there are adult and child positions. By reflecting as a team, discussing what feelings are experienced, or placed on other people, these processes can be identified and addressed. As discussed in other chapters, assertive outreach teams usually function with a democratically organised multi-professional approach. Teams in which there are internal divisions, in which some workers are excluded from important decision making processes, may also exclude service users and their carers from decisions about treatment, care and other service interventions. Language can be powerful and teams often need help in avoiding stigmatising or judgemental talk. When they are struggling, workers sometimes use stereotypical ideas as a kind of short-hand in simplistic communications; describing carers as; 'co-dependent', 'neglectful', 'over-involved', or talking about the cared for person as; 'burdensome', 'ungrateful' or 'needy'. Reflective practice can help with this and a more sophisticated understanding will be more valuable to the team in the long run. We have found that it can be helpful for part of the team to have a conversation about the dilemmas or formulations that people in a family or other systems face, whilst the rest of the team acts as a reflecting team where they observe the conversation and then have a positive conversation offering reflections and different ideas (Andersen, 1987; 1992). Within this framework we have also found it useful for different people to listen from the standpoint of each member of the family or system.

Reflection point

Is your team currently making time to reflect as a group? If not, has this been suggested and why do you think that the team has not committed to this activity. If it has, does everyone attend? Every team will struggle at times to maintain effective and appropriate internal communications, so what can your team do to proactively manage these problems?

How can we manage confidentiality?

Workers often experience a dilemma. On one hand the individual who is served by the team has a right to confidentiality and might ask that no information concerning them

---

Box 7.8 Working around confidentiality

Kwame believed that people were out to get him. He accounted for his paranoia by describing difficult life experiences and asked our team not to disclose information about him to anyone, including his mother, although he was aware that the team would be assessing her needs as a carer. It was found that Kwame's mother felt depressed and stressed. She spent a lot of time with him while he spoke about MI5 and political oppression. She neglected her own social life, while encouraging Kwame to go out, but often got into arguments with him instead. Our team supported Kwame and his mother by taking him out and thereby giving her time for herself. We gave her information leaflets and helped her to understand her son's behaviour in the context of what we know about psychosis generally. We helped her to feel that she was not to blame and she realised that she could help them both by looking after herself and modelling enjoying going out. Kwame became more trusting as he realised that our workers had not given his mother any specific information about him. We helped them to organise a respite break and their relationship improved.

is to be disclosed, while on the other, relatives might struggle to cope with the feelings and actions of their relative and would benefit from conversations with the team. Carers report that confidentiality has been used all too often as an excuse not to include them (Wynaden & Orb, 2005; Cleary et al., 2006; Askey et al., 2009). The dilemma is commonly seen as dichotomous; should we serve the service user or their carers? However, we find that it is possible to meet both agendas (see Box 7.8). A distinction can be made between information that is personal about the client themselves, such as what they have said or are doing, and general information about mental health problems and services (Slade et al., 2007).

Workers must attend to their duties of confidentiality, as required in their various professional and employment roles, but policy or guidance cannot cover all the complex issues which assertive outreach teams will encounter and sometimes they offer conflicting instructions. Whenever possible, the limits of confidentiality and legal parameters must be explained and discussed during engagement, at the start of each new piece of work and at regular reviews. Team members will need to bring complex issues to supervision or team discussion. By meeting requirements for confidentiality in a thoughtful manner, we allow people to choose what they wish to disclose to us, maintaining an awareness of how that information may be used (see Box 7.9). Statutory regulations (in England and Wales) such as Safeguarding Vulnerable Adults, Child Protection and Mental Health Law can provide a framework. The nearest relative may need to be consulted if someone is being compulsorily admitted to hospital, for example, yet confidentiality may later be upheld during a period of recovery. Carers could be confused by this and they need to be informed about the requirements of different laws and policies. Individual plans can be agreed. For example, someone may want their family to be informed if they are becoming unwell, while not wanting them to be informed about psychological work on sexual abuse. Policies have been co-authored with carer groups, highlighting the use of advance statements to record preferences for crisis management (Henderson et al., 2004).

Box 7.9   A confidentiality code of practice

- Patient information is generally held under legal and ethical obligations of confidentiality. Information provided in confidence should not be used or disclosed in a form that might identify a person without his or her consent.
- A duty of confidence is a legal obligation that is derived from case law, a requirement established with professional codes of conduct and it must be included within NHS and Social Services employment contracts as a specific requirement linked to disciplinary procedures.
- In the UK, Caldicott Guardians are senior staff in the NHS and Social Services, appointed to protect patient information and teams need to liaise with these workers to ensure that local protocols are appropriately set up, correctly interpreted and understood.
- As a general principle, the sharing of information must always be purposeful; in the interests of the service user and only overridden if there is a greater duty of care or risk to be addressed. (Department of Health, 2003)

Making families our priority

In England and Wales, government policy initiatives have made families and 'carers' a high priority. The Carers (Recognition and Services) Act 1995 (Department of Health, 1996) established carers' rights to an assessment and required local authorities to provide services for carers. The National Service Framework for Mental Health (Department of Health, 1999: 69), standard six, 'caring about carers', recognises the impact that caring for someone with a mental health problem can have on carers' own physical and mental health and that they also have a right to access services in their own right. This legislation responds to research in which it is found that family environment has a greater impact on recovery from psychosis than does medication (Vaughn & Leff, 1976). Family therapy is as effective as medication (specifically Clozapine) in reducing relapse in psychosis, reducing it by about 30% (see reviews in Burbach, 1996; Fadden, 1998). The National Institute for Clinical Excellence guidelines recommend that family interventions should be offered to all families of people diagnosed as suffering from schizophrenia where they are in close contact with the family, at risk of relapsing or have persisting symptoms (NICE, 2009).

'Helping carers is one of the best ways of helping the people they are caring for' (Department of Health, 1999: 12). In the UK, approximately 55–60% of people receiving treatment for psychosis live at home, often with a family member (MacMillan et al., 1986). It is estimated that up to 1.5 million people in the UK care for a relative or friend with a mental illness (Pinfold & Corry, 2003). In contrast to this, many service users who are referred to assertive outreach describe experiences of surviving alone, disconnected from family as well as services (Lukeman, 2003). In our assertive outreach teams we have found that, 68% of our service users are single, with just 5% being married, in a civil partnership or other stable relationship. We also found that 65% did not feel that they have someone they called a close friend and 31% said they did not have any significant other person that they could confide in (Meddings et al., 2007). It is recognised that people who are referred to assertive outreach present particularly challenging difficulties which can cause complex problems in families, leading to greater isolation and distress. Also, people who are served by these teams are three times as likely as those using standard Community Mental Health Teams to show aggression towards family members (Schneider et al., 2006). Thus, family and social network interventions are especially important in assertive outreach, both to support people in retrieving and developing social support networks and as an aspect of the team's risk assessment and management strategies.

The Policy Implementation Guide (Department of Health, 2001) suggests that within assertive outreach, there should be provision of psycho-education, family therapy, practical support and care plans for carers. Teams can work with relatives on an individual basis, or hold support meetings for relatives and friends. They can provide more formal National Institute for Clinical Excellence guided interventions (Meddings et al., 2010), or work in partnership with carer support services, which are often run by volunteers or charities. Educational material is available and families can be encouraged to support each other, perhaps contributing to service development and review or engaging in political lobbying. When relatives and friends are informed about the sorts of behaviours and problems associated with a mental health difficulty, and ways of coping, they are more able to predict and manage issues in their relationship with the cared for person. Family work needs to be adapted in relation to young carers, the service user's children and younger siblings, being both careful to work in age appropriate ways and to protect against parentification. Where our service users struggle to meet their needs, all kinds of people might be drawn in and some of these carers might find themselves inappropriately carrying worries and responsibilities, so teams need to act to inform and educate.

Engagement and relationships are paramount in assertive outreach and these are enhanced by core elements of family interventions for psychosis, such as:

- Recognising that the family is a resource and that relatives try to do their best for one another.
- Supporting families to deal with the grief and loss involved when a family member develops psychosis.
- Reducing blame and guilt.
- Sharing information and learning.
- Problem solving and developing coping strategies.
- Finding ways to communicate, listening to one another and respecting boundaries.
- Externalising and seeing the psychosis as the problem rather than the person as the problem.
- Developing new scripts about how the family and its members are and might be.
- Developing balance between supporting one another and having independence.

For a more detailed exploration see Kuipers et al. (2002); Smith et al. (2007) and, as applied to assertive outreach, Burbach et al. (2007); Meddings et al. (2010) (see Box 7.10 for what is found helpful about family interventions).

As Meddings et al. (2010) argue, in assertive outreach it may be necessary to adapt and reach out to families by spending time engaging with them and acknowledging their experiences with services; offering appointments at times and in venues which are more suitable to an individual family, including home visits; arranging transport; accepting that some family members may not want to be involved. In an 'Open Dialogue' approach (Seikkula & Arnkil, 2006), professionals, families, employers, friends and other members of people's social networks can be brought together, alongside the person with a diagnosis

---

Box 7.10   What do relatives find helpful about family interventions?

- Increased knowledge/understanding of schizophrenia.
- Relatives felt supported.
- Useful to have a contact point in case of emergencies.
- Relatives felt reassured/encouraged.
- Relatives found the therapeutic alliance helpful.
- Patient encouraged to increase activity levels.
- Advice on managing symptoms.
- Increased caregivers' tolerance of problem behaviour.
- Improved communication between family members.
- Increased relatives' acceptance of illness.
- Increased understanding about medication. (Budd & Hughes, 1997: 344)

of psychosis, to generate dialogues about the experiences, explanations and ways of supporting the person with the diagnosis, as well as each other. It is important that a carer has someone in the team to turn to, a 'carers' champion', someone who will give them time and help them express their views. Alternatively, teams may use separate dedicated family support workers, from partnership organisations.

Managing power and conflict

Irena, a family carer interviewed in Hughes (2007), explained how the team coming to see the family at home gives that family more power; puts them at ease and enables a more natural interaction, which helps the team to really get to know them. This is in comparison to the family attending meetings at the team base where the atmosphere is more formal and they feel more guarded.

> you're more relaxed in our own home and seeing that I think is really important and having that sense of the difference, because we behave differently when we go out of our house… you're more able to say what you want to say. Whereas if you go out to the meetings it becomes like the authority, they become the authority and then the authority feels like the authority knows better and it's like you have to justify yourself all the time and try to explain yourself more. (Irena)

It is observed in Chapter 9 that being identified as a mental health patient is associated with stigma and discrimination; expressed through imbalances in the use of power. This inevitably causes conflict in family or friendship groups. When viewed as an aspect of common rhetorical disputes, stereotypical ideas about mental illness and dependence in relationships can act to place participants in 'subject positions' (Davis & Harre, 1990), or give them access to different 'power bases' (Dallos & Dallos, 1997). People often try to resolve disputes over their status in families by attempting to define 'reality'; by seeking agreement over 'what actually happened'. However, participants will have experienced past encounters differently. Each time the contentious issues are discussed, further conflicting positions might be promoted. This usually leads to participants taking up entrenched positions.

Assertive outreach workers will be trying to bring about fair and impartial decisions that are acceptable to many interested parties. They may themselves be accused of bias and self interest in encounters that can often be hostile. Assertive outreach teams respond to this, as described by Aggertt & Goldberg (2005), by achieving a kind of cognitive flexibility; holding contrasting views in mind. This is necessary because, any attempt to establish who is 'right', is merely exercising power rather than clarifying what happened. It can also leave some participants feeling resentful at having their reality defined for them. So, assertive outreach work is 'team based', fostering an open and accepting culture. While they are held by their team culture, using supervision, reflective practice and team formulation, workers are less likely to be pulled into everyday dramas and conflicts.

In serving the conflicting needs of service users and others who are involved, workers can view all parties as protected by the Human Rights Act. Where one person's rights conflict with another's, a solution is found that is proportionate to the significance of these

---

Box 7.11   Different kinds of power

- People using services may be physically stronger, especially if they are male or their relatives are elderly.
- Some people may have greater power due to intelligence, language, information or education, physical and mental health, money and access to resources.
- People may have power as a result of dominant gender, class, race, or sexual orientation.
- Mental health workers will interrelate with the above and also have statutory powers.

---

rights and the degree to which infringement is occurring in each case. When a service user is known to have become violent while distressed, for example, their right to a private family life needs to be balanced with their family's right to be protected from violence. Through ongoing work, rights and duties can be discussed with the service user, their family and other parties, in an ethical exploration, informed by Systemic Family Therapy, enabling communication based ethics (Willette, 1998; Donovan, 2003). In helping members of the system to work together and agreeing ways forward we may want to support those with least power (often our service users) to express their wants and needs (for examples of different types of power, see Box 7.11).

Treating people for short periods in psychiatric hospital has been part of assertive outreach work and progressing from detention under mental health law to voluntary admission is often a first step to recovery. However, inpatient treatment is another setting in which difficult encounters with families can occur. At such times power dynamics may be played out, so reflection and analysis are important. Psychiatrists or social workers are seen as powerful figures in decisions that impinge on freedoms and liberties. Work in the community can also involve power when investigations are instigated (in England and Wales) under Safeguarding Vulnerable Adults legislation. Plans can be quickly agreed in which the authority of the police or other agencies can be enacted. Strategy meetings will be held with key agencies, such as 'domestic violence support' or 'sheltered housing'. However, the service user and their family members or friends are invited to case conferences and discharge planning meetings, where efforts are made to involve and empower.

There may be dilemmas where teams are aware that people might be doing their best in difficult circumstances, but there are problems such as physical violence, abusive sexual contact, financial abuse, or when the person who uses our services, or others, are deprived of their liberties. Also, social nuisance problems can be addressed in the UK through the use of various powers and police forces dedicate officers to the duty of public protection. The protection of children always takes priority and when the service user has parental responsibilities teams are pulled into complex interactions with other statutory agencies. (See Box 7.12 for a statutory framework for joint decision making.) The main role of the team is often to enable the service user to be the best parent that they can. Support can be extended to children who might be thought of as a 'young carer', but the needs of the child still come first.

Who is assertive outreach for? These teams aim to promote the recovery and social inclusion of people with serious mental health problems who have not engaged with traditional services. In this chapter we have seen how, additionally, teams are required to

---

Box 7.12   Using a statutory framework for joint decision making

Alex has a flat in a pleasant suburban road, but in his mind, he lives in an urban ghetto with gang violence and social oppression. His neighbours complain that he plays loud, aggressive music, that local vagrants use drugs in the flat and that sometimes there are violent arguments. Alex's mental health often breaks down and he is detained against his wishes. However, during these inpatient stays, Alex's parents clean his flat, redecorate and re-furnish it. Alex's physical and mental health problems are addressed in hospital, where he has a better diet and he regains some weight.

The assertive outreach team accepts a referral and through regular contacts they begin to improve Alex's compliance with treatment. This reduces the regularity of his admissions, but Alex then lives in squalor for increasing periods and loses more weight. His parents contact the team repeatedly, complaining that services are neglecting to care for their son. The team investigate these claims using Safeguarding Vulnerable Adults legislation. Assessments are made of Alex's ability to make decisions around substance misuse, budg-eting and allowing people to stay at his flat. In 'family liaison meetings' Alex's life-style choices are discussed and he is encouraged to be more assertive; although his parents are initially mistrustful and dismiss the claim that their son is capable of making decisions or learning from the consequences of his actions.

A further investigation is held when Alex is found to have bruises and cuts on his body. He is brave enough to talk about the threats and physical assaults that he has endured and he gives the name of the perpetrator to the police. Although Alex wants to continue to see this man, who is a drugs dealer, he does not like being threatened and beaten. The police gather evidence, court proceedings are held and this drugs dealer is sent to prison for as-sault and other related crimes that the police had previously been investigating.

Alex's relationship with his parents and with the team, improve through this collaborative work, along with his quality of life. Although he continues to express his interest in music and urban youth culture and he occasionally uses illicit substances.

---

support the relatives and acquaintances of the people who are referred to us. Thereby reducing their stress and health difficulties which result from caring, and also because, by supporting carers, we also have a great impact on the recovery of people using our serv-ices. Again, children may be deemed to take priority and indeed, where children are at risk, all health and social services teams are required to prioritise the needs of those chil-dren. Finally, it could be said that part of the role of teams is to protect families and the public on occasions where people using assertive outreach are assessed to be a risk to others and this may result in compulsory treatment and/or hospital admission even when this is against the express wishes of the person using the services. In order to balance these competing priorities, teams need to protect time for reflective practice, supervision and formulation. Together they can then weigh up the priorities and concerns of everyone who is involved so as to decide how to proceed. They may need to think together about these on a daily basis and in relation to each client.

Conclusion

Families are clearly our most life enhancing form of support but they can easily be labelled as toxic. For many service users, achieving a stable life with some quality of life would not be possible without many hours of support provided by family members and other informal carers. Assertive outreach workers find ways to help service users and their families communicate better and they encourage a better management of risk that enables stability and social inclusion.

Recovery work and social inclusion are only possible where risks are adequately managed. So, assertive outreach teams must achieve a kind of engagement in which all parties feel that they are consulted and involved in important decisions, while the right of confidentiality must also be respected. However, questions remain over whether these teams are providing therapy, education, advice, just a listening ear, or how can they claim to be offering support when they are sometimes required to intervene against the wishes of a service user or their family? Fostering open debate is important so as to support everyone involved, but, at the same time, teams must find some means of exercising authority. It is essential that team cohesion is maintained through the barrage of these conflicting demands.

Acknowledgements

With thanks to: all the families we have worked with and also to Helen Hughes whose in-depth interviews and research with relatives of assertive outreach users provided such a rich source of information to this chapter.

References

Andersen, T. (1987) The reflecting team: dialogue and meta-dialogue in clinical work. *Family Process*, **26**, 415–428.

Anderson, H. & Goolishian, H. (1992) The client is the expert: a not-knowing approach to therapy. In G. McNamee & K.J. Gergen (eds.) *Therapy as Social Construction* (pp. 25–39). Sage, London.

Aggett, P. & Goldberg, D. (2005) Pervasive alienation: on seeing the invisible, meeting the inaccessible and engaging 'lost to contact' clients with major mental illness. *Journal of Interprofessional Care*, **19**(2), 83–92.

Askey, R. Homshaw, J., Gambie, C. & Richard, D. (2009) What do carers of people with psychosis need from mental health services? Exploring the views of carers, service users and professionals. *Journal of Family Therapy*, **31**(3), 310–331.

Barrowclough, C. & Tarrier, N. (1998) The application of expressed emotion to clinical work in schizophrenia. *In Session: Psychotherapy in Practice*, **4**(3), 7–23.

Budd, R.J. & Hughes, I.C.T. (1997) What do relatives of people with schizophrenia find helpful about family intervention. *Schizophrenia Bulletin*, **23**, 341–347.

Burbach, F. (1996) Family based interventions in psychosis – an overview of, and comparison between, family therapy and family management approaches. *Journal of Mental Health*, **5**, 111–134.

Burbach, F., Carter, J., Carter, J. & Carter, M. (2007) Assertive Outreach and Family Work, In: *Changing Outcomes in Psychosis: Collaborative Cases from Practitioners, Users and Carers*, (eds. R. Velleman, E. Davis, G. Smith and M. Drage). pp. 80–97. Blackwell, Oxford.

Cleary, M., Freeman, A. & Walter, G. (2006) Carer participation in mental health service delivery. *International Journal of Mental Health Nursing*, **12**, 189–194.

Coldwell, J., Meddings, S. & Camic, P. (in press) How people with psychosis positively contribute to their family: A grounded theory analysis. Forthcoming publication.

Dallos, S. & Dallos, R. (1997) *Couples, Sex and Power: the Politics of Desire.* The Open University Press, Milton Keynes.

Davis, B. & Harre, R. (1990) Positioning: the discursive production of selves. *Journal for the Theory of Social Behaviour,* **20**, 43–63.

Department of Health (1996) *The Carers (Recognition and Services) Act 1995.* Department of Health, London.

Department of Health (1999) *The National Service Framework for Mental Health.* Department of Health, London.

Department of Health (2001) *The Policy Implementation Guide for Assertive Outreach Services.* Department of Health, London.

Department of Health (2003) *The Confidentiality: NHS Code of Practice.* Department of Health, London.

Donovan, M. (2003) Family therapy beyond postmodernism: some considerations on the ethical orientation of contemporary practice. *Journal of Family Therapy,* **25**, 285–306.

Enns, R.A., Reddon, J.R. & McDonald, L. (1999) Indications of resilience among family members of people admitted to a psychiatric facility. *Psychiatric Rehabilitation Journal,* **23**(2), 127–165.

Fadden, G. (1998) Family Intervention in psychosis, *Journal of Mental Health,* **7**, 115–122.

Fisch, R., Weakland, J.H. & Segal, L. (1982) *The Tactics of Change.* Jossey-Bass, London.

Franklin, R.R., Sarr, D., Gueye, M., Sylla, O. & Collignon, R. (1996) Cultural response to mental illness in Senegal: reflections through patient companions – Part I. *Social Science and Medicine,* **42**(3), 325–338.

Graley-Wetherell, R. & Morgan, S. (2001) *Active Outreach: An Independent Service User Evaluation of a Model of Assertive Outreach Practice.* Sainsbury Centre for Mental Health, London.

Greeff, A.P., Vansteenwegen, A. & Ide, M. (2006) Resiliency in families with a member with a psychological disorder. *The American Journal of Family Therapy,* **34**, 285–300.

Greenberg, J.S., Greenley, J.R. & Benedict, P. (1994) Contributions of persons with serious mental illness to their families. *Hospital and Community Psychiatry,* **45**, 475–480.

Harvey, K., Catty, J., Langman, A., Winfield, H., Clement, S., Burns, E., White, S. & Burns, T. (2008) A review of instruments developed to measure outcome for carers of people with mental health problems. *Acta Psychiatrica Scandinavica,* **117**, 164–176.

Hayward, M., Ockwell, C., Bird, T., Pearce, H., Parfoot, S. & Bates, T. (2004) How well are we doing? *Mental Health Today,* Oct, 25–28.

Henderson, C., Flood, C., Leese, M., Thornicroft G., Sutherby K. & Szmukler G. (2004) Effect of joint crisis plans on use of compulsory treatment in psychiatry: single blind randomised controlled trial. *British Medical Journal,* **329**, 136–140.

Hoenig, J. & Hamilton, M.W. (1966) A new venture in administrative psychiatry. *American Journal of Psychiatry,* **123**, 270–279.

Hughes, H. (2007) Relatives' Experiences of Assertive Outreach, unpublished thesis, University of Surrey.

Kavanagh, D.J. (1992) Recent developments in expressed emotion and schizophrenia. *British Journal of Psychiatry,* **160**, 601–620.

Kuipers, E., Leff, J. & Lam, D. (2002) *Family Work for Schizophrenia: A Practical Guide,* 2nd edn. Royal College of Psychiatrists, London.

Lake, N. (2008) Developing skills in consultation 2: a team formulation approach. *Clinical Psychology Forum,* **186**, 18–24.

Lukens, E.P., Thorning, H. & Lohrer, S. (2004) Sibling perspectives on severe mental illness: reflections on self and family. *American Journal of Orthopsychiatry,* **74**(4), 489–501.

McFarlane, W.R., Dushay, R.A., Stastny, P., Deakins, S.M. & Link, B. (1996) A comparison of two levels of family-aided assertive community treatment. *Psychiatric Services*, **47**, 744–750.

McFarlane, W.R. (1997) FACT: integrating family psychoeducation and Assertive Community Treatment. *Administration and Policy in Mental Health*, **25**(2), 191–198.

MacMillan, J.F., Gold, A., Crow, T.J., Johnson, A.L. & Johnstone, E.C. (1986) Expressed emotion and relapse. *The British Journal of Psychiatry*, **184**, 133–143.

Meddings, S., Perkins, A., Wharne, S., Ley, P., Collins, T. & Wilson, Y. (2007) Being assertive effectively. *Mental Health Today*, May, 34–37.

Meddings, S., Gordon, I. & Owen, D. (2010) Family and Systemic Work. In: *Reaching Out: The Psychology of Assertive Outreach*, (ed. C. Cupitt). pp. 163–185. Routledge, London.

Meddings, S., Shaw, B. & Diamond, B. (2010) Community psychology. In: *Reaching Out: The Psychology of Assertive Outreach*, (ed. C. Cupitt), pp.207–228. Hove, Routledge.

NICE (2009) *Schizophrenia: Core Interventions in the Treatment and Management of Schizophrenia in Primary and Secondary Care (update).* National Institute of Health and Health and Clinical Excellence, London.

Noble, L. & Douglas, B. (2004) What users and relatives want from mental health services. *Current Opinion in Psychiatry*, **17**, 289–296.

Ohaeri, J.U. (1998) Perception of the social support role of the extended family network by some Nigerians with schizophrenia and affective disorders. *Social Science and Medicine*, **47**(10), 1463–1472.

Pinfold, V. & Corry, P. (2003) *Under Pressure: The Impact of Caring on People Supporting Family Members or Friends with Mental Health Problems.* Rethink, London.

Pilgrim, D. & Rogers, A. (1993) *A Sociology of Mental Health and Illness.* Open University Press, Buckingham.

Rapp, C.A. & Goscha, R.J. (2006) *The Strengths Model: Case Management with People with Psychiatric Disabilities*, 2nd edn. Oxford University Press, New York.

Repper, J. & Perkins, R. (2003) *Social Inclusion and Recovery.* Balliere Tindall, London.

Rosenfarb, I.S., Bellack, A.S. & Aziz, N. (2006) A sociocultural stress, appraisal, and coping model of subjective burden and family attitudes towards patients with schizophrenia. *Journal of Abnormal Psychology*, **115**(1), 157–165.

Schneider, J., Brandon, T., Wooff, D., Carpenter, J. & Paxton, R. (2006) Assertive outreach: policy and reality. *Psychiatric Bulletin*, **30**, 89–94.

Schwartz, C. & Gidron, R. (2002) The impact of altruistic behaviors for children and grandchildren on major depression among parents and grandparents in the United States: a prospective study. *Journal of Affective Disorders*, **107**(1), 29–36.

Seikkula, J. & Arnkil, T.E. (2006) *Dialogical Meetings in Social Networks.* Karnac Books, London.

Seloilwe, E.S. (2006) Experiences and demands of families with mentally ill people at home in Botswana. *Journal of Nursing Scholarship*, **28**(3), 262–268.

Shepherd, G., Murray, A. & Muijen, M. (1995) Perspectives on schizophrenia: a survey of user, family care and professional views regarding effective care. *Journal of Mental Health*, **4**, 403–422.

Singleton, N., Aye Maung, N., Cowie, A., Sparks, J., Bumstead, R. & Meltzer, P. (2002). The Mental Health of Carers. H.M.S.O., London.

Slade, M., Pinfold, V., Rapaport, J., Bellringer, S., Kuipers, E. & Huxley, P. (2007) Best practice when service users do not consent to sharing information with carers. *British Journal of Psychiatry*, **190**, 148–155.

Smith, G., Gregory, K. & Higgs, A. (2007) *An Integrated Approach to Family Work for Psychosis: A Manual for Family Workers.* Jessica Kingsley Publishers, London.

Smith, J. & Birchwood, M. (1990) Relatives and patients as partners in the management of schizophrenia: the development of a service model. *British Journal of Psychiatry*, **156**, 654–660.

Stern, S., Doolan, M., Staples, E., Szmukler, G. & Eisler, I. (1999) Disruption and reconstruction: narrative insights into the experience of family members caring for a relative diagnosed with serious mental illness. *Family Process*, **38**, 353–369.

Vaughn, C.E. & Leff, J.P. (1976) The influence of family and social factors on the course of psychiatric illness. *British Journal of Psychiatry*, **129**, 125–37.

Wane, J., Larkin, M., Earl-Gray, M. & Smith, H. (2009) Understanding the impact of an assertive outreach team on couples caring for adult children with psychosis. *Journal of Family Therapy*, **31**, 284–309.

Warner, R. (1994) *Recovery from Schizophrenia: Psychiatry and Political Economy*, 2nd edn. Routledge, London.

Warner, R. (2000) *The Environment of Schizophrenia: Innovations in Practice, Policy and Communications*. Brunner-Routledge, London.

Whomsley, S. (2010) Team Case Formulation. In: *Reaching Out: The Psychology of Assertive Outreach*, (ed. C. Cupitt). pp. 95–118. Routledge, London.

Willette, C. (1998) Practical discourse as policy making: an application of Habermas's discourse ethics within a community mental health setting. *Canadian Journal of Community Mental Health*, (**17**)2, 27–38.

Wynaden, D. & Orb, A. (2005) Impact of patient confidentiality on carers of people who have a mental disorder. *International Journal of Mental Health Nursing*, **14**, 166–171.

Zubin, J. & Spring, B. (1977) Vulnerability: a new view of schizophrenia. *Journal of Abnormal Psychology*, **86**, 103–124.

Chapter 8

Service user experience: engagement and recovery

Simon Wharne and Kamal Spilsted

With contributions from Natalie Darby (N.D.), James Rose (J.R.) and thanks to Nadine Diggins

Introduction

There are many contradictions inherent in the practical work of achieving engagement and promoting recovery in assertive outreach. Service users who meet the criteria for these services often disagree with the interpretations of mental health workers, frequently refusing to accept diagnostic labels and related treatments. Why, many of them have asked, would they choose to engage with services which they do not believe that they need? Workers might also be reluctant to impose services and treatments, but can be obliged because of the risks that have been observed, to take the drastic action of detaining service users under mental health law. This action of denying service users their autonomy or choice and imposing treatment on them, is paradoxically, justified by the belief that treatment is necessary to enable choice and recovery. Following this treatment we usually see better communication and less distress, but many service users feel bullied and abused. Given these constraints on freedom and imbalance in power, this chapter cannot give fair representation to the views or interests of service users, but will instead, combine observations from many different and contrasting narratives.

Many of the people who assertive outreach teams engage and help have been living very isolated lives in which they have become estranged from family and friends. They are often trapped in self-destructive cycles of distress, substance misuse and psychotic illness. Therefore, this chapter will include a discussion of social inclusion as a process through which workers try to foster relationships, build bridges and bring people back into their communities, thereby recovering their mental health. Multi-professional team based processes of engagement are discussed, in which service users are not just understood as passive consumers, giving feedback on the service they receive. They are understood as active citizens with rights, who do not experience services within the terms that workers expect. Recovery is defined as a direct, positive re-engagement and involvement with the community; an involvement that is different for each service user, built on their individual strengths, their aspirations and goals. Although workers might have an essential role, this recovery work will be achieved by service users. So, it is a further paradox that although the worker's initial goal is to engage with the service user, they must then become redundant in that service user's life.

Assertive Outreach in Mental Healthcare: Current Perspectives, First Edition. Edited by C. Williams, M. Firn, S. Wharne and R. Macpherson.

Engagement

Several chapters in this book consider the continuing effectiveness of assertive outreach. In Chapters 1 and 13, both positive and negative observations are made about value for money and the delivery of outcomes. However, engagement is one outcome, the success of which has rarely been disputed. This successful engagement is achieved with that small minority of service users whose needs are not met through standard clinical interventions in secondary mental health services. A simplistic analysis might assume that, because assertive outreach teams work with smaller caseloads, the more effective engagement that they achieve is merely an outcome of a more intensive approach. But this would place the assertive outreach worker in the paradoxical position of attempting to impose more of something on their service users, which had not previously worked for them (Gray & Johanson, 2010). Spindel & Nugent (2000) for example, make this assumption in characterising assertive community treatment as the 'polar opposite' of empowerment philosophy. This concern is also implied when assertive outreach is described as 'therapeutic stalking'. So this chapter will consider whether these teams are pushing standard care and treatment more effectively, or offering something more. It will be argued that the quality of the relationship between the worker and the service user acts as the central mediating factor in the difference between oppression and empowerment (also discussed in Chapter 8). Contrasting understandings of empowerment and recovery will then be considered.

It has been suggested that some assertive outreach interventions, such as more frequent contacts and an interest in all aspects of the service user's life, are oppressive (Smith, 1999). So it is a counter intuitive outcome that these are not the interventions which service users most often complain about; see Box 8.1. It is the intensity of contact which is

---

Box 8.1   Research into service user views on assertive outreach services

- McGrew et al. (2002) found that 44% of those who were asked had no complaints about their assertive outreach style service; while 16% said that they were actually dissatisfied with an under-implementation of interventions commonly provided within this approach, such as more frequent visits (obviously 66% did have some complaints!). 'Compared with clients of programs with low levels of fidelity to assertive community treatment, clients of high-fidelity programs had fewer complaints over-all and fewer complaints about features considered to be specific to assertive community treatment.' (McGrew et al., 2002: 438).
- Service users explained their better engagement with assertive outreach as a consequence of the extra time and commitment provided by workers. They regarded the offering of social support without a focus on medication, and a partnership model of the therapeutic relationship as a positive improvement. They also explained their disengagement as brought about by poor therapeutic relationships and with a loss of control due to medication effects. (Priebe et al., 2005)
- In an independent evaluation of an assertive outreach team, The Sainsbury Centre for Mental Health found that; 'There was very little that the service users disliked, except one or two did say that they would like to have a 'little bit' more contact or visits at the weekend or in the evenings ... Many of the interviewees commented on the fact that the workers did not put them under pressure, and worked at a pace that was comfortable for them. Other positive comments included that the workers were easy to get along with and were very friendly.' (SCMH, 2001a: 331)

Box 8.2   A definition of engagement

As a therapeutic concept, engagement has an established meaning which is mainly derived from psychodynamic theory. Gillespie et al. (2004) observe related terms such as therapeutic alliance, working alliance and helping alliance which date back over many decades. They define this concept of engagement as; 'the client and therapist working collaboratively on treatment tasks, towards mutually endorsed and valued goals. There is also an emotional bond between the client and therapist that includes issues such as mutual trust, acceptance and confidence.' (Gillespie et al., 2004: 440)

---

most often valued by service users, but only when it is delivered within a positive therapeutic relationship. The value that service users place on the relationship that they develop with workers is associated with positive outcomes in ways that compliance with treatment is not (Meaden et al., 2004). It seems that the persistence of workers leads to the development of a trusting and effective relationship and this is the main catalyst for positive change (Chinman et al., 1999).

Workers from different professional groups meet daily in assertive outreach teams to discuss their work and formulate plans, so as to improve engagement with their service users. These teams usually provide a seven day service within which extended hours and daily handovers are a means of achieving 'continuity of care'. So, a team-based commitment to remaining engaged with service users is fostered and a positive team culture is central to this work (Aggett & Goldberg, 2005). Ware et al. (2003) have developed a measure identifying five mechanisms or domains that are thought to be essential to this continuity. 'Knowing' the service user is essential in maintaining engagement and this allows for a degree of 'flexibility' in providing a service which is tailored to the interests, needs and peculiarities of each service user. Workers must be 'available' so that they may respond to contacts that are initiated by the service user, but this needs to be 'co-ordinated' so that other workers can provide cover, without implementing conflicting or contradictory interventions. This co-ordination is also needed so that important interventions are not missed out, or duplicated. When a team is functioning effectively, periods of transition such as admission or discharge from hospital, or hand over of work from one worker to another, are smooth and trouble free. So, *knowledge, flexibility, availability, co-ordination* and the *management of transition*, are key elements in effective team engagement. (See Box 8.2 for a definition of engagement.)

Aggertt & Goldberg (2005) identify a number of techniques for achieving engagement with service users who are particularly isolated. The team maintains a knowledge base which includes many skills across professional roles, such as identifying symptoms and risk, to understanding the welfare benefit and housing systems and an awareness of local community resources. The team works at developing rapport with service users, their carers and their neighbours, if appropriate. The team also achieves a kind of cognitive flexibility, in holding many contrasting and competing views and discourses in mind simultaneously. In doing so it avoids being caught up in blame or scapegoating. Frequent planning meetings are held at different levels of the support network, at which goals are agreed and paced at the right level for everyone involved. Workers are persistent in 'talking up' service users, finding and sharing positive stories of hope and optimism that promote an enthusiasm for effective engagement. In this way, workers own the dilemmas inherent in this engagement process, working as much as possible with confidentiality, but sharing essential information on risk.

By developing an understanding of the service user's life, workers are able to formulate relapse management plans (Burns & Firn, 2002). To achieve these ends, some service providers have employed previously engaged service users as support workers. This has been shown to improve compliance with care and treatment, as reflected in improved attendance at appointments, higher levels of participation in structured social care activities and better access to benefits (Dixon et al., 1997; Craig et al., 2004). Modern technology enables more creative communication and 'text messaging' is often an effective means of maintaining contact. Although this kind of initiative can reduce distance and conflict, there will always be a tension between workers and service users. For example, it is part of the role of assertive outreach teams to monitor service users who are believed to present a risk to themselves or others. So the wariness of those who are being watched is not always an inappropriate paranoia.

Caring means that when I feel upset by something, my worker is upset too. J.R. (service user)

It is important that workers should not be discouraged by a slow engagement. Taking time to really know someone enables the formation of a more effective therapeutic alliance. The importance of time is recognised both in quantitative research (Frank & Gunderson, 1990) and in qualitative research approaches (Addis & Gamble, 2004). For example, some service users who endure psychotic symptoms are quickly engaged when these frightening experiences are effectively treated by medication, but they might then experience psychological distress as their cognitive functioning improves and they become more aware of the deprivations that they have suffered due to their untreated illness. When relieved of their symptoms, they might be more emotionally connected with past traumas and current isolation. So, successful treatment can paradoxically lead to greater risk of suicide (Lysaker et al., 2003) and if workers do not understand the broader picture they can increase the level of this risk. Some service users manage the risk and distress that they experience by 'escaping back into their illness', by disengaging from treatment. Other service users might seek relief from their distress and their isolation through the use of alcohol and illicit substances. Some might reverse their day time night time waking pattern to avoid facing other people. This means that it is not effective to solve just one aspect of a service user's difficulties. Only by understanding the life of the service user as a whole system, will the team be able to provide adequate support (team formulation is discussed in Chapter 7).

In team based work, assessment and diagnosis are not just a technical exercise. It is not just explaining the service user away, so that their concerns, their distress and their complaints can be dismissed as unfortunate effects of their illness. Formulation in assertive outreach is a process through which insights are gained which enable empathy to develop and opportunities are found to improve the service user's quality of life. This approach can be contrasted with clinic based appointments. It has been observed that it is difficult for participants to form mutual understandings in outpatient appointments; the expression of delusional ideas can raise a hurdle to engagement; so that workers fail to develop empathy, ignoring and talking over the concerns of the service user (McCabe et al., 2002). In contrast, an emphasis on understanding and flexibility enables a trusting relationship to develop. The engagement process develops into a mutual relationship in which the assertive outreach team and the service user both feel empowered and more able to take positive risk, supported by trust and sharing mutual goals.

Reflection point

Consider the degree to which you feel at ease in the company of a service user with whom you have successfully engaged. Do you remember how you felt when you first met them? If you have come to feel more comfortable with this particular service user, what happened in your relationship to bring this change about?

The therapeutic relationship

Assertive outreach teams have been able to employ flexibility in maintaining therapeutic relationships, while other services have been required by government initiatives to use standardised forms of care and treatment, often delivered in an 'off the self' manner (Speed, 2007). In this kind of commercialisation, engagement might be thought of as just another outcome that is deliverable, along with other medical and psychological interventions. However, this kind of understanding places the service user in the passive position of the customer and their resistance can be understood as a 'customer relations problem'. In Box 8.10, we discuss our contrasting experiences of a healthcare system into which commercial market principles have been introduced. This 'commercialisation' was intended to place service users in the role of consumers, but it can make them feel like commodities, and within this 'free market' paradigm, the success of competing providers might depend on their willingness to use 'hard selling' strategies. The use of leverage and coercion, for example, is explored in Chapter 12.

Service evaluation is important in a 'healthcare economy.' So quantitative measures of engagement, as developed by Hall et al. (2001), or Tait et al. (2002), are used as audit tools in assessing team effectiveness (measurement is discussed in Chapter 13). However, these measures are recording aspects of the service user, such as their reliability in keeping appointments, along with the openness of their communication and their collaboration or compliance with treatment. Unfortunately this can mean that a failure to engage might be thought of as a negative quality of the service user rather than an outcome of providing a poor service. This 'objectification' is stigmatising for the service user, but also, opportunities to work creatively and understand resistance in therapeutic work are missed (see Meddings et al. (2010)).

My beliefs come from experience of life, not from an illness: illness comes from caring too much. J.R. (service user)

Box 8.3 'Being yourself' to achieve engagement

Assertive outreach workers;

> described 'trying to understand what the client had previously rejected', relaying their efforts to not only try and show a different approach, but also 'be different' from previ- ous nursing roles by 'showing a more human side of myself', discarding their walls of professionalism to reveal their desire to know the client as a person. The nurses ar- ticulated their attempts to be the confluence between an ordinary caring individual and a professional in order to embody themselves in the client's world. (Addis & Gamble, 2004: 453)

Effective teams develop supportive internal communication, in which workers feel more able to 'be themselves'. So, while working within appropriate boundaries, profes- sionals have more time and freedom in assertive outreach to be creative in their interac- tions with service users. They can move outside the rigidity of their roles, to 'be more real', in their interaction with service users, see Box 8.3. Working to achieve engagement can be a very difficult and demanding experience for workers and there is a greater need for supervision and reflection, particularly if 'self-disclosure' is used (Gray & Johanson, 2010). However, a greater sense of work-related satisfaction is experienced when a closer therapeutic alliance is achieved (Addis & Gamble, 2004).

Achieving team cohesion

Working with socially excluded people creates controversy. Some stakeholders, such as neighbours, family or other service providers will claim that the visits of assertive outreach workers are ineffectual in reducing risk and the lack of more robust intervention constitutes a form of neglect. In contrast, other commentators will argue that in making these unwanted and intrusive visits, workers are imposing an unnecessary and oppressive nuisance. An effective team will be constantly debating and regulating the amount of contact in the hope that a path can be taken that is neither oppressive nor neglectful. This requires sensitivity to power in relationships, as understood in psychological approaches to working with rela- tionship conflict (Dallos & Dallos, 1997) (carers and family work are discussed in Chapter 7). Knowledge and skills in working with couples and families are very useful, but workers must also be comfortable when talking about the use of power within their own teams and service systems. Teams must be able to clarify roles within the team and they must be clear about their position and responsibility within an overall service structure (Overtviet et al., 1997; West, 2004) (See Box 8.4 on the importance of consistency.).

In a healthcare climate that has short-term financial pressures, it can be difficult to sup- port the long-term commitments of assertive outreach work. It usually takes about a year for an effective therapeutic relationship to become established and 18 months is a key point by which positive changes should be expected (SCMH, 2001b). Workers can sometimes find themselves unsupported in trying to commit to longer-term work against the flow of management systems that cut budgets and target resources at shorter-term goals. However,

---

Box 8.4   The importance of consistency

Some team members might argue that a particular service user is experiencing symptoms of an untreated illness, leading to risk, such as a delusional belief about a neighbour. However, other team members might argue that the service user is being deliberately abusive towards this neighbour and must be held to account for their behaviour. It is a key feature of an effective team that these differences of opinion are resolved within the team, with one or the other view being adopted by everyone as a working hypothesis. Only then will the service user gain a consistent approach from the team, through which coherent interventions can be made. It is not helpful if the service user gets a visit from one member of the team who warns that police action could be taken against them if they do not treat their neighbour respectfully, while another worker turns up for a following visit and fosters the idea that the service user is unable to control their aggressive behaviour, which must therefore be resolved through changes to the treatment regime.

Box 8.5   Observations on team working from independent research

Most of the interviewees had at some point had a change in workers, but they all said that this was not too problematic because they all have a minimum of two workers at any one time. They also liked having more than one worker, because it means that if at any time one is sick or on leave, they can still see someone they know and who knows their situation. (SCMH, 2001a: 29)

Box 8.6   Therapeutic relationships; from service user led research

She doesn't let me get away with anything – she's not too soft. (SCMH, 1994: 10)

---

the use of care management systems, such as the Care Programme Approach (Department of Health, 1990), has been effective, both in gaining knowledge through a structured assessment and in achieving agreement in care plans (or recovery plans). But, on the other hand, plans cannot be too rigid as the relationship between each service user and the team is a unique and dynamic process in which spontaneous and reactive interactions occur (see Box 8.5). More frequent review is required and rather than calling a room full of people together every six months, strategies and interventions are often re-considered by smaller groups, targeted at each area of need, such as housing, psychological therapy, or medication.

In contrast to the contained world of the hospital or clinic, assertive outreach workers cannot expect their service users to attend regularly or comply with prescribed treatment plans, but must respond immediately to many different kinds of risk (Wharne, 2005). Assertive outreach workers meet service users in their homes and communities, having daily contact with angry relatives, noisy and abusive neighbours, or even the local drug dealers. There can be acquaintances who claim to be owed money, greedy landlords, neglected children or pets and dodgy employers who offer 'a bit of cash-in-hand'. Therapy in this setting does not reflect the expected image of the expert practitioner offering advice to the compliant patient. Where, several decades ago, the individual service user would have been overwhelmed by the total institutional control of the psychiatric hospital system, now it is the worker who can be overwhelmed by the seemingly chaotic life of the temporarily housed benefit claimant. There is a greater need, therefore, to maintain professional standards in the face of these challenges (more often using Safeguarding Vulnerable Adults legislation (in England and Wales) or mental health law). Problems will constantly come to light, as the team works through a process of engagement and assessment, getting to know the service users who would otherwise have been 'lost in the gaps between services'. In the process of entering the world that these excluded people experience, workers take the risk that they might compromise their own values and understandings, encountering realities far removed from their own.

Those of us who work in assertive outreach teams get to know service users who continue to hold beliefs that are at odds with ours, people who have effectively resisted our attempts to make them see things our way (see Box 8.6). Although this might be perceived as an obstacle to therapeutic progress, this resistance is also a sign of resilience, a tenacious and determined holding onto a personal perspective. Assertive outreach workers often express an admiration for their service users who appear to battle on alone against social pressures and expectations. Following the Strengths Model (Ryan, 2002; Rapp & Goscha, 2006), workers try to find means of helping service users to harness their determination and drive, directing it towards positive goals through a series of manageable steps. So where other services have found these independently minded people to be 'problematic', assertive outreach teams often view them as determined and strong individuals. A personal disposition which might be labelled as 'non-help-seeking', is for some a reasonable response given their life experiences (Biddle et al., 2007). On the other hand, there are people who resist pressure by taking a passive stance. They simply 'go with the flow' and might be thought of as vulnerable and deficient in will power. This lack of rational agency and apparent suggestibility will present further difficulties which can be very hard to make sense of (Motzkau, 2009).

While standard services tend to separate out specific problems that can then be targeted with recommended treatments and therapies, assertive outreach teams are confronted with entrenched complexities. Problems can be life-long and Read et al. (2003) observe how the people who develop enduring mental health problems have often suffered abuse in childhood. Due to these traumatic experiences, these service users might not expect anyone to care for them or invest in maintaining their safety, or try to improve their quality of life. The efforts of workers to achieve these ends might be viewed with suspicion or even hostility. Those of us who have had professional training, are the same kind of workers who failed to meet their needs in childhood. On the other hand, workers might be viewed as the ideal parents that they never had. They place us on a pedestal, but, it is then expected that workers will meet their every need, while they remain child-like and helpless. These are barriers to effective engagement which could be understood as a consequence of 'personality disorder' or, they might be viewed as an outcome of social processes (Meddings et al., 2010). People who have endured particular hardships and distressing abuse often share values and beliefs that are 'normal' responses to their experiences. Assessment and engagement across cultural divides are discussed in Chapters 10 and 11. The varying attitudes of different cultural groups to health and illness, along with expectations of what health or social care services should provide are important factors that need to be considered.

> 'Assertive outreach workers are more considerate and reliable. It seems to me that workers in some services only turn up to get paid. They fob you off or put you on the back burner. Workers in assertive outreach genuinely seem to like the work they do and want to find a way to help. N.D. (service user)

Empowerment

This chapter has emphasised the key theme of the quality of the relationship between the service user and their workers. This is a theme identified in most research into service user views (Hodgetts & Wright, 2007) and the therapeutic relationship in assertive outreach can be the service user's main connection with a seemingly uncaring society (Ware et al., 2004). Because this is a professional relationship, it is possible to respect autonomy in a manner that cannot be replicated in more informal relationships (Coffey, 2003). In this section, a discussion of empowerment will lead on to 'recovery philosophy', which then leads on, in Chapter 9, to the notion of social inclusion.

When service providers have used mental health law to detain and treat service users against their wishes, obvious questions arise about the balance of power in the therapeutic relationship. The exercise of choice has become particularly important in our modern Western societies, where a pluralistic political model dominates our thinking. We see ourselves as a collective, in which different groups compete with each other to gain power and influence. However, isolated service users do not have an organised voice in this society, other than through a loose confederation of interested parties including, service users, carers and some workers, who have promoted ideological notions such as 'recovery philosophy' (Anthony, 2000) or 'citizenship' (Barnes & Shardlow, 1997). Through this work, the idea that democratic processes can bring service users more power and freedom has become established (Fitzsimons & Fuller, 2002). The rise of this ideology can be traced back to commentators such as Szasz, Basaglia and Laing. See Box 8.7.

Despite an early enthusiasm for political change and empowerment in mental healthcare, these ideologies have been put into practice more effectively for other service user groups. The work of authors such as Oliver (1990) has reframed the notion of incapacity and we have seen significant changes over recent decades as institutionalised systems of care have closed down. Where disabled people had in the past been obliged to live and work in segregated communal settings, adaptations are now made so that they have their own homes and work in mainstream settings with the rest of society. However, this reframing is only possible due to a separation of a 'whole and healthy personality', from an 'incomplete or unhealthy body' (Mulvany, 2001). This separation is far more difficult to achieve in mental healthcare where service users often report a kind of 'loss of self' (Wisdom et al., 2008) and their identity is regularly defined by an illness category. Awareness raising campaigns have been more effective in other areas of discrimination. People are now described as visually impaired, suffering from learning difficulties, or physically disabled. However, service pro-

---

Box 8.7   Influential ideas from the mental health service user movement

- Thomas Szasz argued that mental illness is a form of deviance which people should have the right to choose. His observations were co-opted by radical conservative who upheld neo-liberal ideas about personal freedoms and responsibilities, rejecting the notion that the state should provide extensive welfare interventions. (Szasz, 1974)
- Franco Basaglia pioneered democratic decision making within clinical groups in a mental health hospital setting. The movement which he inspired embraced ideas associated with communism. So, service users might be considered to have an equal ownership and responsibility for the resources which have traditionally been managed by professional workers and administrators, such as the hospital, its land and maintenance budget. All decisions about the running of the institution and even clinical decisions about treatment and leave from the hospital would be made by the whole community. (Basaglia et al., 1987)
- R. D. Laing observed how phenomena which appear to be symptoms of illness could actually be understood as rational responses to our distressing existential realities in a failed democracy. He inspired a therapeutic approach, in which workers foster relationships with service users that are more naturalistic and ordinary. (Laing, 1969)

---

viders will still define people as schizophrenic, or depressive, for example, making the confusion between person and illness far more difficult to unpick.

Social exclusion is not just a secondary disability for mental health service users, but in some ways the original stumbling block (as discussed in Chapter 9). Problems usually arise from the common everyday disputes between people, which have been played out long before professional workers became involved. Families and friends are the first to diagnose and mental health services are commonly drawn in to conflicts where different parties demand that workers label, control and manage their unfortunate relative or friend. Where mental health problems do clearly reside in the individual, processes of social exclusion and isolation are likely to have been part of the etiological process and by the time that the service user gets referred to assertive outreach teams, disputes are entrenched, positions are isolated and labels stick like glue.

Empowerment is very difficult in mental healthcare and the notion of participation in enforced care and treatment is very paradoxical (Aggertt & Goldberg, 2005; Priebe et al., 2005). In various attempts to resolve this problem, the phenomenon of 'participation' has been interpreted differently (Gillespie & Meaden, 2010). For example, Hickey & Kipping (1998) identified two models of participation related to 'consumerism' and 'democratisation'. With consumerist models, the intention is to promote a plethora of service providers, so that service users have more choice. Costs would be driven down and standards increased in response to competition, so that performance can be improved by measuring and responding to consumer satisfaction. However, choice in the context of imposed treatment might be reduced to contemplating the menu in the hospital dining room, or where to sit in the lounge. Service users almost never have any say over which hospital they are treated in or which members of staff will work with them. Decisions about how much leave they can have, even when they can sleep, or generally what they can do with their time, are often only offered as an inducement to take medication.

In comparison with the impossible fusion of the 'detained consumer', democratisation provides a model in which people can be involved in decision making at a group or community level. This citizen model has a strong tradition in longer stay hospitals and Therapeutic Communities, but in assertive outreach, decision making usually takes place in the community. Service users are supported in a manner that enables them to make decisions, to make mistakes and to learn from the consequences of their choices. This is a positive risk taking strategy (Morgan, 2004) which requires a confident belief in the potential of the service user to grow and develop as a person (Ryan, 2002; Rapp & Goscha, 2006). In the area of employment, for example, assertive outreach teams are more likely to adopt a supporting role in direct placements in ordinary working environments. This approach has been found to be more successful than 'sheltered' work support or segregated vocational training (Rinaldi & Perkins, 2007).

In recognising the autonomy of service users, who want to live 'ordinary lives' with homes, jobs and friends, workers are trying to give back some of the power that they have lost, or simply never gained, in lives which may have been very troubled. The very human relationships that develop in assertive outreach encompass a sharing of power, in which contacts can be informal and unstructured (Addis & Gamble, 2004). It has been observed that users of intensive community mental health services value workers for the 'non-clinical contact' they provide, such as 'a ride somewhere, sharing a joke or just having a coffee.' (Buck & Alexander, 2006: 472). This kind of participation is emphasised in the ethnographic studies of Ware et al. (2003, 2004) and identified in independent service user evaluation such as SCMH (2001a). So the service user's engagement with their worker is a step towards engagement with others and participation in their community (Marshall et al., 2007).

Reflection point

This chapter has mentioned the need for a team formulation, which workers achieve by getting together and talking about the service user. However, relationships work both ways; do the people who use your service get together and talk about you and your team? Consider for a moment what they might say to each other and think about what this means in terms of their power to refuse your service or question its efficacy.

Recovery

There are many ways in which people who suffer from mental health problems might overcome stigma and achieve social inclusion. Liz Sayce identifies four strategies which are discussed in Chapter 9. The most obvious of these routes to recovery is through the treatment of symptoms. Andreasen et al. (2005) claim that this is a necessary step, but Perkins (2001) disagrees. She believes that recovery does not depend on a reduction in symptoms and she points out the reality that for many service users, symptom reduction is not a priority. Service users wanted 'better family relationships', 'better physical health'

Box 8.8   Remission can be defined, but is recovery measurable?

- Remission is; '... a state in which patients have experienced an improvement in core signs and symptoms to the extent that any remaining symptoms are of such low intensity that they no longer interfere significantly with behaviour and are below the threshold typically utilised in justifying an initial diagnosis of schizophrenia.' (Andreasen et al., 2005: 422)
- But; 'There is also no necessary connection between reduction in severity of symptoms and service users' sense of control or engagement in activities.' (Perkins, 2001:9)

Box 8.9   Three dimensions of symptoms identified in schizophrenia

1   A negative symptom dimension (also referred to as psychomotor poverty), includes poverty of speech, decreased spontaneous movement, unchanging facial expression, paucity of expressive gesture, affective non-response, and lack of vocal inflection.
2   A disorganization dimension includes symptoms of inappropriate affect, poverty of content of speech, tangentiality, derailment, pressure of speech, and distractibility.
3   A psychoticism dimension (also called 'reality distortion'), includes hallucinations and delusional ideas. (Andreasen et al., 2005: 446)

---

and the ownership of 'decent clothes and possessions' (Shepherd et al., 1995; Meddings & Perkins, 2002). So, although psychiatric research has achieved an effective measurement of symptoms, the same levels of validity are not found in the measurement of functioning (Fossy & Harvey, 2001). Andreasen et al. (2005) define remission (see Box 8.8) and Andresen et al. (2006) formulate a 'stages model of recovery', but it is important to remember that the idea of recovery has been popularised by service users and, in their view, it is an individual and very personal journey. By employing 'evidence based practice' professional workers can confidently record observations of symptoms or define deficits, here and now, recommending treatments that have worked in the past. However, to become open to 'recovery philosophy', they must accept that they cannot know or measure the future. Workers and their service users must work with the unknown as they take steps forward into new opportunities and possibilities.

Andreasen et al. (2005) refer to three dimensions of schizophrenia which have been identified in studies using factor analysis. They observe cross-scale correspondence relationships to historical constructs of psychopathology dimensions and DSM-IV criteria for schizophrenia. When data is brought together in this way, symptoms tend to cluster into three areas (see Box 8.9). Different treatments can be used to target each area of symptoms and engagement strategies can be used to tackle each dimension differently (Tait et al., 2003). However, as in the measurement of engagement, this categorisation sets aside the service user's own interpretations of their situation. The social context is also edited out of this kind of empirical observation. Many assertive outreach teams achieve a more sophisticated understanding of the way that behaviours are 'managed' through detention and treatment in an institutional setting and recognise that the service user may have adapted to an existence which lacks stimulation, supports isolation and maintains an unreal, unconnected and encapsulated state of being. Many teams 'in-reach' into hospital settings as a part of their engagement strategy.

Many service users have shared their stories of recovery, which emphasise individuality and variation. However, the influential writer and service user Deegan (1996) describes five (non-linear) stages of recovery. The first stage is a shock reaction to the trauma of acute symptoms and associated diagnosis and stigma. The second is denial and rage, as service users hold onto the belief that what is happening to them is a mistake, or a bad dream. Family and friends often get caught up in emotive conflicts, leading to a third stage of despair and self-pity. Service users and their families or friends feel an overwhelming sense of hopelessness and powerlessness. However, the next stage is 'the turning point of hope'. Because it is with a spark of hope that motivation and a willingness to try again are ignited, leading to the fifth stage of finding new meaning and purpose in life, discovering and exploring new possibilities and moving on. Service users might get stuck at any of these stages and the interventions of services might exacerbate their problems leading to an impasse. These person centred ideas have been promoted within the service user movement, inspiring sympathetic workers and policy makers, who have included recovery philosophy in service models and therapeutic approaches. But we must not assume that recovery can be led by services and their workers, who do have other agendas.

Unfortunately the degree to which a particular assertive outreach team is able to provide empathic care or socially inclusive interventions is difficult to observe. These teams have been measured against fidelity scales (see Chapters 3 and 13), but variation in the use of coercion to achieve compliance with treatment, or the quality of therapeutic relationships, or the attitudes of staff are not recorded (Drake & Deegan, 2008). So a team could achieve high fidelity to the assertive outreach model, but still act in an oppressive manner towards service users (Saylers & Tsemberis, 2007). Fidelity must therefore be flexible. For example, although the 'whole team approach' is essential to aid engagement, when the service user is working towards recovery, it might be appropriate to offer a choice of workers, or allocate one worker who can provide specialist support (Saylers & Tsemberis, 2007).

Although service users do not have the power to resist mental health law, they might have the ability to exercise power much more effectively in other areas of their lives, in their social networks, hobbies and employment settings. Service user participation in assertive outreach is, therefore, most often a supported access to participation in the community through good housing, social networks and, where possible, employment. Workers are limited in the degree to which they can involve service users when they are detained under mental health law, but they can try to consult them in any decisions that are made and can try to maintain their contact with family and friends; while ensuring the safety of their housing and possessions and protecting their finances and work opportunities (Roberts et al., 2008). It is important to note that empowerment is actually a rather strange concept. Workers cannot force powerfulness on their service users. As Mahatma Gandhi demonstrated, passive resistance is paradoxically, a very effective way of exercising power. So, it must be stated again that, recovery philosophy is not an approach or intervention that can be provided by workers (Anthony, 2000; Repper, 2000; Allott & Loganathan, 2002; Repper & Perkins, 2003). However, workers can dramatically improve the chance that service users will recover, by adopting a positive and hope-inspiring approach (Shepherd et al. 2008).

Case study 8.1   The Hindu Cow Syndrome
(an email exchange)

Kamal writes: I have been asked to write this synopsis on the Service User Experience of Engagement and Recovery, and have entitled it as above, 'The Hindu Cow Syndrome'. The title may not be appropriate, but I find it somewhat applicable. The form this synopsis shall take is what has caused me personal offence and confusion in this chapter, (excluding minor grammatical errors as believe these purposeful). I also feel it important to express that I have no prior knowledge of the inner workings of assertive outreach, so my views may not be as proactive as a mental health team worker to the point that I may appear totally ignorant or even arrogant. However, it should be remembered that I am relating the chapter to my own personal experience.

Simon writes: I welcome this opportunity to exchange views. You have picked up on my statement in the introduction where I say 'following this treatment workers usually see better communication and less distress, but service users feel bullied and abused.' (Introduction, paragraph 1)

Kamal writes: I feel neither bullied or abused but I feel neglected. However, if being abused is moving into accommodation that I believe unfit for human habitation, with inadequate furnishing then I do feel abused. So the reason that I feel neglected is that I think that this should have been resolved after leaving hospital by assertive outreach but was not. This resulted in a court case carried out by myself of which I still have the papers, and was successful. Therefore, the abuse was unlawful, but, due to my mental condition was unaware that this was the case, hence my distrust and obstructive attitude towards assertive outreach, resulting in communication breakdown.

Simon writes: I understand that living in that horrible flat has been difficult for you and perhaps our assertive outreach team could have done more. However, it is a credit to you that you managed to stand up for yourself and face your landlords in court. We would not want to take over and do things for you that you can do yourself, but would, instead want to help in your own efforts to overcome difficulties and improve your quality of life. You have picked up on the statement that I made; 'they are often trapped in self-destructive cycles of distress, substance misuse and psychotic illness.' (Introduction, paragraph 2)

Kamal writes: Whilst I suffer from distress and psychotic illness these are not self-destructive. In fact I feel that this is the opposite and that I am being taken advantage of. It is this fact that could result in self-destructive cycles.

Simon writes: Yes, unless we can find some way of helping you that does not make you feel that you are being taken advantage of, it would be better for the team to stand back and not interfere too much. You have picked up on the statement that I made; '... both positive and negative observations are made about value for money and the delivery of outcomes.' (Engagement, paragraph 1)

Kamal writes: 'value for money'? Whilst I appreciate that I am a commodity, being treated as such is non-productive when suffering from mental health conditions. However, I am happy to contribute to and comment on this chapter in this dialogue.

Simon writes: I have written here about the inappropriate use of the 'consumer model' in mental healthcare where in day to day practice, service users are not often offered meaningful choice. Thank you Kamal for contributing and commenting in this way.

Although assertive outreach workers can only gain a second hand or vicarious understanding of the service user's quandary with issues of identity, normality and difference, this knowledge is an essential part of the helping process. Respect is central and workers must resist the urge to rush in to help when service users struggle, even when they complain about the lack of support they get. When workers know their service users they trust that they will be able to find ways to manage and they offer support, rather than pushing it at them. For some service users, professional understandings enable an inclusion in society with the aid of ongoing community care, in which decisions about care and treatment are shared (Deegan & Drake, 2006). Sayce (2000) favours a 'disability model' approach to recovery, in which it is acknowledged that full functioning will not be achieved, therefore, adaptations are needed to support service users in living to their full capacity. This thinking is also supported in the Strengths Model (Ryan, 2002; Rapp & Goscha, 2006), in which the idea of finding the right niche for service users is promoted. Where service users are unable to organise some aspects of their lives, such as finances, medication compliance, transport and so on there is no reason why service providers should not continue to meet these needs, so that optimum functioning can be achieved in areas where capacity is still intact, maintaining treatment 'in the least restrictive environment'.

Sometimes workers can make an intervention that transforms the life of the service user, directing them along a clear path towards recovery. For example, dramatic turning points might include, finding stable accommodation, prescribing medication that is effective, moving away from known drug dealers, gaining a voluntary or paid employment role, providing a particular psychological therapy such as Cognitive Behaviour Therapy (CBT), forming a stable and intimate relationship with a new more suitable life partner, or regaining a supportive relationship with a family from whom they have been estranged. However, most of the time, workers will be standing by the side of service users, who continue to endure distressing cycles of failure, facing evictions, financial hardship, isolation, detention under mental health law, imprisonment with repeated patterns of risk to others, self-harm or neglect. But this ongoing support through difficulties can be the most productive. Workers are helping their service users to understand what is happening for them. They can be a sounding board for ideas, while providing acceptance and relief from isolation. It is through the intensity of living through hard life experiences that service users learn and grow, becoming more able, achieving greater self-understanding and self-reliance.

Conclusion

The interventions and general approaches that are commonly used in assertive outreach teams are often different from those of other service providers. Not only are they responsive and strategically managed by the team, with varying levels of intensity, but they are enacted through a mutual and reciprocal team-based relationship with the service user. There are philosophies and ideas that are important in maintaining this relationship, such as consumerism, democracy, citizenship, empowerment, involvement, social inclusion and recovery. It has been observed in this chapter that assertive outreach teams are trying to hold onto important themes from their professional understandings, such as 'therapeuitc alliance' and 'person centred care', while adapting to new ways of evaluating services in health and social care markets. Those of us who work to 'recovery principles', find that it is nice to receive grateful thanks and acknowledgement from service users, but the receipt of this praise is not our main goal.

In the commercial world, many service providers promote their products by including positive customer feedback in their advertisments. Many providers of care and treatment can work within this consumer model, providing eloquent examples of 'customer statisfaction'. This chapter has highlighted particlar aspects of assertive outreach work which should raise our suspicions about using service users in this way. Although it is important to gain service user feedback, this needs to be part of ongoing work, not just 'window dressing'. If workers only ever received possitive feedback then this would suggest that they have made their service users so passive and dependent on them that they dare not say anything negative. In assertive outreach, workers cannot always do what their service users want, they have a duty to protect and serve others, such as their families and the community. Workers do not always have simple and easy answers to problems. Service users are likely to remain distressed, isolated and very dissatisfied. We might actually celebrate their healthy mistrust of workers and their assertive refusal to comply with their wishes. So, on the occasions when risks are adequately resolved, perhaps the most positive feedback workers can get from their service users is when they say (along with their families and friends); 'go away, we don't need you anymore'.

References

Addis, J. & Gamble, C. (2004) Assertive outreach nurses' experience of engagement. *Journal of Psychiatric and Mental Health Nursing*, **11**, 452–460.

Aggett, P. & Goldberg, D. (2005) Pervasive alienation: on seeing the invisible, meeting the inaccessible and engaging 'lost to contact' clients with major mental illness. *Journal of Interprofessional Care*, **19**(2), 83–92.

Allott, P. & Loganathan, L. (2002) A new paradigm for delivering recovery oriented services for people with serious mental illness: implications for service delivery. *The Mental Health Review*, **7**(2), 6–13.

Andreasen, N.C., Carpenter, Jr., W.T., Kane, J.M., Lasser, R.A., Marder, S.R. & Weinberger, D.R. (2005) Remission in schizophrenia: proposed criteria and rationale for consensus. *American Journal of Psychiatry*, **162**, 441–449.

Andresen, R., Caputi, P. & Oades, L. (2006) Stages of recovery instrument: development of a measure of recovery from serious mental illness. *Australian and New Zealand Journal of Psychiatry*, **40**, 972–980.

Anthony, W.A. (2000) A recovery-orientated service system: setting some system level standards. *Psychiatric Rehabilitation Journal*, **24**(2), 159–168.

Barnes, M. & Shardlow, P. (1997) From passive recipient to active citizen: participation in mental health user groups. *Journal of Mental Health*, **6**(3), 289–300.

Basaglia, F., Scheper-Hughes, N. & Lovell, A. (1987) *Psychiatry Inside Out: Selected Writings of Franco Basaglia*. Columbia University Press, New York.

Biddle, L., Donovan, J., Sharp, D. & Gunnell, D. (2007) Explaining non-help-seeking amongst young adults with mental distress: a dynamic interpretive model of illness behaviour. *Sociology of Health & Illness*, **29** (7), 983–1002.

Buck, P.W. & Alexander, L.B. (2006) Neglected voices: consumers with serious mental illness speak about intensive case management. *Administration and Policy in Mental Health and Mental Health Services Research*, **33**(4), 470–481.

Burns, T. & Firn, M. (2002) *Assertive Outreach in Mental Health: A Manual for Practitioners.* Oxford University Press, Oxford.

Chinman, M., Allende, M., Bailey, P., Maust, J. & Davidson, L. (1999) Therapeutic agents of assertive community treatment. *Psychiatric Quarterly*, **70**(2), 137–162.

Coffey, D.S. (2003) Connection and autonomy in the case manager relationship. *Psychiatric Rehabilitation Journal*, **26**(4), 404–412.

Craig, T., Doherty, I., Jamieson-Craig, R., Boocock, A. & Attafua, G. (2004) The Consumer-Employee as a member of a mental health assertive outreach team. 1. Clinical and social outcomes. *Journal of Mental Health*, **13**(1), 59–66.

Dallos, S. & Dallos, R. (1997) *Couples, Sex and Power: the Politics of Desire.* The Open University Press, Milton Keynes.

Deegan, P.E. (1996) Coping with: recovery as a journey of the heart. *Psychiatric Rehabilitation Journal*, **19**(3), 91–97.

Deegan, P.E. & Drake, R.E. (2006) Shared decision making and medication management in the recovery process. *Psychiatric Services*, **57**(11), 1636–1639.

Department of Health (1990) *The Care Programme Approach for people with mental illness.* Department of Health, London.

Dixon, L., Hackman, A. & Lehman, A. (1997) Consumers as staff in assertive community treatment programs. *Administration and Policy in Mental Health*, **25**, 199–208.

Drake, R.E. & Deegan, P.E. (2008) Are Assertive Community Treatment and recovery compatible? Commentary on 'ACT and recovery: integrating evidence-based practice and recovery orientation on Assertive Community Treatment Teams.' *Community Mental Health Journal*, **44**, 75–77.

Fitzsimons, S. & Fuller, R. (2002) Empowerment and its implications for clinical practice in mental health: a review. *Journal of Mental Health*, **11**(5), 481–500.

Fossey, E.M. & Harvey, C.A. (2001) A conceptual review of functioning: implications for the development of consumer outcome measures. *Australian and New Zealand Journal of Psychiatry*, **35**, 91–8.

Frank, A.F. & Gunderson, J.G. (1990) The role of the treatment alliance in the treatment of Schizophrenia. *Archive of General Psychiatry*, **47**, 228–236.

Gillespie, M., Smith, J., Meaden, A., Jones, C. & Wane, J. (2004) Client's engagement with assertive outreach services: a comparison of client and staff perceptions of engagement and its impact on later engagement. *Journal of Mental Health*, **13**(5), 439–452.

Gillespie, M. & Meaden, A. (2010) Psychological processes in engagement. In: *Reaching Out: The Psychology of Assertive Outreach*, (ed. C. Cupitt). pp. 15–42. Hove, Routledge.

Gray, A. & Johanson, P. (2010) Ethics and professional issues: the universal and the particular. In: *Reaching Out: The Psychology of Assertive Outreach*, (ed. C. Cupitt). pp. 229–247. Hove, Routledge.

Hall, M., Meaden, A., Smith, J. & Jones, C. (2001) Brief report: the development and psychometric properties of an observer-rated measure of engagement with mental health services. *Journal of Mental Health*, **10**(4), 457–465.

Hickey, G. & Kipping, C. (1998) Exploring the concept of user involvement in mental health through a participation continuum. *Journal of Clinical Nursing*, **7**, 83–88.

Hodgetts, A. & Wright, J. (2007) Researching clients' experiences: a review of qualitative studies. *Clinical Psychology and Psychotherapy*, **14**, 157–163.

Laing, R.D. (1969) *The Divided Self: An Existential Study in Sanity and Madness.* Tavistock, London.

Lysaker, P., Lancaster, R. & Lysaker, J. (2003) Narrative transformation as an outcome in the psychotherapy of schizophrenia. *Psychology and Psychotherapy: Theory, Research and Practice*, **76**, 285–299.

Marshall, S.L., Crowe, T.P., Oades, L.G., Deane, F.F. & Kavanagh, D.J. (2007) A review of consumer involvement in evaluations of case management: consistency with a recovery paradigm. *Psychiatric Services*, **58**(3), 396–401.

McCabe, R., Heath, C., Burns, T. & Priebe, S. (2002) Engagement of patients with psychosis in the consultation: conversation analytic study. *British Medical Journal*, **325**, 1148–1151.

McGrew, J.H., Wilson, R.G., & Bond, G.R. (2002) An exploratory study of what clients like least about assertive community treatment. *Psychiatric Services*, **53**, 761–763.

Meaden, A., Nithsdale, V., Rose, C., Smith, J. & Jones, C. (2004) Is engagement associated with outcome in assertive outreach? *Journal of Mental Health*, **13**(4), 415–424.

Meddings, S. & Perkins, R. (2002) What 'getting better' means to staff and users of a rehabilitation service: an exploratory study. *Journal of Mental Health*, **11**(3), 319–325.

Meddings, S., Shaw, B. & Diamond, B. (2010) Community Psychology. In: *Reaching Out: The Psychology of Assertive Outreach*, (ed. C. Cupitt). pp. 207–228. Hove, Routledge.

Morgan, S. (2004) Risk Taking. In: *Assertive Outreach: A Strengths Approach to Policy and Practice*, (eds. P. Ryan & S. Morgan). pp. 223–246. Elsevier Health Sciences, Oxford.

Motzkau, J.F. (2009) Exploring the transdisciplinary trajectory of suggestibility. *Subjectivity*, **27**, 172–194.

Mulvany, J. (2001) Disability, Impairment or Illness? The Relevance of the Social Model of Disability to the Study of Mental Disorder. In: *Rethinking the Sociology of Mental Health*, (ed. J. Busfield). pp. 39–57. Blackwell, Oxford.

Oliver, M. (1990) *The Politics of Disablement*. MacMillian, London.

Overtviet, J., Mathias, P. & Thompson, T. (1997) *Interprofessional Working for Health and Social Care*. MacMillan Press, London.

Perkins, R. (2001) What constitutes success? The relative priorities of service users' and clinicians' views of mental health services. *British Journal of Psychiatry*, **179**, 9–18.

Priebe, S., Watts, J., Chase, M. & Matanov, A. (2005) Processes of disengagement and engagement in assertive outreach patients: qualitative study. *British Journal of Psychiatry*, **187**, 438–448.

Rapp, C.A. & Goscha, R.J. (2006) *The Strengths Model: Case Management with People with Psychiatric Disabilities*, 2nd edn. Oxford University Press, New York.

Read, J., Agar, K., Argyle, N. & Aderhold, V. (2003) Social and physical abuse during childhood and adulthood as predictors of hallucinations, delusions and thought disorder. *Psychology and Psychotherapy Research, Theory and Practice*, **76**, 11–22.

Repper, J. (2000) Adjusting the focus of mental health nursing: incorporating service users' experiences of recovery. *Journal of Mental Health*, **9**(6), 575–587.

Repper, J. & Perkins, R. (2003) *Social Inclusion and Recovery*. Balliere Tindall, London.

Rinaldi, M. & Perkins, P. (2007) Implementing evidence-based supported employment. *Psychiatric Bulletin*, **30**, 244–249.

Roberts, G., Dorkins, E., Wooldridge, J. & Hewis, E. (2008) Detained – what's my choice? Part 1: discussion. *Advances in Psychiatric Treatment*, **14**, 172–180.

Ryan, P. (2002) *Assertive Outreach: A Strengths Approach to Policy and Practice*. Churchill Livingstone, Edinburgh.

SCMH (1994) *AOT Service User Evaluation*. Sainsbury Centre for Mental Health, London.

SCMH (2001a) *Active Outreach: An Independent Service User Evaluation of a Model of Assertive Outreach Practice*. Sainsbury Centre for Mental Health, London.

SCMH (2001b) *Keys to Engagement: Review of Care for People with Severe Mental Illness who are Hard to Engage with Services*. Sainsbury Centre for Mental Health, London.

Sayce, L. (2000) *From Psychiatric Patient to Citizen: Overcoming Discrimination and Social Exclusion.* MacMillan Press, Basingstoke.

Saylers, M.P. & Tsemberis, S. (2007) ACT and recovery: integrating evidence-based practice and recovery orientation on assertive community treatment teams. *Community Mental Health Journal*, **43**, 619–641.

Shepherd, G., Murray, A. & Muijen, M. (1995) Perspectives on schizophrenia: a survey of user, family care and professional views regarding effective care. *Journal of Mental Health*, **4**, 403–422.

Shepherd, G., Boardman, J. & Slade, M. (2008) *Making Recovery a Reality.* Sainsbury Centre for Mental Health, London.

Smith, M. (1999) Assertive outreach: a step backwards. *Nursing Times*, **95**(30), 46–47.

Speed, E. (2007) Discourses of consumption or consumed by discourse? A consideration of what 'consumer' means to the service user. *Journal of Mental Health*, **16**(3), 307–318.

Spindel, P. & Nugent, J. (2000) Polar opposites: empowerment philosophy and assertive community treatment. *Ethical Human Science and Services Journal*, **2**(2), 93–101.

Szasz, T. (1974) *The Myth of Mental Illness: Foundations of a Theory of Personal Conduct*, Revised edn. Harper and Row, New York.

Tait, L., Birchwood, M. & Trower, P. (2002) A new scale (SES) to measure engagement with community mental health services. *Journal of Mental Health*, **11**(2), 191–198.

Tait, L., Birchwood, M. & Trower, P. (2003) Predicting engagement with services for psychosis: insight, symptoms and recovery style. *British Journal of Psychiatry*, **182**, 123–128.

Ware, N.C., Tugenberg, T. & Dickey, B. (2003) Ethnography and measurement in mental health: qualitative validation of a measure of continuity of care (CONNECT). *Qualitative Health Research*, **13**, 1393–1406.

Ware, N.C., Tugenberg, T. & Dickey, B. (2004) Practitioner relationships and quality of care for low-income persons with serious mental illness. *Psychiatric Services*, **55**, 555–559.

West, M.A. (2004) *Effective Teamwork: Practical Lessons form Organizational Research.* Blackwell Publishing, Oxford.

Wharne, S. (2005) Assertive outreach teams: their roles and functions. *Journal of Interprofessional Care*, **19**(4), 326–337.

Wisdom, J.P., Bruce, K., Saedi, G.A., Weis, T. & Green, C.A. (2008) 'Stealing me from myself:' identity and recovery in personal accounts of mental illness. *Australian and New Zealand Journal of Psychiatry*, **42**, 489–495.

Chapter 9

Assertive outreach: stigmatising treatment or social inclusion?

Simon Wharne

With contribution from Rebecca Owen

Introduction

Many of the service users who have been referred to assertive outreach teams perceive psychiatric services as stigmatising. They experience imposed treatment as demeaning, with uncomfortable and distressing side-effects, while detention under mental health law is often isolating and traumatic. These reluctant service users might resent the implication that they are unable to control themselves or make competent decisions. They resist the processes whereby they are 'managed' through the authority of state sponsored healthcare. They often report a desire for a kind of freedom which they are not experiencing while they are under the care of these services (Krupa et al., 2005). In contrast, workers want to maintain treatment because they believe that medication enables service users to think clearly, to overcome distressing or distracting symptoms and to be more effective in their social functioning, thereby enhancing the possibility of social inclusion. Workers can achieve a superficial engagement by uncritically accepting the service user's views, but the opportunity to build a stronger relationship might be lost when prescribed medication or psychological therapy are refused. Encouraging compliance with treatment that enables people to live a fulfilling life is a far more tolerable proposition than the notion that we need to 'control our service users by forcing medication on them'.

Everyone in our modern societies will be familiar with the negative stereotypical images of mental illness, as promoted in sensationalised popular culture. These 'lay understandings' feed the social processes behind stigma (see Box 9.1 for a definition of stigma), in which discrimination, prejudice and exclusion act to heap more distress on those who are already struggling. While exclusion appears to be a normal part of everyday interactions, this is a very challenging problem in mental healthcare. So this chapter will describe the task of assertive outreach workers and their service users as more complex than just overcoming problems in treatment and adjustment. There will be an exploration of our stubborn determination to overcome rejection by mainstream society and our hope of finding a niche where there is acceptance. In order to be 'well' people need valued social roles through which to contribute to society and thereby receive affirmation.

This chapter will refer to social psychology research into social exclusion. The difficulties that teams and their service users face, due to negative perceptions, will be discussed.

Assertive Outreach in Mental Healthcare: Current Perspectives, First Edition. Edited by C. Williams, M. Firn, S. Wharne and R. Macpherson.
© 2011 Blackwell Publishing Ltd. Published 2011 by Blackwell Publishing Ltd.

Box 9.1   A definition of stigma

... we define stigma as the co-occurrence of its components – labeling, stereotyping, separation, status loss, and discrimination – and further indicate that for stigmatization to occur, power must be exercised. (Link & Phelan, 2001: 363)

Box 9.2   Three aspects of subjective experiences of stigma

Judgement is something that service users encounter in their anticipated or actual experience of prejudice and discrimination by others, such as friends, family, health workers or the police. This kind of judgement is clearly associated with stereotypical ideas about mental illness, risk and difference, along with common beliefs about morality and responsibility for one's problems.

Comparison highlights a stark contrast between how lives are lived for people who are accepted as 'normal' and those who are believed to be mentally ill. This includes the 'might have been' ruminations which develop when people have been denied life opportunities; people who perhaps have every right to feel bitter when reviewing their life situation. Recovery can remain a distant hope for people who do not believe that their lives will ever be the way that 'they should have been if only they had not been ill'

Personal understanding of the issue offers some hope in the recognition that steps can be taken to minimise stigma, but also, that facing difficulties leads to the development of inner strength and deeper understanding. (Adapted from Knight et al., 2003: 214–218)

Then, the key question of whether assertive outreach interventions are stigmatising or socially inclusive will be addressed. This will lead on to an exploration of the kinds of strategies that teams and their service users might adopt in their attempts to gain social acceptance and inclusion. There will be a discussion of both service user narratives and Health Promotion research.

From stigma to understanding

It is important to understand the lived experience of stigma and Knight et al. (2003) identified three themes expressed by service users, who are diagnosed as suffering from schizophrenia, see Box 9.2.

There is perhaps a trend in England where attitudes towards people who suffer mental health problems are increasingly negative; see Box 9.3 (this is also observed in the United States (US) (Hinshaw & Stier, 2008)). So it is fortunate that most people will still agree with positive statements about people who suffer mental health problems, but this sympathy is significantly reduced when it comes to practical and personal interaction. For example, will landlords rent accommodation to people who disclose that they suffer from mental health problems? (see Box 9.4). So attitudes are more than just abstract ideas which people express in interview situations (Cowan, 1994; see Box 9.5) and we need to consider the manner and context in which attitudes are expressed.

Box 9.3   Attitudes towards mental health service users

Negative attitudes toward mental health service users as a burden and a source of risk in society have increased since 1994. 13% of those asked in 2007 agreed with the statement 'people with mental illness don't deserve our sympathy'; this is an increase from 8% in 1994. Similarly, 12% of people agreed with the statement 'people with mental illness are a burden on society', up from 9% in 1994. Then again, only 58% of those asked agreed that 'people with mental illness are far less of a danger than most people suppose', down from 62% in 1994. These surveys suggest that more respondents are expressing negative views, such as; people who suffer severe mental health problems are not welcome in community neighbourhoods, they cannot be trusted and they should not have the same rights and jobs as anyone else. (Care Services Improvement Partnership, 2007)

Box 9.4   Discrimination in the private rented accommodation market

Telephone calls were made to 160 landlords. Disclosures of mental health problems were made in half of these enquiries and these disclosures led to a significant reduction in the offer of a viewing. (Page, 1995)

Box 9.5   Constructing different versions of the mentally ill

… it has been shown that people do not simply use language to describe the mentally ill as a predefined 'out there' reality, but rather, they actively draw upon a variety of culturally available resources to construct different 'versions' of the 'mentally ill' in order to perform different discursive functions. For example, people construct different versions of the 'mentally ill' depending on whether they are advocating or challenging the move of ex-psychiatric patients into local communities. (Cowan, 1994: 21)

Negative attitudes might be related to the stereotypes that are promoted in the print media; which go to press with much more negative stories than positive, particularly in the United Kingdom (UK) (Huang & Priebe, 2003). There are tragic stories in which mental health service users have committed serious crimes, or put themselves in danger. These are thought to have influenced government policy, as well as having a negative impact on public perceptions, and individual mental health workers are now more likely to be held to account for the actions of the small minority of service users who behave in a dangerous and unpredictable manner (Hallam, 2002). These issues can create a kind of 'blame culture' and a dilemma is created for workers who may understandably try to avoid risks by taking a more paternalistic and controlling approach to providing care, although this is likely to contribute to stigmatisation by labelling, separating and stereotyping people who have already been subject to discrimination and loss of status in society. It is common for people to neglect to seek help because they view the status of 'mental health service user' as stigmatising (Vogel et al., 2006).

Exclusion is an ordinary part of a competitive social dynamic.

> An important point is that, to some extent, exclusion is liable to be a natural product of sustaining coherent social units. Thus, it is not always useful to pathologise either the excluders or the excluded, but rather to focus on the social psychological processes at work. (Hutchinson et al., 2007: 46)

Groups sustain themselves by highlighting and controlling dissenters or breaking links with those who will bring them into disrepute. People maintain their power in our society by grouping together with other powerful people. In this competitive networking, influence and access to resources are gained, perhaps at the expense of those who are more vulnerable (Hinshaw & Stier, 2008).

Exclusion within our own organisations

Workers can find the disorganised behaviour and impaired cognitive functioning of some service users challenging and this leads to rejection (Heresco-Levy et al., 1999). So, when mental health services screen referrals or review progress, assertive outreach teams can be placed under pressure to take on service users who have been documented as 'difficult', or 'treatment resistant'. Then if the team fails to change or control these service users, stigma can be transferred, so that the team is portrayed as failing and ineffectual. It is important, therefore, that these specialist teams maintain close working links with referrers. It is unfortunate that workers can find themselves associated with an excluded service user group. A team might be seen as a kind of ghetto, or treated as a scapegoat; as a place to further exclude (or 'dump') people. These teams should have sufficient resources and status so as to maintain relationships with many partner organisations, in just the same way as they encourage their service users to remain integrated within their communities. If resources are not adequately managed, responsibility for high risk and complex work might be left to workers who do not have sufficient experience, expertise or professional support, thereby increasing stigma, isolation and staff burnout (see Box 9.6).

Box 9.6 Three consequences of hiding stigmatising problems

Pachankis (2007) describes three consequences of hiding stigmatising problems:

- First, people who conceal a stigma fail to receive the valuable feedback from others that can be gained when problems are disclosed.
- Second, people who are concealing do not gain the protective benefits of joining with other stigmatised group members and their distress is heightened by isolation.
- Third, distress occurs not only as a consequence of possessing a stigma but also from the fears that the stigma will be discovered and punished.

Reflection point

In social encounters, do you hesitate before telling people about your employment in mental health services?

Some researchers take the view that mental illness comes first and then social exclusion is a kind of 'additional social handicap' (Crisp et al., 2000), while for others the relationship between mental health problems and social exclusion is more complex (Penn & Wykes, 2003). Experimental trials show that when participants (who are mentally well) believe that they have been excluded, they are more aggressive towards other people, less willing to assist or cooperate and more likely to engage in risky, unhealthy and self-defeating behaviours (Hutchinson et al., 2007). When participants in these trials are excluded from desired relationships or groups, they feel sadness, frustration, disappointment, jealousy, anger and shame. In addition to this emotional distress, they feel less satisfied with their life, their sense of meaningful existence is diminished; self-efficacy and hope are reduced (Hutchinson et al., 2007). So perhaps some of the challenging behaviours that service users display, or the levels of emotional distress that they feel, are a consequence of their exclusion rather than their mental health problems. Also, experimental trials have found that personal rejection is experienced by the body in just the same way as physical pain (MacDonald & Leary, 2005). Participants experience involuntary stress responses and this has been accounted for as a fear that the value of their social identity is at risk (Major & O'Brien, 2005). Experiencing this fear has been shown to have a negative effect on well-being and the 'identity threat' model helps to explain some of the complex interactions between discrimination, stigma and internalised feelings of exclusion, see Box 9.7.

People feel 'out of control' when they are losing important social networks. They need these networks to gain access to group resources, information and means of affirmation (Abrams & Houson, 2006). 'Stigma and discrimination can have a greater impact on people's lives than the mental health problems themselves' (ODPM, 2004: 33; also see Jenkins & Carpenter-Song (2008)) and social exclusion can be self-perpetuating as excluded people often lack the confidence and motivation to seek acceptance (Hutchinson

---

Box 9.7 An 'identity threat' model of the effects of exclusion

Identity threat results when an individual appraises the demands imposed by a stigma-relevant stressor as potentially harmful to his or her social identity, and as exceeding his or her resources to cope with those demands. Identity threat leads to involuntary stress responses such as anxiety, vigilance to threat, and decreased working memory capacity, and motivates attempts at threat reduction through coping strategies such as blaming negative events on discrimination, identifying more closely with the threatened group, and disengaging self-esteem from threatening domains. These involuntary stress responses and voluntary coping efforts have implications for important outcomes such as self-esteem, academic achievement, and health. (Major & O'Brien, 2005: 411–412)

et al., 2007). They are more often subject to harassment in the community (Berzins et al., 2003). In responding to social exclusion, it is sometimes enough for assertive outreach workers to stand beside their service users through difficult experiences of stigmatisation and isolation. However, in contexts where anger and blame are commonly expressed, workers walk a difficult line in positioning themselves as experiencing distress with their service users, rather than imposing it on them. These workers might empathise with service users who do not want to undergo treatment that is uncomfortable and demeaning, but, where there is unacceptable risk, they cannot collude with this avoidance. Workers are, therefore, patiently persistent in their efforts to support compliance; trying to appeal to reason rather than using emotional pressure or coercion (see Chapter 12).

Assertive outreach workers take the brave step of showing solidarity with the excluded person, expressing acceptance where others have rejected. While there is little professional prestige in spending time with 'difficult and rejected' service users, as Addis & Gamble (2004) observe, achieving engagement with service users who have been understood in this negative manner can be extremely rewarding. It is a joy to be with someone who has recovered their trust in their fellow human beings, where there is renewed hope that other people can understand difficult experiences and will share their time with them. So workers in assertive outreach are more likely to find the extreme emotional and psychological responses to exclusion understandable and they will be motivated to share that understanding.

Assertive outreach work can be emotionally draining (Billings et al., 2003), so many teams organise reflective practice meetings and socially inclusive work can also be more formally evaluated (Berry et al., 2008). In a culture where greater value might be placed on our rational professionalism than on our capacity to care, it is important that team members are able to take time to discuss and organise their work. In Chapter 8 it is observed that effective engagement is achieved through an emotional connection with service users. So workers can use the feelings that they experience in their therapeutic work to help them understand complex emotional processes. Paranoia, for example, is understandable as an emotional response to exclusion (Cromby & Harper, 2009). People are perhaps clinging onto the desperate hope that their lives are meaningful and that other people are interested in them, even if this interest is from a remote and persecutory source. Similarly, when we do feel empathic towards someone, we are more likely to find meaning in their eccentric beliefs (Harper, 2004) and there are complex relationships between psychotic illness and the person's beliefs about that illness (Kinderman et al., 2006). So workers will be trying to engage and support recovery by understanding distressing symptoms, rather than dismissing them as meaningless. However, this can be a challenging emotional experience (Hayward et al., 2010) (see Box 9.8). Supporting each other in a team approach and making visits in pairs are, therefore, essential elements of assertive outreach.

Even though workers might not want to reject service users at a personal level, their position as professional workers might be devalued in an institutional system, so that they cannot step outside of rigid boundaries (Hinshaw & Stier, 2008: 384). On the other hand, boundaries can be blurred when workers have a duty of care both to their service users and to the community, see Box 9.9. Teams can be just as caught up in institutional processes as their service users and although workers might want to allocate resources so as to promote inclusion, or express their support or sympathy, they are not always free to do so. Resources are managed in social and healthcare systems through allegiances that are established between

---

Box 9.8   The consequences of feeling disconnected or connected to others

A feeling of not belonging or of being disconnected from others, a sense of isolation alienation abandonment, rejection and lack of support networks have all been shown to correlate with suicide rates in different societies ... 'Similar trends emerge in research on self-harm ... In contrast, strong family ties ... religious affiliations ... and engagement in collective leisure activities ... are all associated with a sense of belonging or connectedness, which can buffer negative thought processes and self defeating behaviours. (Hutchinson et al., 2007: 35)

Box 9.9   Ethical dilemmas which are qualitatively different

Assertive outreach presents us with complex ethical dilemmas, such as:

Boundary diffusion in terms of both the relationship with the client and the mode of service delivery, conflicting allegiances both to the client and to the community in terms of risk and safety, and issues of confidentiality are all identified as posing ethical dilemmas for assertive outreach that are qualitatively different from those that arise in clinic-based or hospital-based care. So problematic are the ethical conflicts inherent within these issues, in relation to the traditional principles of ethical care that Stovall proposes adoption of three further principles drawn from earlier work by Christensen: compassion, humility and fidelity (the latter meaning maintenance of commitment to the client). (Williamson, 2002: 545; also see Stovall, 2001)

Box 9.10   Do our services collude with processes of social exclusion?

As a hospital manager... I see first hand how quick we are to remove people from society and how reluctant we often are to return them because we worry about the harm they may do to themselves. Yet we do not view the isolation, exclusion and removal of rights as harmful. (Social Exclusion Unit, 2004: 34)

---

powerful groups. Ideas about 'the deserving and the undeserving poor' have circulated in our Western societies for several centuries and these notions are particularly influential in the management of limited resources, such as housing for example (Clapham, 2007: 79).

Effective teams face a dilemma in maintaining their prestige and professionalism, particularly when powerful managers can dismiss the opinions of workers by describing them as 'over involved' and 'emotive'. Teams need strong supportive management and their ability to function will be lost if they become isolated and insular (socially excluded). It is important to reflect on the ordinary everyday manner in which exclusion occurs at intra-group and inter-group levels (see Box 9.10). We will all exclude people who appear 'different' or 'difficult' from our friendships and work contact networks. We strengthen the bonds within our own groups by blaming outsiders who threaten us. So, complex processes of exclusion occur in our society, which can be so emotive that we fail to take a rational position from which to adequately observe or account for them.

Treatment and therapy or stigma and labelling?

This chapter addresses the central question of whether assertive outreach is imposing unwanted treatment which is associated with stigmatising labels, or is promoting a kind of recovery that enables social inclusion. Concerns had been expressed prior to the setting up of teams in England, related to a potential return to more oppressive systems of psychiatric care. It was suggested that service users would avoid workers by 'going underground' (Smith, 1999). However, with hundreds of assertive outreach teams functioning across the country, effective engagement has been maintained. Concerns about just what 'assertive' would mean included the suggestion that more coercion would be applied to maintain compliance with prescribed medication and that this would be experienced as punishment rather than treatment, but also, that no exit from assertive outreach had been planned and that workers would be inappropriately intrusive, having keys so that they could gain entry to service user's accommodation, for example (Smith, 1999). However, changes to mental health law have given more structure to mutual decision making (Department for Constitutional Affairs, 2007). Also, where there are powers to 'recall to hospital' in England and Wales, there are rights of appeal. The notions of capacity and consent are defined in these developments and workers cannot just assume that someone lacks capacity, or that they have given consent to receive treatment just because they acquiesce to implicit pressures (see Chapter 12).

Many of the service users who are referred for assertive outreach will suffer memory problems and live disorganised lives so as to be unable to remember appointments or plan activities. Extra efforts is needed to engage when many of these elusive service users live in poorer neighbourhoods, renting small rooms in multi-occupancy buildings, where the intercom systems are broken and the mail is regularly stolen. Trying to find and engage with these service users is a very different kind of work from appointment based clinics. The practical nature of assertive outreach means that workers may well arrange to hold a spare key for some service users who can be forgetful and this is only intended to save the expense of employing a locksmith. The 'no-closure' aspect of assertive outreach had been designed to ensure that workers did not give up on service users in the US, where there has been a lack of secondary services in some areas. So, where there are adequate resources there is an easier step-up from and step-down to other teams. Transitions are more fluid and the work of assertive outreach is often completed when engagement is achieved and practical means of resolving living problems have been found.

How should we talk about problems?

Using language sensitively is a key aspect of maintaining engagement. Workers will be developing a mutual understanding, starting with the service user's perspective, rather than imposing a professional interpretation. This work might involve a kind of 'identity politics' (Sampson, 1993). While the different forms of professional knowledge that we use in assertive outreach can enable us to effectively measure and predict the behaviours of our service users, these understandings can also act as 'self-fulfilling prophesies.' By emphasising one interpretation of a person's behaviour more than another, we steer them

---

Box 9.11   The roots of social inclusion and recovery philosophy

Good ideas are not forgotten in mental health services, they just get recycled, repackaged and renamed. Many of the principles of social inclusion and recovery philosophy were expressed in the 'Normalization' movement several decades ago (Flynn & Nitsch, 1980). These ideas were expressed again in the concept of 'Social Role Valorization' (Thomas, 1994), which became popular in the 1990s.

Wolfensberger (1980) traces principles of normalisation in work with schizophrenia back to the 1950s and he talks about the 'right not to be different'. He observes that 'When we recall that the overwhelming response of society to devalued people is segregation ... we realise that the right not to be segregated and institutionalised (which is almost equivalent to being made different, or more different) is really a bigger issue than the restriction of individual choice' (Wolfensberger, 1980: 93).

---

into different 'life courses', 'care pathways', 'recovery journeys' or 'oppressive institutionalisation'. If we hope to reduce stigma, we must practice a 'reflexive use of knowledge'. Service users might have experienced a kind of loss of identity through the course of their illness (Wisdom et al., 2008). However, by surviving this illness and associated intrusive treatments, they can adopt different or more complex identities (Speed, 2006). It is in our talk that processes of exclusion and inclusion are brought about.

Rather than working to 'recruit people into devalued mentally ill identities', workers can define those people in less stigmatising ways, constructing 'healthy but different identities', although this might also impinge on their right to receive services (Griffiths, 2001). Attention must be paid to the rhetorical manner in which knowledge is expressed and the consequences that this has for different social groups. Social exclusion can act in complex and contradictory ways, for example, when an assertive outreach worker is sat beside their service user, in a meeting with the local authority housing services, they will choose their words very carefully. Their task is to support that service user in gaining housing and they may need to overcome discrimination. They must provide information on any significant risks, particularly when the service user has failed to maintain independent accommodation in the past. For a favourable impression of the service user to be gained, a degree of disablement must be demonstrated, but a potential competency in managing a tenancy must also be established. (See Box 9.11 for the roots of social inclusion and recovery psychology.)

Like other professional groups, mental health workers are experts in applied science. However, unlike other professional groups, the knowledge that they use has filtered out into the consciousness of the general public. Much of the technical language and modelling of mental healthcare is expressed in popular culture. A model of 'Folk Psychiatry' (Haslam et al., 2007), is useful in understanding 'lay knowledge'. Supported by Attribution Theory, this modelling suggests that people employ a number of different dimensions in their explanations for the causes of social behaviours. They will consider, for example, whether the behaviour is normal or deviant; or whether the behaviour is under the person's control, or the outcome of a disease process within them; they will ask whether the behaviour is intended or influenced by emotions or irrational thoughts, related to a personal history and current social difficulties. The particular way that behaviours are understood will mediate the attachment of stigma to the social actor and the degree of social distance that other will seek.

In promoting social inclusion, workers must consider the complex actions of discriminating attributions. Deviations that are chosen are generally subject to a greater degree of moral judgement and condemnation (Corrigan et al., 2003). So, criminal behaviours for example, which are both deviant and chosen are very stigmatising, as is excessive alcohol or substance misuse. However, when bizarre behaviours are not thought to be under the person's control, as in severe mental illness, the attachment of stigma is even greater. Negative cultural images exacerbate these processes and Sayce (2000) discusses the stereotypical character of the 'psycho-killer' in popular drama; an identity that is both criminal and 'mentally disordered'. Assertive outreach teams must consider these common sense and implicit forms of knowledge which underpin stigma and discrimination, along with popular social representations of mental illness.

Surveys suggest that the majority of the public can identify conditions such as schizophrenia and major depression as mental illnesses and they give multi-causal explanations, in which stressful circumstances are combined with biological and genetic factors (Link et al., 1999). However, there remains a strong connection in public fears between mental illness and potential violence. There is also an expressed desire for social distance from people who suffer mental illnesses. Given these beliefs, assumptions and preferences, the use of 'Health Promotion' to improve public awareness, should be an essential aspect of mental healthcare (Read et al., 2006). So, how can teams use their professional knowledge to promote social inclusion, promoting particular understandings, for example, in their dealings with lay persons, such as colleagues in partner organisations, families and other agencies who share in their work? The following discussion will describe four pathways by which service users might achieve social inclusion, borrowing heavily from the work of the author, campaigner and service user Liz Sayce.

'Just like any other illness'

Traditional psychiatry has used rational scientific arguments, claiming, for example, 'that a disease of the brain is no different from a disease of any other bodily organ' (Sayce, 2000; 87), but the 'just like any other illness' message does not promote social inclusion. Biomedical and genetic explanations for mental illness have been found to trigger negative perceptions; that 'mental patients' are dangerous, antisocial and unpredictable. Research participants in experimental trials state that they do not want to develop relationships with people who have been presented to them as suffering from a 'disease of the brain', while in comparison, when problems are explained as psychosocial – related to negative life events – participants are then more accepting of potential social contact (Mehta & Farina, 1997; Read & Harre, 2001). (See Box 9.12 for an example of a Rethink poster campaign.)

Biomedical explanations tend to set aside social inequality and misfortune in the development of mental health problems and might therefore 'blame the victim'. Given the prevalence of negative attitudes in society, perhaps it is a better strategy to promote an understanding of the problems of service users, as 'difficulties that anyone might face'. This would involve placing more emphasis on social and environmental causes. Assertive outreach workers achieve their more effective engagement by listening to the stories of service users with an open mind, rather than imposing a dogmatic medical interpretation

> **Box 9.12**   Mental health awareness campaign
>
> My problem is schizophrenia. What is yours? It's time to rethink mental illness.
> Rethink poster

of their presentation. While recognising the role of social problems in the development of mental health problems, we can still recommend that these problems can be resolved, or managed, though treatment, therapy and support. However, when we are engaging with a service user, accompanying them in an activity with the aim of increasing their social contacts for example, we would use socially inclusive language.

Reflection point

Joe is diagnosed as suffering from schizophrenia and he has been detained several times under a Section of the Mental Health Act. He goes with his assertive outreach worker to the local college to sign on for a course. He falls into conversation with other students and he explains that he needs to find something to do, having been bored and fed up since he broke up from his partner. As people begin to share their stories, he says with bravado, that he had a drugs and alcohol binge and 'lost it for a while'; so he needs to get his life sorted out.

Joe does not mention his diagnosis. So does this mean that he lacks insight into his condition, is he minimising or denying the reality of his illness, should his worker be worried that he might not comply with treatment? Or, is he working to manage his identity? Is he telling his story in a manner that draws people to him, as an 'interesting character', rather than scaring them away? Does he have insight into the reality that diagnostic labels are stigmatising?

'We all have problems'

If we want to promote social inclusion, it might be effective to understand mental health problems as falling on a continuum. Rather than promoting the idea of distinct disease categories, we could talk about a single line, stretching from mental and emotional well-being at one end and severe problems at the other. We are all somewhere on this line and we move up and down it as we face life's challenges. An interest in personal psychological growth has been prompted by popular culture, perhaps making interventions such as counselling and psychotherapy more acceptable. When mental health service users are asked, they express a desire for more psychological therapy (Rose, 2001).

The continuum model of mental well-being is not accepted by everyone and the idea that there is a difference in kind between neurosis and psychosis remains firmly fixed in the public consciousness (Sayce, 2000). Also, as Sayce (2000) observes, if social and psychological problems are largely a consequence of social inequality and the lack of opportunities experienced by minority groups, then promoting therapy could be another form of 'blaming the victim'. Instead of redressing the inequalities that impinge on those who suffer, we offer therapy or other treatments in the hope that we can make them more able to endure distressing exclusion and victimisation (Cromby et al., 2007). At the same time, we are supporting the view that they cannot cope without a form of expertise that can only be provided by our services. So the resilience and autonomy of our service users could actually be undermined (Pilgrim, 1997). Assertive outreach teams will be mindful of these different interpretations as 'barriers to effective engagement' and blind alleys that cause service users to remain in isolated and disempowered social positions.

'Bad, not mad'

Good practice in mental healthcare requires that, when a service user has mental capacity and is responsible for a crime, then, processes of criminal investigation and associated legal proceedings should be facilitated. However, sometimes our caring lapses into paternalism. When we divert service users from the criminal justice system into mental healthcare, for example, we are actually excluding these people from full participation in society. Assertive outreach teams have developed an expertise in working with service users who have multiple problems and it is understood that illegal actions can be the outcome of both mental illness and criminal intent. So when we do refuse to excuse their behaviours, we are not abandoning our service users. When supporting them through police interviews and court processes, we are taking the opportunity to assess and engage. Meanwhile many service users might prefer a custodial sentence of a given duration, rather than an indefinite detention under mental health law.

Service user groups have objected to the use of mental health laws, by which their members are detained and treated against their will (James, 2001). The campaigns and protests that have been organised to challenge detention and enforced treatment can be described as an expression of a 'libertarian model'. In Britain, however, the general public often associate this model with a supposed (but not actual) increase in homicides committed by the mentally ill. This model is also associated with a perceived reduction in resources, as long-stay institutions are closed and care in the community is thought to be under funded (Sayce, 2000). Also, the justified anger of service users is rarely taken seriously, society tends to emphasise 'the meaninglessness of "mad" people's opinions – discrediting views and voices as unworthy by definition, thereby neutralising effective challenges to discrimination' (Sayce, 2003: 626). Assertive outreach workers face a dilemma; should they empathise with and thereby legitimise the anger of their service users, or should they remind them that expressing anger often leads to social exclusion and, in many circumstances, to criminal conviction. We must confess that in mental health services, when our service users express anger, our usual response has been to increase the sedative effect of their prescribed medications.

'Disability rights'

As discussed in Chapter 8, the disability rights movement has transformed the lives of many people, but as a group, mental health service users have not benefited as much as other disadvantaged minorities. Sayce (2000) argues that users or survivors of mental

---

Box 9.13   Independence or normal dependence?

Recovery is not about being independent from services; it is about taking control, living our lives the way we want to live them, pursuing our ambitions and dreams, doing the things that give our lives meaning.

  If, with continuing help and support, a person is able to maintain a home of their own, get a decent job, go out with friends … is 'dependence' really such a bad thing? And if the cost of 'independence' is not doing the things that give us pleasure and purpose in life, but results in isolation or devoting all our energies to be basic necessities of survival, can this really be a good thing? (Perkins, 2003: 6)

Box 9.14   Individual placement in employment

Individual placement support involves integrating employment specialists into community clinical teams and ensuring vocational issues are a core component of the care planning process. The approach requires that there is a primary focus on helping people to gain jobs in open employment, in line with their preferences, as quickly as possible, without protracted pre-vocational training. Support is provided to anyone who wishes to work, without any selection based on their 'employability' or 'work readiness'; advice on welfare benefits is provided and time-unlimited ongoing support enables people to maintain employment and develop their careers. (Rinaldi & Perkins, 2007: 244)

---

health services need to overcome a 'moral shame', a shame at not being accepted as 'reasonable' people. This might be achieved if mental health problems are understood as incapacitating. Unreasonableness is then understandable as an outcome of the extreme difficulties that some people endure and these people could be seen as having a right to the resources that they need to bring their capacity back up to the same level as other people in society. The tired old notion of 'dependence' is often used to justify attitudes that would deny service users access to the same resources as everyone else, but it can be argued that we all depend on each other, see Box 9.13.

  In England and Wales, the disability rights model underpins local government initiatives such as 'Direct Payments' and 'Self Directed Services'. Service users can apply for funds that are paid into a bank account, which they manage. They can use this money to employ personal assistants, for example, to help them get out and about, so that they are less socially excluded. By purchasing products or services that would help them to participate more fully in society, service users contribute more and function at a more effective level. Assertive outreach teams are helping service users to take control of their lives by encouraging them to meet their own needs, while advocating for them to receive the practical support that is necessary to make this happen. The quality of life of these service users can be dramatically improved when they have access to adequate resources. The slogan 'homes, jobs and friends' reminds us of the practical priorities of service users. Holding down a job, for example, would enable a service user to have an aspect of their life that is 'normal', even though they might require a lot of support to maintain that role, see Box 9.14.

From rehabilitation to recovery

The psychological internalisation of discrimination and social exclusion is a particularly difficult problem to solve. Although assertive outreach workers will express acceptance, their offers of help might be rejected or misunderstood, particularly when they are at odds with the service user's life experiences. Research has even found that experiences of discrimination can lead to the development of psychotic symptoms in their own right (Janssen et al., 2003). Many service users experience derogatory auditory hallucinations, which constantly reaffirm their difference and undermine their confidence, making them feel worthless. As discussed in Chapters 8, 10 and 11, workers need to understand the ethnic background and culture of their service users. They need to work with communities and groups, because 'affiliation with similarly devalued others provides an opportunity to receive and benefit from social support, which itself can buffer the ill effects of perceived discrimination on well being' (Schmitt & Branscombe, 2002: 39). When people suffer from mental health problems they feel singled out and different, but this problem is heightened where the person is also from a minority ethnic background and already experiencing discrimination (Cognitive Behaviour Therapy (CBT) techniques might be useful in helping service users overcome these problems (Corrigan & Calabrese, 2005)).

Assertive outreach teams and other related service providers face a dilemma in promoting social inclusion through group work. Ideally, service users would be supported in engaging with groups in their communities, as appropriate to their interests and cultural background, following a recovery model (Shepherd et al., 2008). However, because of the widespread discrimination described above, mental health services have provided group based interventions in which service users are encouraged to provide each other with social support. It has to be accepted, however, that this is a compromise and although segregated services often provide a successful pragmatic approach, there is a risk that service providers will find themselves colluding with damaging processes of social exclusion.

Service users who are referred to assertive outreach teams have often disputed their diagnosed condition and have failed to engage with these services; why, they have asked, would they attend services for the mentally ill when they do not have these problems themselves. Very often they use stigmatising language to describe their fellow service users. As discussed in Chapter 8, mental health workers sometimes use the concept of 'lack of insight' when service users dispute their diagnosis, but this might be just a strategy that is being used as an attempt to gain social inclusion (see Box 9.15 for research).

Service users face a dilemma; 'There appears an evident struggle between belonging, and keeping oneself separate from a group that does not have a positive social identity' (Knight et al., 2003: 216). The ambivalence of reluctant service users is an understandable response to old 'slow stream' rehabilitation wards and day centres, which have been very depressing places. Funding priorities would have meant that furnishings in these institutional environments have been old, drab and neglected. Once service users had adjusted to life in these institutions, moving on became very difficult. With the popularisation of 'Recovery Philosophy', it is increasingly expected that therapeutic work should take place in the community, see Box 9.16. In contrast to traditional rehabilitation,

Box 9.15 Research into social integration and use of support services

One hundred participants who had a diagnosis of schizophrenia and attended community psychiatric services were interviewed. Five groups were identified:

- The first group consisted of 24 persons who had regular social contacts in different social settings. They had at least one close emotional relationship; they felt able to establish new social contacts with persons who were not mentally ill if they wanted. Most of the persons in this group did not want to have contact with other patients.
- The second group consisted of 21 persons who had regular social contacts in different social settings and these contacts were not limited to fellow service users. However, they wanted more opportunities to engage in 'normal' social activities. Lack of money, along with a fear of stigmatization, were cited as barriers to social integration and some members of this group used segregated mental health support services.
- The third group consisted of 22 persons who had regular social contact exclusively with other service users. The most important problem mentioned by these patients was a lack of close emotional relationships. Persons in this group expressed a lack of confidence in their ability to maintain social relationships and many used segregated mental health support services.
- The fourth group consisted of 18 persons who only had contact with members of their family and had a close emotional relationship to at least one family member. Persons in this group felt that they were incapable of establishing new social contacts, but did not want to have contact with service users who have similar problems.
- The fifth group consisted of 15 persons who either had no contact with other people, or only sporadic contact. Persons in this group felt unable to establish contact with other people on their own. They continued to suffer from isolation and rejected the option of social relationships with other service users. (Adapted from: Kilian et al., 2001)

Box 9.16 The ward on a bus!

Rebecca Owen, a worker giving a presentation at a training event, described the development of a Continuing Needs Service (including Assertive Outreach, Rehabilitation and Recovery Services).

These services were originally provided through an eight bedded unit, where service users were rehabilitated from their enduring mental health problems. The unit also provided short-term respite for those who had been discharged to community placements. A day programme was offered, including a full-weekly programme of groups, such as physical activities, coping skills, leisure group, communication skills, creative writing, art therapy, health promotion, self help groups (male/female), psychosocial intervention for family members, and individual therapy for users. All staff attended case reviews, lead by the consultant psychiatrist. Service users were involved in decision making and taking responsibility for the day to day running of the unit. Many of the groups offered would be based in the community with the aim of integration and broader socialization.

Despite the success of this service, the local Trust decided to close the inpatient beds, reducing the service to day attendance. Assertive outreach and other recovery services are now provided. As with many other assertive outreach teams, social activities now take place in public places and attendees travel by public transport. Social inclusion is facilitated through activity groups, such as taking a picnic to the park, or visiting an art gallery or museum. Many service users attend, who had formerly been inpatients and Rebecca referred to the strange sight of seeing a group of familiar people all sat on a bus, as opposed to sitting or pacing about in a psychiatric ward.

assertive outreach workers meet service users in ordinary community settings, engaging in everyday social activities. It is recognised that mental health services are stigmatised. Their clinics and office bases are viewed as toxic; only slightly better than sewage plants and prisons (Knight & Moloney, 2005). Meanwhile service users have found mutual support by joining together in their own right outside of the context of mental healthcare. When they have set up more formal support networks for themselves it is often useful to contract with these groups who can provide independent advocacy or service evaluation. Self-help groups are a valuable resource for both service users and service providers.

Some service users continue to struggle to achieve therapeutic change and it must be noted that where rehabilitation is organised by service providers, recovery cannot be guaranteed. Recovery, as discussed in Chapter 8, is an individual journey that the service user chooses to take and it cannot be imposed. What has happened for the service users described in Box 9.16 is that services have changed their environment instead (this has been described as 'nidotherapy'; see Tyrer et al. (2007)). These former inpatients live in their own accommodation with support services coming in to help them maintain their domestic routines and self-care. They may need reminding and collecting when there is a 'recovery activity', which will be led by workers. However, under law and within the policies of service providers, these people are living in the community. Perhaps by living a life that appears more 'normal' these service users might gain the opportunity to make choices that will enable a genuine inclusion in society. By bringing the control and management of resources down to the level of the individual service user, each of these service users can then take whatever path they choose on their individual journey towards recovery.

Conclusion

It is just as easy to portray assertive outreach teams as oppressive and disempowering, as it is to portray their service users as deviant and dangerous. However, these stereotypical views are not only imprecise but are representing really in specific ways, maintaining imbalances in the distribution of power and resources. In order to achieve social inclusion, assertive outreach teams and their service users must understand and work with commonplace rhetorical disputes over rights, freedoms, access to resources and obligations. The work of these teams is not limited to treating psychiatric or psychological problems, but must extend into 'identity politics', 'health promotion' and 'disability awareness'. While social exclusion is an everyday and very normal discrimination, it's devastating impacts are both a cause and a consequence of mental health problems. Social exclusion is just as traumatic as any related mental health problems and perhaps, even more difficult to overcome.

This chapter has described how effective teams will not be imposing professional understandings on their service users, but will instead be listening to them and helping them form positive identities. Many service users will have experienced extensive and distressing social exclusion and will have taken the self protective step of avoiding difficult social encounters which have the potential to confirm rejection and thereby re-traumatise. When they are brave enough to move on from this isolated position they might initially only socialise within groups of fellow service users, where there is a greater chance that they will experience understanding and acceptance. Alternatively, service users might choose not to disclose their mental health problems and to form other identities, deviant or conventional, within which to express themselves. Taking up employment is a direct route to social acceptance, but the use of a disability model has also been discussed as enabling a more managed process of social involvement in which statutory resources are used to directly purchase support.

References

Abrams, D. & Houson, D.M. (2006) *Equality, Adversity and Prejudice in Britain*. Equalities Review, Cabinet Office, London.

Addis, J. & Gamble, C. (2004) Assertive outreach nurses' experience of engagement. *Journal of Psychiatric and Mental Health Nursing*, **11**, 452–460.

Berry, C., Hayward, M. & Porter, A. (2008) Evaluating socially inclusive practice: part 1 – a tool for mental health services. *Journal of Mental Health Training, Education and Practice*, **3**, 31–41.

Berzins, K.M., Petch, A. & Atkinson, J.M. (2003) Prevalence and experience of harassment of people with mental health problems living in the community. *British Journal of Psychiatry*, **183**, 526–533.

Billings, J., Johnson, S., Bebbington, P., Greaves, A., Priebe, S. & Muijen, M., et al. (2003) Assertive outreach teams in London: staff experiences and perceptions. *British Journal of Psychiatry*, **183**, 139–147.

Clapham, D. (2007) Homelessness and Social Exclusion. In: *Multidisciplinary Handbook of Social Exclusion Research*, (eds. D. Abrams, J. Christian & D. Gordon). pp. 79–94. John Wiley & Sons, Chichester.

Corrigan, P.W., Bodenhausen, G., Markowitz, F., Newman, L. Rasiski, K. & Watson, A. (2003) Demonstrating translational research for mental health services: an example from stigma research. *Mental Health Services Research*, **5**(2), 79–88.

Corrigan, P.W. & Calabrese, J.D. (2005) Strategies for Assessing and Diminishing Self-Stigma. In: *On the Stigma of Mental Illness: Practical Strategies for Research and Social Change*, (ed. P.W. Corrigan). pp. 239–256. American Psychological Association, Washington, DC.

Cowan, S. (1994) Community attitudes towards people with mental health problems: a discourse analytic approach. *Journal of Psychiatric and Mental Health Nursing*, **1**, 15–22.

Crisp, A.H., Gelder, M.G., Rix, S., Meltzer, H.I. & Rowlands, O.J. (2000) Stigmatisation of people with mental illness. *British Journal of Psychiatry*, **177**, 4–7.

Cromby, J., Diamond, B., Kelly, P., Moloney, P., Priest, P. & Smail, D. (2007) Questioning the science and politics of happiness. *The Psychologist*, **20**(7), 422–425.

Cromby, J. & Harper, D. (2009) Paranoia: a social account. *Theory and Psychology*, **19**, 335–361.

CSIP (2007) *Attitudes to mental health 2007: Report*. Care Services Improvement Partnership, London.

Department for Constitutional Affairs (2007) *Mental Capacity Act 2005: Code of Practice*. Department for Constitutional Affairs, London.

Griffiths, L. (2001) Categorising to exclude: the discursive construction of cases in community mental health teams. *Sociology of Health & Illness*, **23**(5), 678–700.

Hallam, A. (2002) Media influences on mental health policy: long-term effects of the Clunis and Silcock cases. *International Review of Psychiatry*, **14**(1), 26–33.

Harper, D. (2004) Delusions and discourse: moving beyond the constraints of the rationalist paradigm. *Philosophy, Psychiatry and Psychology*, **11**, 55–64.

Haslam, N., Ban, L. & Kaufmann, L. (2007) Lay conceptions of mental disorder: the folk psychiatry model. *Australian Psychologist*, **42**(2), 129–137.

Hayward, M., Holford, E. & Kinderman, P. (2010) Social Inclusion. *The Psychologist*, **23**(1), 20.

Heresco-Levy, U., Ermilov, M., Giltsinsky, B., Lichtenstein, M. & Blander D. (1999) Treatment-resistant schizophrenia and staff rejection. *Schizophrenia Bulletin*, **25**(3), 457–465.

Hinshaw, S.P. & Stier, A. (2008) Stigma as related to mental disorders. *Annual Review of Clinical Psychology*, **4**, 367–393.

Huang, B. & Priebe, S. (2003) Media coverage of mental health care in the UK, USA and Australia. *Psychiatric Bulletin*, **27**, 331–333.

Hutchinson, P., Abrams, D. & Christian, J. (2007) The social psychology of exclusion. In: *Multidisciplinary Handbook of Social Exclusion Research*, (eds. D. Abrams, J. Christian & D. Gordon). pp. 29–58. John Wiley & Sons, Chichester.

James, A. (2001) *Raising our Voices: An account of the Hearing Voices Movement*. Handsell Publishing, Gloucester.

Janssen, I., Hanssen, M., Bak, M., Bijl, R., De Graaf, R. & Vollebergh, W., et al. (2003) Discrimination and delusional ideation. *British Journal of Psychiatry*, **182**, 71–76.

Jenkins, J.H. & Carpenter-Song, E.A. (2008) Stigma despite recovery: strategies for living in the aftermath of psychosis. *Medical Anthropology Quarterly*, **22**(4), 381–409.

Kilian, R., Lindenbach, I., Löbig, U., Uhle, M. & Angermeyer, M.C. (2001) Self-perceived social integration and the use of day centers of persons with severe and persistent schizophrenia living in the community: a qualitative analysis. *Journal of Social Psychiatry and Psychiatric Epidemiology*, **36**(11), 545–552.

Kinderman, P., Setzu, E., Lobban, F. & Salmon, P. (2006) Illness beliefs in schizophrenia. *Social Science & Medicine*, **63**, 1900–1911.

Knight, M.T.D., Wykes, T. & Hayward, P. (2003) 'People don't understand': an investigation of stigma in schizophrenia using Interpretative Phenomenological Analysis (IPA). *Journal of Mental Health*, **12**(3), 209–222.

Knight, M.T.D. & Moloney, M. (2005) Anonymity or visibility: an investigation of stigma and Community Mental Health Team (CMHT) service using Interpretative Phenomenological Analysis (IPA). *Journal of Mental Health*, **14**(5), 499–512.

Krupa, T., Eastabrook, S., Hern, L., Lee, D., North, R. & Percy, K., et al. (2005) How do people who receive assertive community treatment experience this service? *Psychiatric Rehabilitation Journal*, **29**(1), 18–24.

Link, B.G., Phelan, J.C., Bresnahan, M., Stueve. A. & Pescosolido, B.A. (1999) Public conceptions of mental illness: labels, cause, dangerousness and social distance. *American Journal of Public Health*, **89**(9), 1328–1333.

Link, B.G. & Phelan, J.C. (2001) Conceptualizing stigma. *Annual Review of Sociology*, **27**, 363–385.

MacDonald, G. & Leary, M.R. (2005) Why does social exclusion hurt? The relationship between social exclusion and physical pain. *Psychological Bulletin*, **131**, 202–223.

Major, B. & O'Brien, L.T. (2005) The social psychology of stigma. *Annual Review of Psychology*, **56**, 393–421.

Mehta, S. & Farina, A. (1997) Is being 'sick' really better? Effects of the disease view of mental disorder on stigma. *Journal of Social and Clinical Psychology*, **16**(4), 405–419.

ODPM (2004) *Mental Health and Social Exclusion: Social Exclusion Unit Report*. Social Exclusion Unit, Office of the Deputy Prime Minster, London.

Pachankis, J. (2007) The psychological implications of concealing a stigma: a cognitive-affective-behavioral model. *Psychological Bulletin*, **133**, 328–345.

Page, S. (1995) Effects of the mental illness label in 1993: acceptance and rejection in the community. *Journal of Health and Social Policy*, **7**, 61–68.

Penn, D.L. & Wykes, T. (2003) Editorial: stigma, discrimination and mental illness. *Journal of Mental Health*, **12**(3), 203–208.

Perkins, R. (2003) The altar of independence. *Openmind*, **119**, 6.

Pilgrim, D. (1997) *Psychotherapy and Society*. Sage, London.

Read, J. & Harre, N. (2001) The role of biological and genetic causal beliefs in the stigmatisation of 'mental patients'. *Journal of Mental Health*, **10**(2), 223–235.

Read, J., Haslam, N., Sayce, L. & Davies, E. (2006) Prejudice and schizophrenia: a review of the 'mental illness is an illness like any other' approach. *Acta Psychiatrica Scandinavica*, **114**, 303–318.

Rinaldi, M. & Perkins, P. (2007) Implementing evidence-based supported employment. *Psychiatric Bulletin*, **30**, 244–249.

Rose, D. (2001) *Users' voices: the perspectives of mental health service users on community and hospital care,* Sainsbury Centre for Mental Health., London.

Sampson, E.E. (1993) Identity politics: challenges to psychology's understanding. *American Psychologist*, **48**(12), 1219–1230.

Sayce, L. (2000) *From Psychiatric Patient to Citizen: Overcoming Discrimination and Social Exclusion.* MacMillan Press, Basingstoke.

Sayce, L. (2001) Social inclusion and mental health. *Psychiatric Bulletin*, **25**, 121–123.

Sayce, L. (2003) Beyond good intentions: making anti-discrimination strategies work. *Disability and Society*, **18**(5), 625–642.

Schmitt, M.T. & Branscombe, N.T. (2002) The meaning and consequences of perceived discrimination in disadvantaged and privileged social groups. *European Review of Social Psychology*, **12**, 167–200.

Shepherd, G., Boardman, J. & Slade, M. (2008) *Making Recovery a Reality.* Sainsbury Centre for Mental Health, London.

Smith, M. (1999) Assertive outreach: a step backwards. *Nursing Times*, **95**(30), 46–47.

Speed, E. (2006) Patients, consumers and survivors: a case study of mental health service user discourses. *Social Science & Medicine*, **62**(1), 28–38.

Stovall, J. (2001) Is assertive community treatment ethical care? *Harvard Review of Psychiatry*, **9**, 139–143.

Thomas, S. (1994) A brief history of the SRV development, training, and safeguarding council. *The International Social Role Valorization Journal*, **1**(2), 15–18.

Tyrer, P., Kramo, K., Miloseska, K. & Seivewright, H. (2007) The place for nidotherapy in psychiatric practice. *Psychiatric Bulletin*, **31**, 1–3.

Vogel, D.L., Wade, N.G. & Haake, S. (2006) Measuring the self-stigma associated with seeking psychological help. *Journal of Counselling Psychology*, **53**, 325–337.

Williamson, T. (2002) Ethics of assertive outreach (assertive community treatment teams). *Current Opinion in Psychiatry*, **15**, 543–547.

Wisdom, J.P., Bruce, K., Saedi, G.A., Weis, T. & Green, C.A. (2008) 'Stealing me from myself': identity and recovery in personal accounts of mental illness. *Australian and New Zealand Journal of Psychiatry*, **42**, 489–495.

Wolfensberger, W. (1980) The Definition of Normalization Update, Problems, Disagreements, and Misunderstandings. In: *Normalization, Social Integration, and Community Services*, (eds. R.J. Flynn & K.E. Nitsch). pp. 71–115. University Park Press, Baltimore.

Chapter 10

Meeting the black and ethnic minority agenda

Simon Wharne and Neil Sanyal

With thanks to Thembela Duri and Val Biggs

Introduction

Assertive outreach teams often develop a multi-professional approach which can mirror the diversity of our pluralistic societies. Team members will be working to overcome the splits, power differences and the narrow points of view that can undermine team cohesion and prevent effective engagement with service users. Meanwhile, very different understandings of ethnic diversity are likely to be expressed, both in our society and within mental health services. For some workers, particular cultural or ethnic differences might be just background detail in a file, while for others, they are often a source of important information that is essential for engagement and for achieving therapeutic outcomes. These details can help teams to formulate their understandings where 'cross-cultural encounters' have contributed to the development of social, psychological or psychiatric problems.

Research has found that people from some ethnic minorities are more likely to be diagnosed as suffering from enduring mental health problems. In formulating their understandings, assertive outreach teams might account for this as an outcome of the stress caused by migration and encounters with new cultures. Alternatively, the possibility that mis-diagnosis might have occurred will be considered, as these teams achieve more accurate assessments. In completing these culturally sensitive assessments it is recommended that workers should first consider their own culture, along with the situated position of their own common assumptions and even their professional knowledge. Theoretical approaches such as humanistic counselling, for example, are built on individualistic philosophies that are particular to Western societies.

The central functions of diagnosis and treatment which are fulfilled by assertive outreach are founded on Western scientific principles, which many service users will find alien or simply incomprehensible. So workers face dilemmas; should they help service users to re-engage with their families and ethnic communities and, thereby, foster solidarity with views that are at odds with mainstream society. Or should they collude with an intrusive process of acculturation through which service users might begin to accept Western interpretations of illness and treatment. As 'agents of the state' assertive outreach

Assertive Outreach in Mental Healthcare: Current Perspectives, First Edition. Edited by C. Williams, M. Firn, S. Wharne and R. Macpherson.

teams have to work within a stratified society, with different levels of access to resources and opportunities which often coincide with ethnic and cultural divides between communities. From a more critical perspective, it must be acknowledged that discrimination and intolerance are expressed in the symptoms that service users suffer and mental health-care cannot be separated from the dynamics of racism.

Ethnicity and mental health problems

Concerns have been raised about differences in the use of mental health services by people from minority ethnic backgrounds. For example, research has found that, in comparison with the White British population in the UK, members of African-Caribbean communities who have mental health difficulties make less use of first-line support services. They are detained under mental health law more often and are more often placed in secure hospital settings. They are prescribed psychiatric medication more often and in higher doses and they are far less likely to receive non-physical interventions, such as counselling or cognitive behaviour therapy. Similar differences are found between members of South Asian communities and the White British population. Both African-Caribbean and South Asian service users express less satisfaction with services than their White counterparts (Bhugra, 2000; Shapley et al., 2001; Bowl, 2007; Dein et al., 2007).

The socio-economic status of different ethnic groups might account for some of the variation in experience of mental healthcare. However, Bowl (2007) observes that there is 'cultural and institutional exclusion' in mental health services. For example, in relation to members of African-Caribbean communities a 'circle of fear' is observed, which operates between mental health service providers and their service users. Inclusion is hindered by language barriers and a lack of understanding of cultural difference. It is thought that because of these factors, workers commonly misinterpret particular behaviours as signs of mental illness, making inaccurate diagnosis and failing to engage effectively with service users. It is also thought that institutional exclusion can also arise from the application of standard procedures, which do not acknowledge differences or the disadvantage of those who have specific needs related to their ethnicity (Fernando, 2002).

In England and Wales, government policy recognises a need for services to be extended to excluded ethnic and community groups (Delivering Race Equality in mental Health Care, 2005; New Horizons, 2009). It seems likely that assertive outreach teams will have a central role in further efforts to deliver mental healthcare to these ethnic groups. However, it is unfortunate that by emphasising ethnicity, we might imply that it is the difference of others that is 'the problem' and segregated services are need. To counter this unhelpful assumption, it is important that mainstream services should accept responsibility for meeting the different needs of ethnic minorities and to aid appropriate engagement. Rather than focusing exclusively on the unusual needs of individuals, services should consider how broader barriers to inclusion can be removed by changing service structures, policies and general attitudes. As discussed in Chapter 9, the impact of stigma, exclusion and discrimination, even when they are self-imposed, is a major hurdle for service users: 'Perceived discrimination may induce delusional ideation and thus contribute to the high observed rates of psychotic disorder in exposed minority populations.' (Janssen et al., 2003: 71)

Box 10.1   Is there a connection between racism and mental illness?

The Fourth National Survey of Ethnic Minorities provided UK evidence of a cross-sectional association between inter-personal racism and mental illness ... A nationally representative sample of 5196 persons of Caribbean, African and Asian origin were asked about racial discrimination in the preceding year. Those who had experienced verbal abuse were 3 times more likely to be suffering from depression or psychosis. Those who had experienced a racist attack were nearly 3 times more likely to suffer from depression and 5 times more likely to suffer from psychosis. Those who said their employers were racist were 1.6 times more likely to suffer from a psychosis. (Chakraborty & McKenzie, 2002: 475)

(see Box 10.1). Perceptions are mediated by our use of language and assertive outreach teams must be attuned to these subtleties. So, this chapter will consider strategies by which workers might gain a more accurate understanding of their service users and how this can be expressed in processes of 'team formulation' and team based interventions.

The use of assertive outreach strategies, in engaging with and improving the quality of life of excluded people from ethnic minorities, is an established and successful approach. Mohan et al., (2006) for example, compared higher and lower intensity community services. They found that intensive community treatment led to a significant reduction in inpatient bed days for African-Caribbean patients compared with White patients in the intensive treatment group and with all patients in the control group. Yang et al. (2005) found that an assertive community treatment team in Toronto, designed to specifically address the needs of people with severe mental illness from various ethnic minorities, was successful in enabling them to live in the community, reduced relapse rates and alleviated psychiatric symptoms (see Box 10.3). Two thirds of their service users had to use languages other than English to communicate with their primary workers, suggesting that bilingual and bicultural workers contributed enormously to effectively serving these individuals. This suggests that simply targeting help at specific groups is effective, but the processes involved in providing that help might actually be quite complex. To illustrate that work, this chapter will introduce ideas from transcultural psychiatry, humanistic psychology and critical theory, through which the dilemmas that assertive outreach teams face in working across different cultures will be identified and discussed. Working with Black and Ethnic Minority diversity will be introduced in this chapter, leading on to the discussion of diversity of gender, class, faith and sexuality in Chapter 11.

Diversity and 'normality'

The first problem that is encountered in describing cultural diversity is that of locating one's own position within a range of different perspectives or varying forms of theoretical analysis. In our post-modern world, we cannot expect to categorise or define all aspects of our shared world within one theoretical model. No single culture holds a value-free or scientific vantage point from which the 'difference of others' can be described. So, assertive outreach

---

Box 10.2   The problem of relativism

Social anthropology and medical anthropology have presented a challenge to the belief that there are universal categories of mental illness. A relativist position would suggest that there are as many categories of mental health (or physical health) as there are languages and culture in which they are expressed. Intermediate arguments suggest that there may be common elements in ideas of mental illness but that cultural expression of syndromes may differ significantly, or that symptoms may cluster in different ways in different cultures. (Fenton & Sadiq-Sangster, 1996: 66)

---

teams cannot stand outside of the cultural diversity that they are trying to comprehend. They are immersed both in their own professional understandings and in the idiosyncratic presentations of the many different service users whom they encounter. They are trying with their service users, to ground themselves in some kind of shared understanding. Somehow, out of this relativity, they must produce an objective observation of human behaviour. There is an expectation that they should identify and treat universally recognised 'classifications of mental illness', which have a consistent and reliable presentation across cultural groups, at all levels of different societies (see Box 10.2). So, can they claim to have an exclusive access to universal truths, or are they reduced to promoting just one more understanding in a world that is already full of alternative opinions?

When different professional groups in assertive outreach teams promote their contrasting forms of expertise, this is not just problematic due to rivalry, segregated supervision or pedantic disagreement. A hierarchy can be observed, not only in the 'scientific' grounding of these different forms of knowledge, but also in the status that each professional holds. An assertive outreach team is not, therefore, a comfortable and neutral position from which to observe or debate the colourful diversity of the 'world out there'. It is very much an expression of the conflicts and splits of that world. Teams can sometimes internalise dynamics of dominance and tyranny. Chapter 2 explores multi-professional working and, the need for teams to reach consensus in their formulations is identified in Chapter 8. This chapter will reflect on the pragmatic experience of assertive outreach teams in their use of different kinds of knowledge and in their attempts to include all views.

In assertive outreach, we do need to resolve our internal disagreements as to whether a medical, psychological or cultural explanation for a service user's difficulty should predominate at any one time. When things go wrong, other agencies will impose their own interpretations on our actions, so it is essential for teams to clearly articulate formulations and coherent understandings in support of their agreed care plans. For example, a simplistic medical model of mental illness is often applied by the general public; in the guise of neighbours, relatives, coroners, magistrates and newspapers; see the discussion of 'folk psychiatry' in Chapter 9. So, we must promote our more sophisticated understandings wherever possible.

Assertive outreach teams are made up of workers who have been socialised into the culture of their different professional groups (Dombeck, 1997). However, an integrated use of their contrasting approaches must be achieved, because when these workers cannot agree amongst themselves, how can they express the necessary authority with which to persuade others outside of the team of the validity of their opinions? However, this chapter

---

Box 10.3   An ethno-culturally focussed assertive outreach service

Dr Yang and his colleagues from the Department of Psychiatry at Mount Sinai Hospital developed an assertive community treatment team with a mandate to serve people from ethnic minority groups in central Toronto. The team has been based on the original PACT model. Surveys identified the main groups needing ethno-culturally focused services in this area have been East and Southeast Asian, African, Caribbean, and indigenous Native Canadian populations. All workers have been bilingual and share the cultural backgrounds of one of these key ethno-minority groups. Workers have been assigned to patients based on language, culture, gender and geographic location. An acculturation assessment is undertaken as part the psychosocial evaluation for all patients. To engage patients, culturally sensitive and meaningful group activities are strongly incorporated into regular programming. Particular attention has been paid to channeling resources into creating liaisons between team members and families and to providing family psycho-education in the patients' native tongue to support and promote family involvement in patients' care. All team meetings and special 'clinical situation' discussions highlight specific cultural issues, such as culturally influenced stigma, a lack of trust of authority, compliance with medication, or use of alternative health practices. Seasonal and festival celebrations from diverse cultures have been incorporated into the activity programmes, so as to enhance cultural understanding and promote mutual respect.

Significant reductions in hospitalisation have been noted, from the year before admission to Assertive Community Treatment, to the year afterwards. Total number of bed days for the sample declined by 5,874 days, from 7,095 days to 1,221 days—an 83 % reduction. (Yang et al., 2005)

---

will not be promoting one single assertive outreach approach through which all cultures and ethnicities can be classified and managed. Diversity is important because it is the pluralistic structure of multi-professional teams and notions of democratic decision making that have enabled mental health services to move on from a dark history including extreme forms of institutional abuse. This is a past that we must not forget and, although it is more difficult to exercise authority in a state of uncertainty, we must remember how easy it is for the use of simplistic understandings to promote dangerous stereotypical ideas.

Reflection point

Consider the way in which you dress in your work role. Do you present yourself in a manner that emphasises your status as a professional worker, or do you manage your appearance so as to blend in within the social world of the service user you are supporting?

Transcultural psychiatry

The work of Littlewood & Lipsedge (1998) is recognised as influential in the development of 'transcultural' approaches. Their analysis has led to an emphasis being placed on the stressful nature of cross-cultural encounters. Psychological difficulties are experienced

---

Box 10.4   Problems in translating understandings of mental illness

The terms that are used in mental health assessments can have a culturally specific meaning. When commonly used terms were translated into Amharic (an Ethiopian language),
Kortmann (1987) found that responses reflected a different meaning structure. 'Do you feel
unhappy?' received the common response of 'No, because no-one has died.' The concept
'unhappy' appears not to exist in this culture in any sense that is separate from a clear
cause or situational context such as recent bereavement. The question, 'Do you cry more
than usual?' was interpreted as asking whether the person had attended more funerals
than usual. The question, 'Is your appetite poor?' was interpreted as a question about the
availability of food. The question, 'Do you sleep badly?' was interpreted as a question about
nightmares or sleep-walking. (Kortmann, 1987)

---

when people migrate from one country to another and these problems have been described
as 'culture shock', or as an 'identity crisis'. The Stress-Vulnerability Model of Psychosis
(Zubin & Spring, 1977) provides a simple means of explaining the relationship between
the three factors of stress, vulnerability and cultural diversity in the development of mental health problems. The implied hypothesis would state that within any society there is a
dominant majority norm. People who migrate will be different from this majority and will
experience more stress, exacerbating existing vulnerabilities, leading to the development
of mental health problems (Cantor-Graae & Selton, 2005). Boydell et al. (2001) found
that 'The incidence of schizophrenia in non-White ethnic minorities increased significantly as the proportion of such minorities in the local population fell' (Boydell et al.,
2001: 1336). (Although, if culturally sensitive assessments had not been achieved, this
'incidence of schizophrenia' might include inaccurate diagnoses.)

Polish culture provides an example of a culturally specific understanding, as 'mental
health problems' hardly exist as a common conversational concept. Those who suffer
psychotic illness have been kept in the 'mental hospital outside town', while husbands
and wives will rarely discuss any psychological problems that occur for each of them and
even depression doesn't translate easily. Similar issues are found with Ethiopian culture,
as described in Box 10.4. Mental health issues are just not discussed in society at all, in
contrast to societies where psychological and psychiatric understandings have become
part of everyday language.

Encountering new understandings in a different culture will be difficult and it has been
observed that although migration can be stressful, first generation immigrants are likely
to have benefited from growing up in a cohesive cultural setting. Community support is a
protective factor that some members of migrating ethnic minorities might lack. So it is
often second generation immigrants, caught between two cultures with conflicting social
expectations who are more likely to use mental health services, but, are less satisfied with
those services (Parkman et al., 1997; Carta et al., 2005) (see Box 10.5). In assertive outreach teams, where an enduring engagement is achieved with service users, there is a
greater opportunity to understand mental distress as an 'ordinary' response to social difficulties. In assertive outreach, helping a person re-engage with their ethnic group, family
or peer group would be an important step in enabling them to transform their individual
distress into a shared, socially inclusive and normal experience.

Box 10.5   African and Caribbean young men – a circle of fear?

It has been observed that alienation from society prevents some African-Caribbean young men from looking at their own health and they engage in denial of any 'strange' thought processes. They are alienated from GPs and preventive services, and often end up being picked up by police under s.136* and then getting sent higher up the tariff of care when they don't cooperate with treatment. Staff in mental health units often have a fear of people who they think of as 'big, black and dangerous' and this reduces the chances of engagement. So when they are discharged these people then begin the circle again. (Keating, 2007)

As discussed in Chapter 8, assertive outreach teams employ specific strategies through which knowledge of the service user's culture is gained; for example, by engaging with families and local minority communities, although some dilemmas associated with engaging family carers are discussed in Chapter 7. Some teams employ workers from ethnic minorities, which enables more accurate assessment and effective formulation (Department of Health, 1999), but it would be very difficult to maintain a workforce within which all isolated groups are represented. So, assertive outreach teams should be incorporating best practice in the use of cultural competence and capability. They do need to incorporate unfamiliar cultural perspectives into their formulations (Alverson et al., 2007) and they will often struggle to comprehend the complexities of their service user's lives. For example, they will be trying to unravel threads in order to decide whether a person's behaviours are understandable as 'healthy and normal within their culture' or whether they are 'an outcome of a biological or psychological problem'.

Distinguishing the social and cultural origins of behaviours from psychological and biological causes is important because radically different interventions are required to address problems in one or the other scenario. Supporting people in understanding and coming to terms with their experiences, perhaps by facilitating a sense of solidarity with others who have experienced similar problems, is one area of intervention. Treating people pharmaceutically, sometimes against their will through the use of mental health law, is a very different approach, often experienced as increasing trauma, isolation and stigma. As described in Chapter 7, a formal structure is often used in assertive outreach to combine the contrasting understandings which are promoted by workers from different professional backgrounds (Lake, 2008). Attempting to understand complexities across cultures adds extra dynamics to these formulation processes, so there will be more questions to answer, as described by Lewis-Fernandez & Diaz (2002), for example, see Box 10.6.

One of the important factors that can help some people from ethnic minorities survive a system that seems stacked against them is strong family support. In a small-scale comparative study of service users of assertive outreach on the South Coast, Sanyal (2008) found that those from Black and Minority Ethnic backgrounds reported a significantly better quality of life than their White British counterparts in the area of family support. Also in current good practice, cultural competence or capability is about the worker learn-

---

* Section 136 of the mental health act enables police officers to detain a person who appear to be vulnerable due to mental health problems in a public place.

Box 10.6   Components of the cultural formulation

- Individual's ethnic or cultural reference group(s).
- Degree of involvement with both the culture of origin and the host culture (for immigrants and ethnic minorities).
- Language abilities, use, and preference (including multi-lingualism).
- Predominant idioms of distress through which symptoms or the need for social support are communicated.
- Meaning and perceived severity of the individual's symptoms in relation to norms of the cultural reference group(s).
- Local illness categories used by the individual's family and community to identify the condition.
- Perceived causes and explanatory models that the individual and the reference group(s) use to explain the illness.
- Current preferences for and past experiences with professional and popular sources of care.
- Stresses in the local social environment.
- Role of religion and kin networks in providing emotional, instrumental, and informational support.
- Individual differences in culture and social status between the individual and the clinician. (Summarised from DSM-IV, pp. 843–844, by Lewis-Fernandez & Diaz, 2002: 275)

Box 10.7   Core beliefs in modern Western psychiatry

Firstly people should function as self-reliant individuals. So, anyone who appears to be 'dependent' on others and those who reject personal responsibility are thought of as psychologically immature or inadequate.

Secondly 'psycho-pathology' is believed to reside in the individual, rather than in the interaction between the individual and physical, historical or spiritual realities, or other people. Therapeutic interventions are designed, therefore, to change individuals, rather than their 'social' problems.

Thirdly it is thought that disorders can be separated into discrete categories. So, attention is directed away from resolving distress, towards strict diagnostic boundaries. Distinctions are formed between 'real biological illness', 'genuine psychological distress' or 'general malingering'.

Fourthly mental disorders have a universal and biological causation; so the role of cultural and social factors in the onset and course of a disorder will be secondary.

Lastly it is thought that the whole world speaks a direct translation of English and the patient's words can be directly transposed in to a list of symptoms. (Adapted from Andary et al., 2003: 19–20)

---

ing to understand their own culture and how it is constructed (see Box 10.7) so that they can better begin to understand others' cultures and not be afraid to ask difficult questions of service users from a different culture than their own. This can involve some uncomfortable 'deconstruction of norms', when a history of imperialism and assumptions about other cultures and populations are exposed. It is hard to face the reality of social phenomena such as the eugenics movement, slavery or economic exploitation. There are hidden histories of oppression in which professional groups such as psychiatry and psychology have been complicit.

Box 10.8   Translating understandings across cultures

In the Asian tradition of Ayuraveda, maintaining good health involves moderation, self-control and personal responsibility. Diseases are not thought of as separate phenomena, whether mental or physical. Although some techniques for 'restraining the mind' are used in various schools of yoga, these are commonly combined with other approaches to 'purification' by purges and enemas; with 'pacification' by herbs that tranquilise or counteract depression. Dietary control is also considered to be important. The 'contemplation of 'self' involves a realisation of that self as it would be when uncontaminated by time or space – not a psychotherapeutic exploration of a lived life.' (Fernando, 2002: 146). So people who come from these cultures do take medicines but would not understand their effects in the same terms as practitioners in Western scientific healthcare.

While some aspects of non-Western approaches to health have translated into our culture, such as meditation, they have lost their connection with an integrated and holistic sense of self, becoming exclusively mental. Similar changes have occurred in the Western use of Japanese psychotherapies, such as 'Morita therapy', which are founded on Zen Buddhism and Shintoism. Traditional approaches, such as meditation, possession rituals and the consumption of health foods are used in these therapies. However, Morita therapy has undergone changes as Japan has been industrialised and influenced by Western culture. It now has a narrow use for specific personality problems and ideas about possession and the influence of spirits are no longer influential. (Fernando, 2002)

Many of the philosophical positions that our workers assume in their therapeutic work will not be shared by people from different cultural backgrounds. So, how do we ensure that our formulation processes reach out to include the perspective of the service user? In assessing mental health problems across cultural divides, we cannot rely on a simple 'fact file' approach (Culley, 2000); ethnic identity is a fluid and complex phenomena and employing stereotypical descriptions of cultural norms will not be adequate. Statutory services have sometimes formed partnerships with organisations which can provide specific ethnic forms of support (Fernando, 1995), but it is not easy to build bridges across multiple shifting understandings of mental distress. However, there will be common experiences across cultures and the difficulty of maturing from childhood and adopting an adult role in society is a transition that, perhaps, everyone struggles with.

Having recently moved on from a long history of institutional care in which patients were in many ways treated like children, workers in mental health services are usually very aware of the need to engage with service users in a respectful manner. Meanwhile, engagement can be facilitated more effectively when we help service users to improve their quality of life in practical ways, such as housing, vocational opportunities, benefit claims and social connectedness. Providing practical help is perhaps universally recognised as a gesture of acceptance and this kind of support has always been a mainstay of assertive outreach interventions. However, to make sure that there is no misunderstanding, it is important to constantly check that the nature of the helping relationship is understood by all parties (see Box 10.8).

Assertive outreach teams, with their emphasis on engagement, have become very skilled in identifying the preferred inter-personal styles of service users, particularly related to the expression of distress and in asking for help. So, rather than viewing the ethnicity of the service user as the cause of non-compliance, for example, it can be accepted that it is the failure of services to communicate effectively and explain the

---

Box 10.9 Different understandings of the causation of illness

Western theories of natural causation

- Infection: invasion of the body by noxious micro-organisms (e.g. the germ theory).
- Stress: exposure to physical or psychic strain (e.g. over exertion, prolonged hunger, fear, etc.).
- Organic deterioration: physical decline with old age; early failure of organs: hereditary defects.
- Accident: unintended physical injury (not supernatural).
- Overt human aggression: wilful infliction of physical injury by another person; attempted suicide.

Non-Western theories of natural causation

- Imbalance in the qualities of yin and yang (in Chinese medicine) or am and duong (in Vietnamese culture).
- Nervous weakness, as in neurasthenia.
- Loss or blocking of vital energies.
- Loss of vital essences (e.g. ch'i), as in semen loss.
- Being 'hit' or 'caught' by external winds which can enter the body making the person vulnerable to harm by spirits.

Mystical causation of illness

- Fate: illness is due to astrological influences, predestination, bad luck.
- Ominous sensation: particularly powerful dreams, sights, sounds or sensations are experienced and are believed to cause not just portend illness.
- Contagion: illness is caused by contact with a supposedly polluting object, substance or person (e.g. a menstruating woman; a dead body).
- Mystical retribution: violation of a taboo or moral injunction directly causes illness. (Adapted from Andary et al., 2003: 104–105)

---

importance of compliance that is the problem. For instance, there are significant variations in the way that people conceptualise illness, see Box 10.9. Observing the way in which people attribute meaning to symptoms is important, as compliance with treatment will be mediated by these understandings (Kirmayer et al., 1994). Ethnographic studies have observed distinctly different patterns in the use of language, as people from different cultural backgrounds talk about illness in sharply contrasting ways (Kortmann, 1987; Stern & Kirmayer, 2004).

While mental health workers might believe that their assessments are a means of gaining information about the service user, their approach to understanding might actually impose meanings in an oppressive manner. A distinction between psychological and physical aspects of our being might be promoted, which people from different cultures do not understand. They might, therefore, appear immature or childlike when seeking help. This impression would be gained because they fail to talk about distress in the manner expected by professional workers.

Many service users complain about pain or tiredness which cannot be accounted for as an outcome of recognised physical illnesses and it might be assumed that this is a 'coping strategy' more often adopted by individuals who have endured trauma, separation and loss in their childhood. Brown et al. (2005), for example, review theoretical models which

---

Box 10.10 What do symptoms actually mean?

In Modern Eurocentric Western culture, a lack of appetite can express many things:

An actual indication of a disease or disorder that has not been identified: unexplained lack of appetite might actually be caused by a depressive disease process.

A symbolic expression of an emotional intra-psychic conflict: a psychotherapist might believe that a lack of appetite represents a defence against feelings of losing control.

As an indication of specific psychopathology: a psychiatrist might believe that a reported lack of appetite is a symptom of dependent personality disorder and, therefore, an inappropriate help seeking behaviour.

As an idiomatic expression of distress: referring to a lack of appetite might be a symbolic means of expressing disgust in response to the greed or gluttony of others.

As a metaphor for experience: someone might say that they have lost their appetite for life when describing their experience of working in a boring job.

As an act of positioning within a local world: an expression of a lack of appetite might emphasise the distressed position of the sufferer and the duty of care that others have to offer more appealing foods.

A form of social commentary or protest: an expression of a lack of appetite might represent a protest against oppression and a threat to wrestle back some control through self-starvation. (Adapted from Laurence et al., 1998)

---

use notions such as 'dissociation', 'hysteria' and 'conversion'. These can be experienced as stigmatising interpretations, as if this is a more 'primitive' means of talking about distress. The depth of knowledge gained by assertive outreach workers, in their longer-term work with service users, can enable more supportive communication. There are many anecdotal accounts of service users reporting symptoms that had previously been dismissed as somatic but, following engagement with an assertive outreach team, a physical health cause has been identified and appropriate treatment provided. More often, however, workers learn to understand talk of various kinds of pain and distress as a part of the complex and multiple levelled communications, which occur in relationships in all social groups in all cultures.

Researchers have found that somatisation is common in all the cultural groups and societies that they have studied (Laurence et al., 1998). This prevalence challenges the notion that it is indicative of some special form of psychopathology. Instead, differences among groups might be understood as cultural styles in expressing distress and different beliefs and practices related to seeking help. When we consider how difficult it is to establish the meaning of a reported symptom, even when there are no cultural differences between the worker and the service user, the importance of taking time to know the service user is clear. Consider the different meanings of 'lack of appetite', as listed in Box 10.10. An assessing mental health worker cannot just record 'a loss of appetite' as a reported symptom of a physical or mental illness. Any number of different meanings could apply, in isolation or combination. So, to record an accurate assessment the worker would need to understand the context in which the service user is using these words. Assertive outreach workers need to assess over a much longer period during which they repeatedly check that there is a shared understanding with the service user.

Humanistic approaches to diversity

In developing complex understandings of their service users, assertive outreach teams often come to see them as active agents who are making decisions. This is, however, another understanding that is specific to our 'individualist' Western societies. In these societies we believe that all people are free to move on from their histories, free to adopt different beliefs and attitudes, behaving in new ways. In contrast there are societies in which it is commonly thought that the future will have a direct continuity with the past, therefore there can only be one set of true beliefs and a limited number of appropriate behaviours. Following the Littlewood & Lipsedge (1998) transcultural approach, it is in encountering the differences between these sharply contrasting cultures, that we experience stress. 'Trans-generational' conflict might occur, for example, as children grow up with experiences of more than one culture and may choose to live in a manner that prompts their parent's disapproval.

Following migration, populations often blend together and inter-marriage will create complex cultural mixes. When viewed from a humanistic perspective, people in these diverse communities are understood as making choices in assuming particular identities and cultural positions. This modern self-actualisation is reflected in the popularisation of humanistic counselling approaches, where an emphasis is placed, not so much on distress or dysfunction, as on helping the person make choices related to their identity; finding out 'who they really are' (a kind of 'lifestyle coaching'). These influential therapeutic models and related practices will be expressed in assertive outreach teams, as workers who are trained in these approaches bring their knowledge to team discussions and clinical reviews. For example, the idea of the 'rational choice-making individual' is central to many of the developing therapeutic interventions, such as CBT, which are used in these teams.

Although personal choice is considered important in healthcare, this individualism is not promoted in all cultures. Hofstede (1991), for example, surveyed up to 88,000 IBM employees in 50 countries. He found that some cultures were largely individualist in the sense that the ties between people were loose with everyone being expected to look after themselves and their immediate family. In contrast, other cultures were largely collectivist, in the sense that people from birth onwards were integrated into strong, cohesive kinship groups, which protected them throughout life in exchange for unquestioning loyalty. Across another dimension he found that some cultures have a strong hierarchical structure, in which those who are in power are respected and obeyed, while those who are powerless can expect that the powerful will look after their interests and protect them. However, in other societies hierarchy was viewed unfavourably. In these cultures, holding power and exercising power over others was considered authoritarian and unjust. Assertive outreach workers will have engaged with service users by becoming sensitive to their cultural expectations. The will have found, for example, that some people believe that 'accepting charity' is stigmatising, or that 'public servants' should serve.

Encountering different cultural expectations in diverse geographical locations is one kind of problem, while growing up with Mixed Heritage is another. Having a Mixed Heritage background can be isolating because each person's particular heritage would be

---

Box 10.11   How healthy is individualism?

A total of 276 first-year students attending an Australian university completed an anonymous survey. As expected, idiocentrism was associated with smaller and less satisfying social support networks, less skill in managing both self and others' emotions, lower intentions to seek help from family and friends for personal and suicidal problems and higher levels of hopelessness and suicidal ideation. Thus, there appear to be social and psychological disadvantages associated with having strong individualistic values and beliefs within an individualistic culture. (Scott et al., 2004: 143)

---

unique, although, paradoxically, this is the fastest growing group within Black and Ethnic Minority classification in the UK. So, many more people will need to find their own personal identity and roots with a reduced sense of belonging. This kind of individualism has been found to be linked with greater social isolation and the loss of the protective factors of family and community (Scott et al., 2004) (see Box 10.11). Meanwhile, it is mainly within modern Western societies that people have come to be understood primarily as 'rational, choice-making individuals'. Understanding the 'mental health consumer', as a rational choice maker, connects neatly with the individualistic tradition of Western psychotherapy (McDonald et al., 2007). However, it has been observed that through our adoption of these philosophies, we have been losing our positions in traditional extended families. Life-long occupational roles in local communities are in decline, as people lose local connections and move away from their extended families. This has been described as a process of 'reflexive modernisation' (Adkins, 2002) and it has been claimed that in promoting humanistic philosophies we might be losing freedoms in subjecting ourselves to a new form of self-government (Rose, 1996). It is argued that while we appear to have so much more choice, playing with life-styles and identity, the context of this choice is diminished as all cultures are recruited into modern Western consumerism, where everyone lives very similar lives, purchasing the same products. Assertive outreach workers face a dilemma. Should they try to re-engaging service users with others from their cultural background, where they are likely to be supported in holding beliefs about the causation or management of illness that are at odds with those promoted by healthcare professionals, or should they encourage the adoption of modern Western values.

It is recognised that when people move to live in a different society, there is a process of acculturation. Glovsky & Haslam (2003) examined the understandings expressed by Brazilian citizens who were living for extended periods in New York. It was found that those who had become acculturated to life in that society held more psychologised understandings of mental disorders than those who remained more connected with the society from which they originate. Acculturated Brazilians more often used concepts such as emotional distress and intrapsychic dysfunction or conflict to explain odd behaviours. In Chapter 8 it is recognised that the service users who are referred to assertive outreach teams are less likely to accept the interpretations of mental health workers than those who are not. These people may have become estranged from their communities, but they have also been unable to access adequate support from mental health services. In engaging with these service users, do assertive outreach teams genuinely reach out into the understandings and values of minority groups, or are they supporting a process of acculturation? The benefits and disadvantages of promoting various understandings of mental illness are also discussed in Chapter 9.

Reflection point

Consider what we mean by the term 'identity'. We assume that the Scottish person who wears a kilt is proud of their national identity and the young man who wears a football shirt wants to be identified with a team and fellow supporters. We make similar assumptions when we see different hairstyles, tattoos or makeup. However, can we assume that a Muslim woman has chosen to wear a veil or that a Jewish man has chosen to be circumcised? What about members of majority cultural groups. In Western societies; has the man in a business suit chosen his social identity?

Consider your social identity: what assumptions will people from different social backgrounds bring to their encounters with you and are these preformed ideas about you correct?

A critical analysis

In a critical analysis, cultural identities are not simply already out there waiting to be discovered. They are constructed by dominant classes, as 'deviant', 'threatening', or somehow 'unjustified' and this is a means to exclude, oppress or control. For example, in an effort to improve the population's health, initiatives might be set up to encourage people to attend for screening, or change their diet and otherwise alter their behaviour. Those who do not follow this 'good advice' might then be labelled as 'difficult'. Service providers might develop a notion of the 'ideal service user', against which others would be judged, when in reality, very few people actually match up to this definition (McDonald et al., 2007). When people are judged unfavourably against a White middle class male norm it is often said that they should take action to improve their situation. But without the privileges of that class, there is often no action that they can take. A critical analysis has observed a political agenda behind the state's support of humanistic psychotherapy, in which social problems can be 're-packaged' as personal problems (Cromby et al., 2007). The paradoxical nature of humanistic empowerment can mean that the interests of disadvantaged people in society are not advanced (Cruikshank, 1993; Baistow, 1995).

Psychiatric services generally tend to be 'colour blind', not only in the sense that culture and ethnic background are only secondary issues in diagnostic formulation, but also in the sense that it is the form of symptoms that is observed, rather than their content (Boyle, 1992). In examining personal experience, we find that ethnicity is not just a background factor that might cause or exacerbate mental health problems; it does not just mediate the expression of those problems; racism is actually expressed in the nature of the mental illness (Brown, 2003). For example, a person from a devalued ethnic group might express understandable nihilistic thoughts and feelings, which are brought about by the systematic blocking of their efforts for personal growth (Akbar, 1991). Clinicians who attempt to treat these people might 'translate' their difficulties into a depressive illness,

---

Box 10.12   Racial discrimination in the work place?

It has been found that in mental health N.H.S. Trusts across the South East Coastal Region of the UK, 37% of job applicants who are short listed are from Black Minority Ethnic groups, but only 13% from these groups are appointed. More employees from these groups are involved in disciplinary hearing and bullying and harassment investigations in comparison with British Whites. (Santry, 2008)

---

but this is missing the point. Living in a society where being White is constantly and subtly constructed as 'better' or 'normal', people from Ethnic Minorities might develop feelings of self-loathing, or they might invest in 'anti-society' political or religious arguments. Being 'other' is expressed though negative thoughts, delusions and paranoia. Mental illness is then enmeshed in racial conflict.

Critical Race Theory puts racial conflict back into our understanding of mental illness (Delgadon & Stefancic, 2000). For example, when discriminatory processes are hidden, the people who are discriminated against cannot express their anger and those who discriminate cannot express their fear of retaliation. If we fail to recognise that opportunities and resources are distributed disproportionately in a form of 'racial stratification', then mistrust, antipathy, indifference and violence are likely to develop (Brown, 2003). On the one hand there will be people who cannot be angry and, therefore, expresses false-affability, passivity, resignation, withdrawal and self-destruction (Case, 1993). On the other hand there will be a delusional denial of the reality of discrimination in our society and paranoia is then expressed by those who explain societal problems as caused by the presence of ethnic minorities (Thompson & Neville, 1999). Workers who are themselves from ethnic minority backgrounds might struggle with the expectation that, because they have taken on a professional role, they must represent the interests of the state in controlling the challenging behaviours of service users from their own community. Those same workers might also be subject to racial abuse (often, but not exclusively by White service users), being caught themselves between different cultures in complex ways (see Box 10.12).

Assertive outreach teams employ enhanced strategies to achieve engagement and use longer-term working approaches. Because of this, social inequalities and conflicts become more than just 'background information on the case file'. As discussed in Chapter 8, assertive outreach teams usually need to engage at a community level with families and groups (Meddings et al., 2010), where the hidden realities of oppression and discrimination must be recognised and articulated (see Box 10.13). Although workers follow legislative policies in managing risk, such as Safeguarding Vulnerable Adults (in England and Wales), they must also be careful not to impose interpretations that inappropriately combine notions of 'otherness' with 'risk'. While these teams might be bringing a more scientific and effective approach to mental healthcare, that is based in modern Western thinking, they might also bring stigmatising attitudes. Positive attitudes towards mental health problems are more often found in cultures where extended kinship networks are important and where there is more tolerance of eccentricity (Warner, 1994; Rosen, 2003). Assertive outreach teams must be careful not to impose values through which service users are only seen as worthwhile if they have employment, for example. They must not

---

Box 10.13   Cultural sensitivity

Ida (2007) writes about the migration of populations due to war, economic forces or natural disaster. The isolation that is caused by language barriers and cultural differences is compounded by multiple discriminations based on ethnicity, sexual orientation and foreign-born status. It is argued that these are not just individual problems; it must be understood that 'This type of historical trauma goes deep and can leave invisible scars that last for generations.' (Ida, 2007: 50). Imposing a strong Western medical interpretation of distress can often re-traumatise service users. Sensitivity is required and creative solutions are needed, for example; 'Recovery may involve the use of traditional healers to help with problems that are viewed as psychological in nature.' (Ida, 2007: 51)

---

overvalue individual decision making if the service user gains acceptance by meeting the needs of others within their community group (Coldwell, 2008).

The history of mental healthcare includes extreme forms of abuse and oppression where narrow understandings have dominated and, only through the heroic campaigning of oppressed people, sometimes in collaboration with sympathetic academics and practitioners, have improvements been achieved. Strong models of biological determinism have been cut down to size by a dogged promotion of psychological and social models. However, balance is still needed. If we did not have the ability to diagnose illness, our detention and treatment of patients would then contravene the Human Rights Act. We would be accused of imprisoning and poisoning our service users. Nevertheless, disputes over diagnostic formulations need not divide teams and in assertive outreach, these are often resolved by the need to achieve shared outcomes. There is little point for example, in treating a person's biological problems, if we fail to motivate and give hope at a psychological level. But also, it is not possible for the service user to develop and express hope, while they are still troubled by distressing symptoms and are unable to eat or sleep. Similarly, there is little point in promoting hopefulness, if the person does not have essential social opportunities, such as contact with friends or family, work or leisure activities, or somewhere safe to live and adequate finances.

Conclusion

In assertive outreach, developing an understanding of service users is not just a categorisation of them as occupying some position in a matrix of stereotypical 'others'. It is more than an engagement with them through which therapeutic interventions enable them to develop 'self-understanding', or manage their 'symptoms'. To achieve a mutual understanding with service users, their families and their communities, workers must keep an open mind about conflicting interpretations. They must maintain sensitivity to cultural differences, rather than imposing meanings. Believing that one interpretation is right and another is wrong would be unhelpful, while neglecting any area of knowledge or expertise can create barriers to recovery. Teams will not always know whether to help service users adopt a more Western form of individual self-understanding, or to facilitate their connectedness with others who share their culture. However, the provision of practical help is an intervention that can usually be understood across different cultures.

Over the past few decades, the knowledge that is held by service users and their carers has been increasingly valued as a timely balance to the expertise of trained professionals. So value must also be placed on understandings that are grounded in different cultures and ethnic minority communities. This enables us to be mindful of the problems created by narrow forms of understanding and teams can formulate a more sophisticated and open kind of awareness. So, although we should be positive and optimistic in applying our different kinds of expertise, we must not forget lessons from our history and we must observe that discrimination and oppression are still with us.

References

Adkins, L. (2002) *Revisions: Gender and Sexuality in Late Modernity*. Open University Press, Buckingham.

Alverson, H.S., Drake, R.E., Carpenter-Song, E.A., Chu, E., Ritsema, M. & Smith, B. (2007) Ethnocultural variations in mental illness discourse: some implications for building therapeutic alliances. *Psychiatric Services*, **58**(12), 1541–1546.

Andary, L., Stolk, Y. & Klimidis, S. (2003) *Assessing Mental Health Across Cultures*. Australian Academic Press, Bowen Hills.

Baistow, K. (1995) Liberation and regulation? Some paradoxes of empowerment. *Critical Social Policy*, **42**, 34–46.

Bhugra, D. (2000) Migration and schizophrenia. *Acta Psychiatrica Scandinavica*, **407**, 68–73.

Bowl, R. (2007) Responding to ethnic diversity: black service user's views of mental health services in the UK. *Diversity in Health and Social Care*, **4**, 201–210.

Boydell, J., van Os, J., MacKenzie, K., Allardyce, J., Goel, R. & McCreadie, R.G., et al. (2001) Incidence of schizophrenia in ethnic minorities in London: ecological study into interactions with environment. *British Medical Journal*, **323**, 1336–1338.

Brown, R.J., Schrag, A. & Trimble, M. (2005) Dissociation, childhood interpersonal trauma, and family functioning in patients with somatization disorder. *American Journal of Psychiatry*, **162**(5), 899–905.

Brown, T.N. (2003) Critical race theory speaks to the sociology of mental health problems produced by racial stratification. *Journal of Health and Social Behaviour*, **44**, 292–301.

Boyle, M. (1992) Form and content, function and meaning in the analysis of 'schizophrenic' behaviour. *Clinic Psychology Forum*, **47**, 10–15.

Cantor-Graae, E. & Selton, J-P. (2005) Schizophrenia and migration: a meta-analysis and review. *American Journal of Psychiatry*, **162**, 12–24.

Carta, M.G., Bernal, M., Hardoy, M.C. & Haro-Abad, J.M. (2005) Migration and mental health in Europe. *Clinical Practice and Epidemiology*, **1**(1), 1–16.

Case, E. (1993) *The Rage of a Privileged Class*. Harper Collins Publishers, New York.

Chakraborty, A. & McKenzie, K. (2002) Does racial discrimination cause mental illness? *British Journal of Psychiatry*, **180**, 475–477.

Coldwell, J. (2008) *Schizophrenia and family burden: past, present and implications for future research*. Research Dissertation.

Cromby, J., Diamond, B., Kelly, P., Moloney, P., Priest, P. & Smail, D. (2007) Questioning the science and politics of happiness. *The Psychologist*, **20**(7), 422–425.

Cruikshank, B. (1993) Revolutions within: self-government and self-esteem. *Economy and Society*, **22**(3), 326–344.

Culley, L. (2000) Working with Diversity: Beyond the Fact File. In: *Changing Practice in Health and Social Care*, (eds. C. Davies, L. Finlay & A. Bullman). pp. 131–142. Sage, London.

Dein, K., Williams, P.S. & Dein, S. (2007) Ethnic bias in the application of the Mental Health Act 1983. *Advances in Psychiatric Treatment*, **13**, 350–357.

Delgadon, R. & Stefancic, J. (2000) *Critical Race Theory: The Cutting Edge*, 2nd edn. Temple University Press, Philadelphia.

Department of Health (1999) *National Service Framework for Mental Health*. Department of Health, London.

Dombeck, M.T. (1997) Professional personhood: training, territoriality and tolerance. *Journal of Interprofessional Care*, **11**(1), 9–21.

Fenton, S. & Sadiq-Sangster, A. (1996) Culture, relativism and the expression of mental distress: South Asian women in Britain. *Sociology of Health & Illness*, **18**(1), 66–85.

Fernando, S. (1995) *Mental Health in a Multi-ethnic Society*. Routledge, London.

Fernando, S. (2002) *Mental Health, Race and Culture*, 2nd edn. Palgrave, Basingstoke.

Glovsky, V. & Haslam, N. (2003) Acculturation and changing concepts of mental disorder: Brazilians in the USA. *Transcultural Psychiatry*, **40**(1), 50–61.

Hofstede, G. (1991) *Cultures and Organizations: Software of the Mind*. Harper Collins, London.

Ida, D.J. (2007) Cultural competency and recovery within diverse populations. *Psychiatric Rehabilitation Journal*, **31**(1), 49–53.

Janssen, I., Hanssen, M., Bak, M., Bijl, R., De Graaf, R. & Vollebergh, W. (2003) Discrimination and delusional ideation. *British Journal of Psychiatry*, **182**, 71–76.

Keating, F. (2007) ARE Foundation – London: A Race Equality Foundation Briefing Paper, http://www.raceequalityfoundation.org.uk

Kirmayer, L.J., Young, A. & Robbim, B.C. (1994) Symptom attribution in cultural perspective. *Canadian Journal of Psychiatry*, **39**, 384–594.

Kortmann, F. (1987) Problems in communication in transcultural psychiatry: the self-reporting questionnaire in Ethiopia. *Acta Psychiatrica Scandinavia*, **75**, 563–570.

Lake, N. (2008) Developing skills in consultation 2: a team formulation approach. *Clinical Psychology Forum*, **186**, 18–24.

Laurence, J., Kirmayer, M.D. & Young, A. (1998) Culture and Somatization: clinical, epidemiological, and ethnographic perspectives. *Psychosomatic Medicine*, **60**, 420–430.

Lewis-Fernandez, R. & Diaz, N. (2002) The cultural formulation: a method for assessing cultural factors affecting the clinical encounter. *Psychiatric Quarterly*, **73**(4), 271–295.

Littlewood, R. & Lipsedge, M. (1998) *Aliens and Alienists: Ethnic Minorities and Psychiatry*, 3rd edn. Routledge, London.

McDonald, R., Mead, N., Cheraghi-Sohi, S., Bower, P., Whalley, D. & Roland, M. (2007) Governing the ethical consumer: identity, choice and the primary care medical encounter. *Sociology of Health & Illness*, **29**(3), 430–456.

Meddings, S., Shaw, B. & Diamond, B. (2010) Community Psychology. In: *Reaching Out: The Psychology of Assertive Outreach*, (ed. C. Cupitt). pp. 207–228. Hove, Routledge.

Mohan, R., McCrone, P., Szmukler, G., Micali, N., Afuwape, S. & Thornicroft, G. (2006) Ethnic differences in mental health service use among patients with psychotic disorders. *Social Psychiatry and Psychiatric Epidemiology*, **41**, 771–776.

Parkman, S., Davies, S., Leese, M., Phelan, M. & Thornicroft, G. (1997) Ethnic differences in satisfaction with mental health services among representative people with psychosis in south London: PRiSM study 4. *The British Journal ofPpsychiatry*, **171**, 260–264.

Rose, N. (1996) *Inventing our Selves: Psychology, Power, and Personhood.* Cambridge University Press, Cambridge.

Rosen, A. (2003) What developed countries can learn from developing countries in challenging psychiatric stigma. *Australian Psychiatry*, **11**, Supplement.

Santry, C. (2008) Minority staff get worse deal on jobs, pay and grievances. *Health Service Journal*, 7 August, 4–5.

Sanyal, N. (2008) Int*ensive Case Management: is there a difference in quality of life outcomes for people from BME backgrounds compared to White British people.* Dissertation for MSc Degree course at Institute of Psychiatry/King's College, London.

Scott, G., Ciarrochi, J. & Deane, F.P. (2004) Disadvantages of being an individualist in an individualistic culture: idiocentrism, emotional competence, stress, and mental health. *Australian Psychologist*, **39**(2), 143–153.

Shapley, M., Hutchinson, G., McKenzie, K. & Murray, R.M. (2001) Understanding the excess of psychosis among the African-Caribbean population in England. Review of current hypotheses. *British Journal of Psychiatry*, **40**, 60–68.

Stern, L. & Kirmayer, L.J. (2004) Knowledge structures in illness narratives: development and reliability of a coding scheme. *Transcultural Psychiatry*, **41**(1), 130–142.

Thompson, C.E. & Neville, H.A. (1999) Racism, mental health and mental health practice. *The Counseling Psychologist,* **27**(2), 155–223.

Warner, R. (1994) *Recovery from Schizophrenia: Psychiatry and Political Economy*, 2nd edn. Routledge, London.

Yang, J., Law, S., Chow, W., Andermann, L., Steinberg, R. & Sadavoy, J. (2005) Assertive Community Treatment for Persons with Severe and persistent Mental Illness in Minority Groups. *Psychiatric Services*, **56**(9), 1053–1055.

Zubin, J. & Spring, B. (1977) Vulnerability: a view of schizophrenia. *Journal of Abnormal Psychology*, **86**, 103–126.

Chapter 11

Diversity and assertive outreach

Simon Wharne and Caroline Williams

With thanks to Neil Thompson

> Diversity. A term increasingly being used to emphasise the differences between individuals and across groups ... Diversity and difference are the roots of discrimination, in the sense that it is through the identification of differences that discrimination (and thus oppression) takes place. Thompson, N. (2006: 41)

Introduction

The society in which we live is diverse. The term 'diversity' is used to describe the differences in society as a positive asset and, therefore, can be viewed as a positive term (Thompson, 2006) and celebrates the contribution 'difference' makes to our society. We can't escape difference, as we all share this commonality; paradoxically difference is, therefore, the one thing we all have in common. For some groups in society, however, difference can be a negative experience and inequalities can exist for groups who deviate significantly from what is viewed as the 'norm' in society. This can be a reality for many people who come into contact with assertive outreach services.

As we know, it is a sad indictment of modern Western society that people with ongoing severe mental health problems can often be viewed upon negatively as 'different' by their local communities; not as a form of celebration, but as a form of abuse. Homicides that catch the media's attention are usually attributed to the 'mad schizophrenic'. Negative media representations of community care can influence public perceptions that community care isn't working and people with mental illnesses receiving care in the community are unpredictable and dangerous (Rose, 1998). However, despite overwhelming evidence over the past 50 years that homicide rates due to mental disorders are low (Taylor & Gunn, 1999; Large et al., 2008) and that it is more likely perpetrators of homicides are not mentally ill, the public still seemingly hold perceptions that people with mental illnesses are dangerous and unpredictable (Crisp et al., 2000). Such stereotypes only serve to alienate and disenfranchise people with long-term psychosis. People with severe mental health problems can experience discrimination and oppression from their community, but also from the caring profession. Service users who are

Assertive Outreach in Mental Healthcare: Current Perspectives, First Edition. Edited by C. Williams, M. Firn, S. Wharne and R. Macpherson.
© 2011 Blackwell Publishing Ltd. Published 2011 by Blackwell Publishing Ltd.

referred to assertive outreach usually report negative experiences of the psychiatric system, hold a distrust and have consequently disengaged.

Very little attention has been given to diversity issues in assertive outreach and to a degree, why should it, after all assertive outreach teams exist within a wider inter-agency multi-disciplinary framework. When we discuss issues of diversity with colleagues a common reaction is to place this as a wider issue outside the scope of assertive outreach practice. However, it could be argued that assertive outreach teams engage individuals who have experienced oppression, discrimination and exclusion in one form or another and, therefore, the need for assertive outreach to contain an individual's distress also involves anti-oppressive practice in order to engage the person in a non judgemental and sophisticated way.

This chapter will draw together some threads from debates and dilemmas that are highlighted throughout this book. Diversity will be considered in the specific areas of gender, class, faith and sexuality to provide examples of the complexity of assertive outreach and examples of both practical and ethical problems will be explored. We will consider diversity and anti-oppressive practice in assertive outreach, for instance, do mental health services impose a dominant cultural view of what 'normal behaviour should be', or is it possible to treat mental illness from a position that is accepting of social diversity? It has been argued that believing everyone in society has the same rights and opportunities is a commonly accepted delusion (Delgadon & Stefancic, 2000). For many people, sharing in this delusion requires an expression of false affability. In contrast, many service users in assertive outreach will express a healthy anger at the lack of opportunity that they experience. Their anger however, might only add to their social exclusion, as they are subject to the atrophy of isolated poverty, punctuated by cycles of crisis and breakdown. Assertive outreach teams attempt to break these cycles by offering many things, including empathetic understanding, practical help, continuity of care and various therapeutic interventions.

Why should equality and diversity and anti-discriminatory practice (ADP) matter to assertive outreach workers?

As soon as we start to think about the relationship between diversity and mental health problems, we have already started to separate a suffering individual from the many different contexts in which that suffering might occur. In Chapter 9, it was observed that we tend to seek close or distant relationships with people, depending on our attribution of positive or negative motivation behind their behaviours. It is thought that the expression of mental distress cannot be separated from stereotypical ideas which confuse difference with both 'dangerousness' and 'vulnerability'. The Strengths Model has been influential in assertive outreach (Rapp & Goscha, 2006) and perhaps we should think about difference as adaptive, as a source of creativity and opportunity. Mental health workers might feel that they are under pressure to define and control that which is different in society, but would it not be better to leave control to law enforcement agencies; we could then celebrate social variation. On the other hand, no matter how hard workers try to be

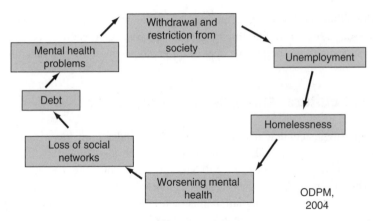

Figure 11.1 A cycle of exclusion. Adapted from ODPM, 2004.

non-judgemental and accepting, it seems inevitable that a moral position must be taken and teams will be debating ethical complexities.

It has been argued that people with severe mental health problems can become isolated from the psychiatric system, from their community and experience further chronicity of psychiatric symptoms and social disability (Figure 11.1, OPDM, 2004). Such exclusion & isolation in the face of severe mental health problems could arguably make such an individual suitable for assertive outreach services and, therefore, these teams are potentially seeing individuals who for one reason or another are socially excluded and hence discriminated against in some way. Social exclusion is borne out of discrimination, amongst other factors (ODPM, 2004); people become excluded as society closes the doors and reduces opportunities that might have previously been there. The experiences of assertive outreach service users are discussed in Chapter 8 and processes of social exclusion receive a more in-depth discussion in Chapter 9. It could be argued that users of assertive outreach services carry the legacy of psychiatric system failures; failures to provide a service that meets the needs of people with severe mental illness and, thus, ends in systematic social exclusion from the very system which seeks to 'care' for the individual.

It is here we come back to our question, why is ADP relevant to assertive outreach teams? As discussed, these teams, attempt to meet the needs of an excluded and disenfranchised population; arguably more so than any other community mental health team. Diversity and anti-discriminatory practice (ADP) are, therefore, core themes in assertive outreach practice as well as therapeutic engagement and should not be seen as an add-on; but should be an integral part of what these services provide. For instance, it has been argued that good engagement provided by assertive outreach teams, is through 'a respectful, enabling partnership that offers time understanding and support' (Gillespie & Meaden, 2010: 18), however is it possible to develop a respectful and understanding partnership without an apprehension of past and present oppressive practices and the need to change such practices? Assertive outreach teams have an opportunity by recognising and celebrating difference to provide a different legacy to the one that has preceded it. It is a complex issue, however, failing to engage with the issue can lead to greater misunderstandings and sometimes perpetuate oppressive practice consciously or subconsciously.

Personal, cultural and structural influences

It has been suggested that discrimination is best understood when examining the phenomena on a personal, cultural and structural level, also known as 'PCS analysis' (Figure 11.2, Thompson, 2006). We will attempt to introduce the reader to PCS analysis, however, for a more thorough discussion and introduction, we would advise the reader to consult Thompson (2003); our aim in this section is to provide an overview in order to provide a relevance to practice. The PCS model was developed by Dr Neil Thompson and disseminated through the social work practice literature and we refer to his work throughout when describing PCS analysis. The 'P' level refers to the personal or psychological level, the 'C' level refers to the cultural level and the 'S' refers to the structural level. To understand discrimination and oppression towards service users in assertive outreach services it makes sense to understand the dynamic of oppression via PCS analysis and understand the complexities of discriminatory practice in assertive outreach practice, and we will provide a closer explanation of the model.

The 'P' level focuses on the personal attitudes, values, assumptions, norms we posses as individuals; our own personal rules for living. When we interact with people who use assertive outreach services, we may hold certain prejudices about their lifestyle choices, sexuality, gender, diagnosis, ethnicity or cultural beliefs. Our individual beliefs and assumptions are shaped by life experiences but also are influenced by the culture in which we inhabit; which is where the 'C' level comes in. The 'C' level refers to a set of shared commonalities we have with others as well as shared norms, beliefs and assumptions (as opposed to individual beliefs and assumptions); we can experience such shared cultural

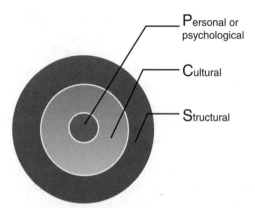

Figure 11.2   PCS Analysis. Neil Thompson, Anti Discriminatory Practice, 1992, reproduced with permission of Palgrave MacMillan.

norms in humour or the sharing of stereotypes with others. In assertive outreach practice, teams may share negative stereotypes relating to certain groups of people they are in contact with, for instance people with personality disorders, or the conduct of carers. Shared custom and practice may engender a culture that unwittingly becomes oppressive towards service users and/or staff members. Such shared cultures may hinder service users reaching their potential as such oppressive cultural values may hinder creative interventions (see Case study 11.1). As can also be seen in Case study 11.1, shared negative views of individual service users and other staff groups can reduce opportunities and can also potentially create inertia and an environment for omitting to act on serious issues. However, in contrast, staff members may hold strong personal negative views of particular groups in society (e.g. sex offenders), but in the work situation they may share very difficult cultural values with their colleagues that are based on support and rehabilitation and they may be able to compartmentalise such views and divorce the personal from the cultural with a dependence on particular roles and work based cultures.

Case study 11.1   A dog's life

Bill has been a user of assertive outreach services for two years, he has a diagnosis of paranoid schizophrenia, uses alcohol excessively and is mostly intoxicated when the team visit. Bill's house is in a poor state of repair and there is rising damp. Bill also has many dogs and reports that he takes pleasure from them; when the team visit Bill they regularly find three dogs in the garden barking at them, there are dogs in the kitchen barking loudly and scratching at the door concealed from view. There are always three cats and two dogs in the lounge, one of which is a puppy. The dogs look thin and Bill says he finds it difficult coping with them at times. Bill has also stated he would like to get another dog. The social worker has become concerned about the welfare of the animals and takes it back to the team meeting. A few stronger members of the team are dismissive and minimise the social workers concerns claiming that the social worker needs to focus on the more pressing aspects of care, such as medication. One of the stronger members of the team states Bill has a possible personality disorder and is manipulative and that the dogs are the least of their concern, highlighting that their focus should be on his symptoms and alcohol misuse rather than issues that aren't a concern for a healthcare team. The team agrees with the stronger members; the social worker feels isolated and Bill continues to find it difficult coping with his dogs.

When shared discriminatory cultural norms become the fabric of the service, this can create an institutional culture that is pervasive, this is where the analysis moves into a structural level, or the 'S' level. A clinical example of the 'C' and 'S' levels can be illustrated via a report published in the early 1990s, entitled 'Big, Black and Dangerous' (Special Hospital Services Authority, 1993) which refers primarily to the death of Orville Blackwood, an African-Caribbean gentleman and an inpatient at Broadmoor Hospital. The report highlighted the shared cultural norms at Broadmoor Hospital operating at the time (the 'C' level); a shared culture in which Black patients were less likely to be offered therapeutic interventions and were more likely to be restrained and administered intramuscular neuroleptic medication. These shared cultural norms became part of the institutional fabric (the 'S' level) and the report title was reference to how Black patients were referred to by the staff. Although this report was some time ago, similar issues have been highlighted again recently in the Rocky Bennett Inquiry (Blofeld, 2003) in which institutions can became racist or discriminatory. As can be seen via PCS analysis, one section can merge into another; personal values can merge into cultural norms and can then merge into structural levels, however, staff members may be also able to hold different views in different levels of the PCS model.

Understanding discrimination is one thing, however, challenging it can be more difficult for many staff members. The reflection point below illustrates the complexities in challenging discrimination, particularly when this comes from a service user to a member of staff. The assumption is that this is a staff to service user issue, however, issues of challenging discrimination have wider implications and can be from staff to service user, user to staff, carer to staff and staff member to staff member.

Reflection point

Mike is a user of the local assertive outreach service. Mike has refused to work with his care coordinator as he has been told he is gay. Mike won't share with the team who has told him, however, he stated to the support time recovery worker, 'I don't like gays and I don't want them in my house'. Mike agrees to accept a depot from the care coordinator, however, he continues making homophobic comments whilst receiving the depot. The care coordinator is anxious about working with Mike and is aware he has a violent past and is now worried about how other clients will view him.

How do you approach this as a team?
How would you support the care co-ordinator?
Would you support Mike in his request? If not, how would you approach this?

Is there a typical assertive outreach service user?

It would be very difficult to attempt to describe a typical assertive outreach service user. There are some patterns of behaviour that are commonly observed by these teams, but generally assertive outreach referral criteria create caseloads of a very diverse nature. In this complexity it is rarely possible to employ one simple form of understanding or give precedence to any particular professional discipline. Some might argue that this cuts against the usual trend of mental health services (Box 11.1) and assertive outreach does seem to be a uniquely integrated multi-professional working environment. Teams have inherited theoretical positions from diverse sources, such as psychological and psychiatric theory, therapeutic community work, recovery philosophy, the politics of social inclusion, humanistic philosophies and many more. There has been a shift from the application of knowledge by specific separate professional bodies to a shared and debated form of complex inter-professional understanding in teams, in other words a shift from individual professional working to generic team working (see Chapter 2 for more on team working). This healthy debate extends into our interactions with service users, their family carers and other support agencies.

Box 11.1   The challenge of complex causation and treatment

Despite over a hundred years of scientific research into the causation and treatment of mental distress, we are still unable to provide any incontrovertible evidence of either what causes mental distress or how it can be treated effectively. There is, though, a considerable body of circumstantial evidence which suggests that mental distress is the product of interplay between various psychological, social, political, environmental and biological factors. Regrettably, few mental health professionals are willing to take account of all these factors. (Coppock & Hopton, 2000: 10)

Since the introduction of more critical theoretical understandings in the 1960s and 1970s, theoretical understanding of mental illness has been located in socio-politics and the power of mental health workers to define 'normality' and 'abnormality' is questioned. The fluctuating, ambiguous and culturally relative nature of professional understandings has been highlighted to reveal how mental disorder is related to social divisions based on gender, class, religion, sexuality, age and ethnic origins.

Whereas differences in patterns of mental health and illness had traditionally been attributed to the inherently flawed 'nature' or vulnerability of certain individuals or groups, attention turned to the significance of oppressive social relations and the social construction of health and illness. (Coppock & Hopton, 2000: 90)

Gender

Contrary to popular belief, gender is not biologically determined. Gender refers to socially constructed roles, attributes and behaviours that a society deems acceptable for men and women to adopt (WHO, 2010). Such roles are not determined by biology, but by societal norms. For instance in Saudi Arabia, women are not permitted to drive, yet in the United Kingdom (UK) women can drive; this is not a biologically determined role but one based on a cultural value. 'Sex' is a medical term which refers to biological sex and takes into account secondary sexual characteristics and biological determinants such as chromosomes for the basis of determining an individual's 'sex'. The difference between 'gender' and biologically determined 'sex' can be seen in the case of individuals who are transgendered; an individual's biological sex from birth will be at odds with the expression of their gender role in society. Therefore, gender, it is argued, is a social construct (Thompson, 2006).

It has been argued that in a patriarchal society where masculinity is privileged and femininity devalued, women are more likely to attract a diagnosis of mental disorder, whether they conform to or depart from their sex-role stereotype (Busfield, 1996). This argument proposes that feminine characteristics are associated with weakness and mental ill health, but if women express traits perceived as 'masculine', such as anger, this can be dismissed as an unhealthy deviation from their natural state. Where women have been brought up with the expectation that they should be socially passive, any

---

Box 11.2   Past abuses

The dominance of medical discourse in women's lives as a whole has been mirrored in the response to women's madness in which biology has legitimated 'treatments' from cliloridectomy, sterilization, hysterectomy, through to lobotomy, insulin therapy, electro-convulsive therapy (ECT) and psychotropic medication. Women are twice as likely to be prescribed psychotropic medication and are more likely to receive ECT. (Coppock & Hopton, 2000: 99)

---

depressive feelings associated with this state can also be dismissed as a lack of adjustment to an expected role (Sheppard, 1991). So it is claimed that complex forms of social positioning and devaluing of personal experience act to place women outside of mainstream society, which has traditionally been a male domain. Reflexive supervision can be useful in helping workers consider their own position in relation to the service user and healthcare systems that can sometimes seem particularly patriarchal (Hawes, 1998). Patriarchy can be seen in the assignment of roles based on gender in society, for example the traditional view of 'women staying at home to look after children while men go to work', such a view is based on a perception that such roles are biologically determined and, therefore, are 'natural', despite evidence to the contrary (Thompson, 2006).

It is difficult to overcome established cultural inequalities. For example, welfare benefits can bring women financial independence from men, but patriarchal ideologies can then trap them in the domestic sphere, where they care for children and the home. Meanwhile unemployed men might then be excluded from both home and work and perhaps the modern stereotype of an 'outsider' is, therefore, an emotionally crippled ineffectual male who loses control; the 'psycho-killer' of popular fiction (Sayce, 2000). However, women with severe mental health problems can be just as excluded, losing parenting roles and associated identity, for example. Children are taken into the care of the local authority during periods when their mother's mental health is thought to put them at risk. So, while men who endure discrimination are expected to exhibit their masculinity through violent and risk-taking behaviour, women are expected to defer to the needs of others and they more often internalise their distress in self-harming behaviours (Rosenfield et al., 2006). In working to support service users in their relationships with other people, assertive outreach workers will encounter ideas about social stereotypes both in the attitudes of the general public and in the policies that govern their work (Hallam, 2002). In working to challenge these stereotypes, assertive outreach workers might collaborate with families and friends, with charities, community development projects or with other agencies where the interest of disadvantaged social groups are advanced. This can be described as 'community psychology' (Meddings et al., 2010). Assertive outreach might employ these principles in their work with women's groups (Holland, 1992), for example (see Box 11.2).

It is inevitable that people will experience difficult life events, but if they have been brought up with patriarchal 'idealised' notions of gender roles, these cultural ideals can act like a double-edged sword (Mahalingam & Jackson, 2007). These ideals provide a

---

Box 11.3   The impact of domestic violence

Domestic violence can include rape, assault, torture, imprisonment, psychological or emotional abuse (this includes continual threats, sleep deprivation, constant undermining of confidence and displays of total power). The violence is carried out by husbands, boyfriends, fathers, brothers, sons and other relations. In many cases this violence is similar to the conditions experienced in concentration camps, which is known to cause hallucinations and thought disorder. Women who experience violence often have to endure many episodes of trauma carried out by men that are known to them. These events can re-occur at anytime that the woman is in contact with the man, and so they can have the constant threat of this violence hanging over them which is extremely stressful. (Meadow, 2001: 86)

---

powerful cultural referent to which men and women aspire, often boosting their self pride, but the pressures of living up to expectations can create a sense of shame, leading to depression. These common 'identity problems' are heightened for individuals who have experienced significant abuse. The experience of hearing voices has been associated with a trauma history (Read & Ross, 2003), such as rape, assault or torture, often in the context of ongoing domestic violence (see Box 11.3). The abuse continues to be 'spoken by different voices, splintered inside yourself, which are memories and beliefs implanted by such constant abuse' (Meadow, 2001: 86).

The gender of a worker does have an impact on the therapeutic relationship (McCabe & Priebe, 2004). However, in assertive outreach there is a whole team approach with contacts made by several workers, so problems can be identified and addressed. Some users of assertive outreach services may reject the services of a worker based on their gender, for instance, we have had experience of instances where service users have requested male only workers or female only workers. On the surface such instances can seem discriminatory, however, negative life experiences have contributed to a negative view of specific genders, and such firm beliefs are hard to modify. An approach that seeks to investigate an individual's view of gender roles and gradually (and sensitively) expose them to either gender can help in developing alternative beliefs of males or females and reduce generalised views based on experiences or culturally inherited beliefs of gender roles. This can also assist an individual in developing skills in interacting with others and developing a flexible view of individuals in their local communities.

Social class

Research has shown that people who were born into deprived families with a father of a lower social class are more likely to develop psychotic illness (Harrison et al., 2001). Other associated indicators of poverty and perceived social exclusion include rented housing, parental unemployment, claiming welfare and single parent households (van Os et al., 2000; Wicks et al., 2005). Previous chapters have highlighted ongoing social exclusion as both a contributing factor and an outcome of suffering severe mental illness.

A question is raised in Chapter 9 as to whether it might not be better to work at resolving inequalities in society rather than simply 'treating the symptoms'. While some people do overcome their difficulties to achieve successful lives in society, social deprivation can have a devastating effect on others. Some of the people who are supported by assertive outreach teams are unable to manage finances or maintain possessions. We find that money is spent or just given away on the day that the welfare payment is made; the person is unable to assertively resist the demands of their peers. If someone has never owned anything of any value for very long and lives from day to day, it is often much simpler for them to subsist on handouts, by begging, or attending charity services.

Survey evidence shows that Britons living in more deprived conditions have lower subjective expectations of life, less interest in their health or in the future, and increased belief in the role of chance in determining health (Wardle & Steptoe, 2003). It is not surprising, therefore, that people living in these conditions are more often admitted to psychiatric hospital (Brooker et al., 2007). However, assertive outreach teams are likely to take referrals where people are isolated and excluded in unusual circumstances. Where teams serve rural commuter populations for example, people who are unable to maintain well paid employment are likely to be priced out of accommodation, unless they have family support. So, although a person might have enjoyed a privileged upbringing, the stigma of failing in social networks where expectations are extremely high increases distress, isolation and uncomfortable reliance on others. People who are different can be more visible and isolated in rural or suburban areas and it is often the assertive outreach team that works to achieve engagement in these difficult settings, mediating complex family and neighbourhood tensions. But if a person who suffers severe and enduring mental health problems is unable to sustain their existence in middle class communities, they tend to drift into urban settings where accommodation is cheaper and again it is likely to be an assertive outreach team that will be looking out for them.

Social stratification is often associated with cultural, religious or racial divides (Muntaner et al., 2004) and links between racial stratification and particular symptoms are discussed in Chapter 10. This is another setting where, assertive outreach teams will be applying principles from community psychology, in establishing their understanding of local settings. These teams have made practical interventions their priority, in helping service users avoid the harsher effects of deprivation, but have also offered psychological therapies. It is important to feel empathy where service users are constrained by their circumstances, but to still have confidence in their ability to make self-empowering choices. It is recognised that although poverty places limits on the options open to an individual, that person can still make choices which will either protect their mental health or undermine it; see Box 11.4 (also see Muntaner et al., 2000). So teams can work to lessen the impact of social deprivation, but following a recovery model, they must encourage service users to make choices that enhance their well-being and improve their quality of life. Care is needed in this work to ensure that service users are able to take up real life opportunities, rather than recording an illusionary choice, as if structural constraints simply do not exist; it is very easy to 'blame the victim' for their failure to succeed.

Poverty is relative and it is often said that due to the availability of welfare benefits, people in our Western societies no longer have any real understanding of deprivation. People are considered to be poor even when they have furniture, electrical goods and food

---

Box 11.4 Exercising constrained choice

The structural constraints-choice issue... refers to whether the effects of social inequalities on mental health are due to free will or to forces beyond individual or
group control. 'Choice' refers to the capacity of individuals or groups to make independent decisions and act upon their environment with consequences for their
mental health (e.g. 'people choose to use heroin'), while 'structural constraints' refer
to the social environment that determines or puts limits on people's mental health
(e.g. 'the stresses of poverty enhance the relative appeal of heroin'). (Muntaner
et al., 2004: 102)

---

to eat. However, many of us who work in assertive outreach teams will have had the experience of helping a service user through their discharge from acute psychiatric hospital;
where their entire 'worldly possessions' are contained within a black dustbin bag provided
by the hospital. We have taken the patient from the hospital to temporary hostel accommodation, wondering how to help this person to start building a life for themselves.

Religious belief

As discussed in previous chapters, assertive outreach teams do not simply record information such as religious belief as background information. Developing an understanding
of the service user and the way that they live their life is important in achieving engagement. Religious belief is also likely to influence a person's attitude towards symptoms,
their coping style, their willingness to accept help and the nature of their recovery. So it
might be useful to employ cognitive theory based psychological therapies in exploring the
pragmatic aspects of religious belief. There is an expectation in the UK that workers
should act to meet the spiritual needs of the people who make use of their services and
people who claim to hold spiritual beliefs achieve better recovery from illness (NHS
Education for Scotland, 2006; Department of Health, 2009). However, religious belief is
more than just an expression of different ways of thinking and teams will not be able to
avoid discussion of moral conduct and the ethics of different interventions (see the section on ethics below).

   Teams face a dilemma in encouraging service users to engage with religious communities. This involvement might strengthen beliefs that act against the scientific rationale for
maintaining compliance with treatment. In our psychiatric understandings we might view
symptoms such as auditory hallucinations as meaningless outcomes of dysfunctional biological systems, (see Case study 11.3). Some religious groups promote different meanings and conflict can develop. Sayce (2000) has been critical of some religious belief
systems, observing that 'Traditionally, Christianity holds that sin and the devil are the
origin of most psychosis' (Sayce, 2000: 53) and 'Christian literature associates mental
illness with sin and it portrays recovery as "turning to God"' (Sayce, 2000: 54). However,
as with other aspects of the service user's life, teams often find themselves working with
religious groups and faith leaders in their efforts to sustain community living (see Box 11.5
for religious coping styles). So it is problematic when a service user experiences symptoms

---

Box 11.5   Religious coping styles

- Collaborative problem solving styles such as membership of a religious community and engagement in regular shared activities, have been linked to greater general psychological competence (Harthaway & Pargament, 1990). In situations of higher stress, this membership has been found to improve symptoms of depression (Bickel et al., 1998). It is associated with greater involvement in recovery-enhancing activities and increased empowerment (Yangarber-Hicks, 2004).
- Deferring religious coping methods such as 'a way forward will be found for me' have been related to lower levels of psychological resourcefulness (Harthaway & Pargament, 1990), but in situations where the individual has little control over stressful circumstances, this can be a helpful coping strategy (Pargament, 1997). This approach is also associated with improved quality of life (Yangarber-Hicks, 2004).
- Self-directing problem solving styles, such as 'we must do something because we will be held to account', have been linked to greater general psychological competence, but have also been associated with anxiety and depression (Bickel et al., 1998).
- Being passive and pleading for 'divine intervention' has been linked to experiencing greater distress (Pargament et al., 2000).

---

such as elated mood and delusions which are expressed in religious terms. Their fellow believers can become very distressed when a service user claims a strange or special religious significance. Assertive outreach workers can find themselves involved in difficult and emotive debates and whether they follow a faith or not themselves, this can be very difficult.

Sexuality

In modern Western societies attitudes toward sexual activity have changed so that unmarried women are no longer placed in asylums for becoming pregnant and homosexuality is no longer considered a mental health disorder for which aversion therapy is an appropriate treatment. Admissions to hospital are now usually brief and patients who have mental capacity continue to have a 'right to family life' along with its associated sexual activities. Progressive modernisation has brought about the closure of the gender segregated Victorian asylums, but now, it is 'mixed wards' that are the target of reformers. In acute wards, it can be difficult to manage the promiscuous or 'predatory' aspects of sexual behaviour, in a setting where service users can be very vulnerable (Thomas et al., 1995). Also, it cannot be assumed that mental health workers will not be drawn into patterns of abuse and exploitation related to sexuality and it is essential that service users are treated seriously when they disclose distressing experiences. These matters should be investigated using structures such as Safeguarding Vulnerable Adults (in England and Wales).

This relationship between sexuality and mental health is another example of social, psychological and biological complexity. In England and Wales, King et al. (2003) surveyed 1086 gay, lesbian and bisexual people. It was found that there were inequalities in mental health and oppressive practices from services (when seeking mental health support) were identified problems. It appeared that these associations were an outcome of discrimination

---

Box 11.6   The use of advanced directives to managed disturbed sexuality

A service user who expressed ambiguous thoughts about her sexuality was particularly distressed by her sexual conduct at times when she suffered from an elated mood. This woman usually enjoyed stable monogamous relationships, but during periods of treatment at the local acute psychiatric hospital, she engaged in sexual intercourse with several other patients. This problem was solved when the assertive outreach team agreed an advance directive. The plan made the statement that hospital staff would intervene to prevent her from engaging in these 'out of character' sexual activities during subsequent admissions.

---

from a personal, structural and/or cultural basis related to sexuality. There is a danger that health professionals may pathologise homosexuality (Neal & Davies, 2003) and gay experiences may be subject to heterosexist judgements (Faria, 1997) when judging the sexual preferences and lifestyles of service users. For instance, one only has to look at the diagnosis of borderline personality disorder to see how sexual orientation can be legitimately pathologised in a diagnostic category (Zucker, 1996), particularly when sexual behaviour and preference doesn't meet our own cultural norms. However, assertive outreach teams are well positioned to develop a therapeutic relationship which is anti-oppressive, non-judgemental and allows users to explore issues with sexuality (see Case study 11.2).

Case study 11.2   A practice example – 'Sandra'

Sandra is struggling with her emotions, she recently attended A&E as she cut herself several times and has been drinking large amounts of alcohol. She finds it difficult discussing issues with the team and there is a risk of disengagement. She developed a good rapport with one worker and has opened up stating she doesn't know whether she is gay or straight and is embarrassed and ashamed of the possibility of being gay, but feels she wants to talk to someone about it. The team discuss Sandra's problem, provide her with psycho-sexual support from the psychologist and then provide her with the number for the local gay and lesbian switchboard, where they run a telephone counselling service. Sandra starts calling the switchboard with some support from the team. In the weeks following this intervention, Sandra starts to gain trust in the team, she is engaging more with the team's visits and her cutting behaviour stops.

As discussed in Chapter 9, a conceptual framework can be developed for understanding increased mental health problems in terms of 'minority stress'. Stigma, prejudice, and discrimination can create a hostile and stressful social environment that causes mental health problems. Complex stress processes might be acting, including expectations of rejection, hiding and concealing, internalised homophobia, and ameliorative coping processes (Meyer, 2003). Again the difficulties associated with sexuality might be linked to other experiences of exclusion such as poverty and ethnic minority origins (Diaz et al., 2001). On the other hand, membership of an oppressed group can bring people together. Sharing experiences can foster a supportive environment in which people become more motivated to resist oppression and advocate for the meeting of specific needs relevant to

---

Box 11.7   The power of group action

The organisations that originally responded to HIV/AIDS were set up by gay men, for gay men. While governments were often obstinate and reticent, or even obstructive, gay men invented and promoted safer sex, providing non-statutory support for those who became ill. The organisations that gay men set up enabled them, as a network of communities to face and overcome both the AIDS epidemic and the associated institutionalised homophobia. (Flowers & Langdridge, 2007: 684)

the lesbian and gay communities have ... found ways of arguing both for 'getting the government out of the bedroom' and for obtaining government funds, and have pushed for anti-discrimination provision in work, insurance and other areas of 'private' life. (Sayce, 2000, 128)

---

the group (see Box 11.7). People who are referred to assertive outreach teams often have difficulties in feeling part of a group and extra support might be needed to help them make use of the advocacy that would be available to them, if they could form relationships with others.

In their response to different sexualities, workers in assertive outreach will again be working against the promotion of negative stereotypical ideas in their work with members of minority groups. Health promotion will be part of their role, however, this will not be just the provision of practical 'safe-sex' knowledge, but also the promotion of political understanding. For example, 'HIV/AIDS is a global epidemic primarily affecting heterosexuals ... It is associated with poverty, war, societal breakdown (often associated with debt-crises), political change ... and the crossboarder movements of peoples in search of greater economic security' (Flowers & Langdridge, 2007: 685).

The ethics of diversity in assertive outreach

The ethics of assertive outreach work are discussed throughout this book and particularly in Chapter 12. Concerns have been highlighted as to whether 'assertive' might sometimes mean intrusive or work against diversity. In the UK, workers follow policy under mental health law for assessing the service user's capacity to choose to refuse treatment and associated services, balanced against the evidence for risk. Human rights are applied with the principle of proportionality, where one right is balanced against another. However, if we are perceived to be delivering some form of psychological therapy, the issue of gaining informed consent is brought to the fore (Gray & Johanson, 2010). 'Choice' and 'consent' are contentious issues in this setting. In using a multi-professional approach it is not always clear whether a team is trying to 'change the individual', or change their 'social environment', or, there might be a process by which a service user from an ethnic minority background is being acculturated to our society.

As discussed in Chapter 10, much emphasis is placed on individual choice in our society and making people choose when they are unaccustomed to this freedom can cause distress. Sometimes we do not know whether a person has chosen to refuse help, or if they

---

Box 11.8   Practice Example – choice and responsibility

Sam tells his assertive outreach workers that he has a problem with voices telling him to do things. He feels that he is being watched and his actions are controlled. In team handovers we agree that it is important for Sam that he should feel more able to make his own choices. It is suggested that the amount of medication that is prescribed should be increased, but Sam says the medication sedates him and he feels that he lacks volition while he is taking it. It is suggested that, because his medication is not effectively treating his symptoms, the team must see him more often, but Sam says that this increases his feelings of being watched and he mentions past occasions when our colleagues have taken his choices away by detaining him and giving him medication against his will. The team tries to agree a 'recovery plan,' but Sam says he does not want to be part of society, he says he is different from other people; he wants to be left alone to 'do his own thing'.

In a formulation meeting, the team considers the fact that Sam has committed minor crimes on several occasions, but because it has been thought that his illness prevents him from making rational decisions, he has not been prosecuted. At a review meeting workers talk with Sam about the issue of criminal responsibility. It is agreed that he can choose to remain on his current treatment but must accept more support in finding ways to manage his symptoms. It is agreed that if he breaks the law again, the team will support him through the processes of arrest, charges and court appearance. It is agreed that if he wants freedom to choose he must accept responsibility for the choices that he makes and this agreement is recorded in his care plan.

---

are just pre-empting what they believe will be a further rejection by society, or, do they simply not understand what we are asking of with them. Patient perseverance, supported by team reflection, is usually the way forward and team reflection often attends to the behaviour of the service user which can be at odds with what that person is saying.

In their efforts to avoid oppressive interventions, teams often try to ensure that service users have choices. However, increased choice also brings increased responsibility (see Box 11.8). There are principles which guide the work of assertive outreach teams. For example, teams might reflect on the question of; 'to whom does the care plan belong'? Or, are the goals recorded in this plan our goals or those of the service user. If workers are left with feelings of anxiety and concern when they go home at the end of the day, then the therapeutic relationship is not working; 'ownership' of these feelings needs to be handed back to the service user. Service users are more likely to achieve recovery goals and remain safe when a strong therapeutic relationship has been fostered and honest discussions can be held. Assertive outreach teams have the luxury of long-term working within which to negotiate genuine recovery goals. By including service users in risk assessments, workers can help them 'contain' their own anxiety and responsibility, which will motivate them to remain safe and work towards achieving their goals.

We face a difficult task in mental healthcare in that we must 'embrace diversity' and value the views of those who are dismissed by mainstream society due to their mental distress. As discussed in Chapter 12, some members of the team might want to take action to 'persuade', 'threaten' or 'compel' Sam (who is described in Box 11.8) into taking more medication. His criminal behaviour may well be an outcome of untreated illness and while we might have hope that recovery is possible, as discussed in Chapter 8, this could remain more of an aspiration than a reality.

Box 11.9   Diverse understandings of the experience of hearing voices

- Hearing voices is just a symptom of illness, so the content of the internal speech has no meaning and should be dismissed. Attending to voices would cause distress and is a disabling distraction (Tyrer & Steinberg, 1993).
- Hearing voices is an experience of Extra Sensory Perception or shared consciousness, through which important messages are communicated in a manner that is only accessible to a few people (de Valda, 2001).
- Hearing voices is a misattribution of the source of an internal dialogue. Attending to voices is unnecessary because they are just random thoughts, but if it helps, a person can listen to them and then challenge the rationality of their contents (Bentall, 2004).
- Hearing voices is caused by experiences of trauma, such as rape, assault or torture, in contexts such as ongoing domestic violence. Different internal voices are splintered memories and beliefs implanted by abusers (Meadow, 2001).
- Hearing voices may be understood as an unconscious attempt to eliminate, in fantasy, the unbearable reality of one's own thoughts (Martindale, 2007).
- Hearing voices is a higher order experience of spiritual guides or a lower order experience of demonic torturers (Steer, 2001).

Many teams will struggle with colleagues who take a firm stance on divisive issues. There is a movement against the power of pharmaceutical companies, for example, in which the promotion of free gifts with drugs company logos is treated with suspicion. There is another movement against the use of the term 'schizophrenia', which it is claimed, is an inaccurate term bringing stigma rather than understanding to our practice. It is not helpful to foster conflict but if teams can adopt an open and accepting approach to their work, these debates can be managed and it is often helpful to service users to feel that they are involved in evaluation and reform of services, part of the debate, rather than just subject to it. (See Box 11.9 for diverse understandings of the experience of hearing voices.)

Conclusion

Assertive outreach teams cannot deliver 'off the shelf' interventions. It is important to remember that the way that we talk, in many ways, constructs the objects that we observe. Our narratives can turn our service users into hopeless victims of social injustice, or determined survivors who resist oppression. Following the strong principles of hope and social inclusion that are expressed in assertive outreach, it need not be assumed that difference equals danger or vulnerability. It could be recognised that everyone has strengths or abilities and can find opportunities for positive growth through which they will improve the quality of their life.

Oppressive practices can be all too familiar for teams and can go unnoticed. However, we have discussed and introduced PCS analysis as a way of understanding how oppressive practices can develop. Such awareness can hopefully assist teams to reflect and develop anti-oppressive practices, which can help teams manage the 'cultural drivers' in their teams. Teams can also provide a supportive culture in which individual interpersonal development can take place and staff can appreciate 'difference' in a positive way. This can arguably contribute to a healthy team culture and healthier relationships with service users in supporting the choices they make in life.

The world in which assertive outreach staff members work is complex. Research can neatly divide subjects into categories, but as we go out to encounter the worlds that our service users inhabit, we can face overwhelming confusion. For example, our experience of ethnicity is gendered and gender relations are ethnically distinct and impacted by social class (Barn, 2008). Assertive outreach teams have a unique opportunity in their long-term work to achieve a more detailed understanding of each different service user. So, rather than imposing simplistic notions, this sophisticated understanding gives value to diverse and contrasting points of view, providing more opportunity to affirm and give positive meaning in our work.

References

Barn, R. (2008) Ethnicity, gender and mental health: social worker perspectives. *International Journal of Social Psychiatry*, **54**(1), 69–82.

Bentall, R.P. (2004) *Madness Explained: Psychosis and Human Nature*. Penguin Books, London.

Bickel, C.O., Ciarrocchi, J.W., Sheers, N.J., Estadt, B.K., Powell, D.A. & Pargament, K.I. (1998) Perceived stress, religious coping styles, and depressive affect. *Journal of Psychology and Christianity*, **17**(1), 33–42.

Blofeld, J. (2003) *Independent Inquiry into the Death of David Bennett. An Independent Inquiry set up under HSG(94)27*. Norfolk, Suffolk, and Cambridgeshire Strategic Health Authority, Cambridge.

Brooker, C., Ricketts, T., Bennett, S. & Lemme, F. (2007) Admission decisions following contact with an emergency mental health assessment and intervention service. *Journal of Clinical Nursing*, **16**(7), 1313–1322.

Busfield, J. (1996) *Men, Women and Madness: Understanding Gender and Mental Disorder*. Macmillan, Basingstoke.

Coppock, V. & Hopton, J. (2000) *Critical Perspectives on Mental Health*. Routledge, London.

Crisp, A.H., Rix, S., Meltzer, H.I. & Rowlands, O.J. (2000) Stigmatisation of people with mental illnesses. *The British Journal of Psychiatry*, **177**, 4–7.

Delgadon, R. & Stefancic, J. (2000) *Critical Race Theory: The Cutting Edge*, 2nd edn. Temple University Press, Philadelphia.

Department of Health (2009) Religion or Belief: A Practical Guide for the NHS. Department of Health, London.

Diaz, R.M., Ayala, G., Bein, E., Henne, J. & Marin, B.V. (2001) The impact of homophobia, poverty, and racism on the mental health of gay and bisexual Latino men: findings form 3 US cities. *American Journal of Public Health*, **91**(6), 927–932.

Faria, G. (1997) The Challenge of Health Care Social Work with Gay Men and Lesbians In: G.K. Auslander, *International Perspectives on Social Work in Health Care*, (ed. G.K. Auslander). pp. 65–72. Haworth Press, New York.

Flowers, P. & Langdridge, D. (2007) Offending the other: deconstructing narratives of deviance and pathology. *British Journal of Social Psychology*, **46**, 679–690.

Gillespie, M. & Meaden, A. (2010) Psychological Processes in Engagement. In: *Reaching Out: The Psychology of Assertive Outreach*, (ed. C. Cupitt). pp.15–42. Routledge, Hove.

Gray, A. & Johanson, P. (2010) Ethics and Professional Issues: The Universal and the Particular. In: *Reaching Out: The Psychology of Assertive Outreach*, (ed. C. Cupitt). pp. 229–247. Routledge, Hove.

Hallam, A. (2002) Media influences on mental health policy: long-term effects of the Clunis and Silcock cases. *International Review of Psychiatry*, **14**(1), 26–33.

Harrison, G., Gunnell, D., Glazebrook, C. Page, K. & Kwiecinski, R. (2001) Association between schizophrenia and social inequality at birth: case-control study. *British Journal of Psychiatry*, **179**, 346–350.

Harthaway, W.L. & Pargament, K.I. (1990) Intrinsic religiousness, religious coping, and psychosocial competence: a covariance structure analysis. *Journal for Scientific Study of Religion*, **29**(4), 423–441.

Hawes, S.E. (1998) Positioning a Dialogic Reflexivity in the Practice of Feminist Supervision. In: *Reconstructing the Psychological Subject: Bodies, Practices and Technologies*, (eds. B.M. Bayer & J. Shotter). pp. 94–110. London, Sage.

Holland, S. (1992) From Social Abuse to Social Action: A Neighbourhood Psycho-Therapy and Social Action Project for Women. In: *Gender Issues in Clinical Psychology*, (eds. J. Usher & P, Nicholson). pp. 66–77. Routledge, London.

King, M., McKewon, E., Warner, J., Ramsay, A., Johnson, K. & Cort, C. (2003) Mental health and quality of life of gay men and lesbians in England and Wales. *British Journal of Psychiatry*, **183**, 552–558.

Large, M., Smith, G., Swinson, N., Shaw, J. & Nielsson, O. (2008) Homicide due to mental disorder in England and Wales over 50 years. *The British Journal of Psychiatry*, **193**, 130–133.

Mahalingam, R. & Jackson, B. (2007) Idealized cultural beliefs about gender: implications for mental health. *Social Psychiatry Psychiatric Epidemiology*, **42**, 1012–1023.

Martindale, B.V. (2007) Psychodynamic contributions to early intervention in psychosis. *Advances in Psychiatric Treatment*, **13**, 24–42.

McCabe, R., & Priebe, S. (2004) The therapeutic relationship in the treatment of severe mental illness: a review of methods and findings. *International Journal of Social Psychiatry*, **50**, 115–128.

Meadow, K. (2001) Violence and Voices. In: *Raising Our Voices: An Account of the Hearing Voices Movement*, (ed. A. James). pp. 86–88. Handsell Publishing, Gloucester.

Meddings, S., Shaw, B. & Diamond, B. (2010) Community Psychology. *In: Reaching Out: The Psychology of Assertive Outreach*, (ed. C. Cupitt). pp. 207–228. Hove, Routledge.

Meyer, I.H. (2003) Prejudice, social stress, and mental health in lesbian, gay, and bisexual populations: conceptual issues and research evidence. *Psychological Bulletin*, **129**(5), 674–697.

Muntaner, C., Eaton, W.W. & Diala, C. (2000) Socioeconomic inequalities in mental health: a review of concepts and underlying assumptions. *Health*, **4**, 82–106.

Muntaner, C., Eaton, W.W., Miech, R. & O'Campo, P. (2004) Socioeconomic position and major mental disorders. *Epidemiologic Reviews*, **26**, 53–62.

Neal, C. & Davies, D. (2003) A Historical Overview of Homosexuality and Therapy In: *Pink Therapy. A Guide for Counsellors and Therapists Working with Lesbian, Gay and Bisexual Clients*, 5th edn, (eds. D. Davies & C. Neal). pp. 11–23. The Open University Press, Berkshire.

ODPM (2004) *Mental Health and Social Exclusion: Social Exclusion Unit Report*. Social Exclusion Unit, Office of the Deputy Prime Minster, London.

NHS Education for Scotland (2006) Spiritual Care Matters: An Introductory Resource for all NHSS Staff. NHS Education for Scotland, Edinburgh.

van Os, J., Driessen, G., Gunther, N. & Delespaul, P. (2000) Neighbourhood variation in incidence of schizophrenic. *British Journal of Psychology*, **176**, 243–248.

Pargament, K.I. (1997) *The Psychology of Religion and Coping: Theory, Research, Practice*. The Guilford Press, New York.

Pargament, K.I., Koenig, H.G. & Perez, L.M. (2000) The many methods of religious coping: development and initial validation of the RCOPE. *Journal of Clinical Psychology*, **56**(4), 519–543.

Rapp, C.A. & Goscha, R.J. (2006) *The Strengths Model: Case Management with People with Psychiatric Disabilities*, 2nd edn. Oxford University Press, New York.

Read, J. & Ross, C.A. (2003) Psychological trauma and psychosis: another reason why people diagnosed schizophrenic must be offered psychological therapies. *Journal of American Academy of Psychoanalysis and Dynamic Psychiatry*, **31**(1), 247–268.

Rose, D. (1998) Television, madness and community care. *Journal of Community & Applied Social Psychology*, **8**, 213–228.

Rosenfield, S., Phillips, J. & White, H. (2006) Gender, race, and the self in mental health and crime. *Social Problems*, **53**(2), 161–185.

Sayce, L. (2000) *From Psychiatric Patient to Citizen: Overcoming Discrimination and Social Exclusion*. MacMillan Press, Basingstoke.

Sheppard, M. (1991) General practice, social work and mental health sections: the social control of women. *British Journal of Social Work*, **21**, 663–683.

Special Hospital Services Authority (1993) *Report of the Committee of Inquiry into the Death in Broadmoor Hospital of Orville Blackwood and a Review of the Deaths of Two other Afro-Carribbean patients: 'Big, Black & Dangerous'* Special Hospital Services Authority, London.

Steer, M. (2001) Creative Voices. In: *Raising Our Voices: An Account of the Hearing Voices Movement*, (ed. A. James). pp. 74–82. Handsell Publishing, Gloucester.

Taylor P.J. & Gunn, J. (1999) Homicides by people with mental illness: myth and reality. *The British Journal of Psychiatry*, **174**, 9–14.

Thomas, C., Bartlett, A. & Mezey, G.C. (1995) The extent and effect of violence among psychiatric in-patients. *Psychiatric Bulletin*, **19**, 600–604.

Thompson, N. (2003) *Promoting Equality*, 2nd edn. Hampshire, Palgrave Macmillan.

Thompson, N. (2006) *Anti Discriminatory Practice*. Hampshire, Palgrave Macmillan.

Tyrer, P. & Steinberg, D. (1993) *Models for Mental Disorder, Conceptual Models in Psychiatry*. Chichester, John Wiley & Sons.

de Valda, M. (2001) Mind as computer. In: *Raising Our Voices: An Account of the Hearing Voices Movement*, (ed. A. James). pp. 83–85. Handsell Publishing, Gloucester.

Wardle, J. & Steptoe, A. (2003) Socioeconomic differences in attitudes and beliefs about healthy lifestyles. *Journal of Epidemiology and Community Health*, **57**(6), 440–443.

WHO (2010) *What do we mean by sex and gender?* Fact Sheet, World Heath Organisation. http://www.who.int/gender/whatisgender/en/index.html

Wicks, S., Hjern, A., Gunnell, D., Lewis, G. & Dalman, C. (2005) Social adversity in childhood and the risk of developing psychosis: a national cohort study. *American Journal of Psychiatry*, **162**, 1652–1657.

Yangarber-Hicks, N. (2004) Religious coping styles and recovery from serious mental illness. *Journal of Psychology and Theology*, **32**(4), 305–317.

Zucker, K.J. (1996) Letters to the editor. Sexism and heterosexism in the diagnostic interview for borderline patients? *American Journal of Psychiatry*, **153**(7), 966.

Chapter 12

Personal autonomy, leverage and coercion

Mike Firn and Andrew Molodynski

Introduction

Issues of public protection, private distress, choice and free will are central to mental health practice and come into particularly sharp focus in acute, intensive and forensic services. In the United States assertive community treatment (ACT) was developed as a way of reaching people who were high users of inpatient care due to frequent relapse and disengagement from standard services. In England the policy to develop assertive outreach was precipitated at least in part by government concerns over highly publicised homicides, involving mentally ill patients in the community who had avoided or been excluded from services. At the heart of assertive outreach practice is the dilemma of delivering a service to people who are ambivalent about receiving it or actively refusing it and are, for the most part, not legally bound to accept it (Williamson, 2002).

Practice has moved beyond mere supervision and monitoring and teams, carers and service users are routinely faced with hard decisions about detention, capacity, best interest and coercion. The new mental health legislation for England and Wales in 2007 (Department of Health, 2007) has strengthened compulsory treatment in community settings, despite the mixed evidence from research carried out in parts of the world where similar powers have been available for some time.

The chapter starts by considering the ethical context of assertive outreach and then discusses the range of formal and informal tactics routinely used in practice, which can impact on a service user's personal autonomy. These have been categorised as a 'hierarchy of treatment pressures' (Szmukler & Appelbaum, 2008), starting with persuasion and proceeding all the way through to coercion. Brief case studies will be used to illustrate this. Studies have shown that treatment expectations and the nature of the therapeutic relationship affect the subjective experience of coercion and that perceived coercion does not simply correlate with applied coercion (Monahan et al., 2005).

How can assertive outreach services negotiate these ethical considerations maturely against a range of ideological and moral stances, within mental health services and across society, while at the same time keeping as their central concern the long-term well-being of service users? When does push become shove? When is concern overly paternalistic?

Assertive Outreach in Mental Healthcare: Current Perspectives, First Edition. Edited by C. Williams, M. Firn, S. Wharne and R. Macpherson.
© 2011 Blackwell Publishing Ltd. Published 2011 by Blackwell Publishing Ltd.

What can we learn from first person accounts from service users and carers and qualitative studies, to inform ethical, humane and defensible practice?

Personal autonomy

Selfishness is not living as one wishes to live; it is asking others to live as one wishes to live. And unselfishness is letting other people's lives alone, not interfering with them. Selfishness always aims at uniformity of type. Unselfishness recognises infinite variety of type as a delightful thing, accepts it, acquiesces in it, enjoys it. (Oscar Wilde)

Some of the most powerful voices from service users making a plea for personal autonomy are expletives and, therefore, unprintable. Mental health practitioners can face abuse in their daily practice and can be perceived as abusive. Assertive outreach can be portrayed as 'aggressive outreach'. It is the 'service that won't go away'. Service users who refuse treatment find themselves being contacted more frequently by professionals. The individual's reasons for refusal of the service may not result from impaired judgement due to the processes of mental illness, but as much from their prior experience of mental health services – what Morgan & Ryan (2004) described as the difference between the 'hard to engage client' and the 'hard to engage service'.

Practitioners are often faced with making decisions that may override the will of an individual in the typical 'intervention versus neglect' dilemma for public services. If you intervene at what point do you intervene? In most secular societies the right of personal autonomy is increasingly and popularly held as paramount. We sometimes selfishly forget that autonomy has two opposing sides. The *principle of autonomy* is that individuals in a given society should be permitted to have control over their own lives, so far as is compatible with other people having similar autonomy over their lives. There are many occasions where we sacrifice some of our own autonomy for the greater good. Taxation is a prime example as are other areas of state proscription and censorship. Our commitment to autonomy as an inviolable right does not hold if we view autonomy as a condition of persons largely constituted by our relations with others (Oshana, 2006). Mental health, child protection and euthanasia are examples where the state allows for personal choice and freedom to be legally overridden and each of these areas is politically and ethically controversial.

Assertive outreach has been described as 'therapeutic stalking' (Macmillan, 2005; Graham, 2006) and characterised as a vehicle for delivering social control to an already marginalised group. Just like a stalker the assertive outreach worker engages in surveillance, repeated and unsolicited letter writing and calling at the home, which may cause the 'target' distress. Just the type of behaviours that the England and Wales Protection from Harassment Act (1997) OPSI (1997) was introduced to criminalise. Fortunately the opening articles of the Act, shown in Box 12.1 to illustrate a legal framework, do allow assertive outreach workers the defence of showing that their behaviour was reasonable under the circumstances.

Similar language is used in other legislation and rests on phrases such as 'reasonable and appropriate' (Department of Health (2007)) in relation to the setting of condi-

---

Box 12.1   Protection from Harassment Act (1997)

Prohibition of harassment

(1) A person must not pursue a course of conduct—
    (a) which amounts to harassment of another, and
    (b) which he knows or ought to know amounts to harassment of the other.
(2) For the purposes of this section, the person whose course of conduct is in question ought to know that it amounts to harassment of another if a reasonable person in possession of the same information would think the course of conduct amounted to harassment of the other.
(3) Subsection(1)doesnotapplytoacourseofconductifthepersonwhopursueditshows—
    (a) that it was pursued for the purpose of preventing or detecting crime,
    (b) that it was pursued under any enactment or rule of law or to comply with any condition or requirement imposed by any person under any enactment, or
    (c) that in the particular circumstances the pursuit of the course of conduct was reasonable. (OPSI, 1997)

---

tions for community treatment orders in England and 'reasonable force' or 'the degree of force used was not disproportionate in the circumstances as he viewed them' (OPSI, 2008: 76(6)) used in defences for people who have fought off burglars when they believed they would be attacked. It has been argued that these imprecise phrases are designed as a source of lucrative employment for lawyers, yet they provide some markers against which to come to a judgement and for teams to debate alternative courses of action.

Shifting values

The values of medical and nursing professional codes of conduct are well known. They are based on ethical and moral optimums. These codes give primacy to the interests of patients, respect for individuals and detail the need to uphold confidentiality. Williamson (2002) concluded that traditional ethical constructs from professional codes are limited when it comes to some of the dilemmas faced in assertive outreach and that a more useful approach would be to consider the values expressed by individuals receiving the service and striving towards practice that meets with their approval and satisfaction. Morgan & Ryan (2004) go further, suggesting that in considering professional codes of conduct: 'an urge to adhere to a universally agreed set of values will only result in the loss of any sense of value diversity.' (Morgan & Ryan, 2004: 73). The concept of engagement, individually tailored care and the 'patient-led' agenda are central in assertive outreach and serve us well for the most part. Indeed it is the only way of ensuring recovery as a self determined outcome. However, if values are not fixed but vary across individuals, groups and contexts, this causes potentially infinite ethical dilemmas. Typically we do not have a clear right and wrong answer and often, in practice, we face making a choice of the 'least worst' alternatives.

Box 12.2   Puzzles problems and mess

- **Puzzles** are the simplest to resolve since there is a clear right answer that requires thought and logic or the application of a discipline specific accepted formula to determine. For example, an uncommon scenario where the team must seek advice on the right approach according to the legislative framework around consent to treatment or detention.
- **Problems** are where assumptions and resources become variables and an element of educated guesswork may be required. Here the value of the team approach in assertive outreach is appreciated. 'Two heads are better than one' is the aphorism. For example, there is a difference of opinion between the treating team and the family as to the suitability of a residential placement. The team is under pressure to discharge from hospital and no other alternatives have been sourced.
- **Mess** is where control and reason are of less use. The complexity is such that there may not even be agreement on definition of the problem and there are many dependent parts of the system contributing to the mess. (Gammack et al., 2007)

Box 12.3   Independent inquiry into the care and treatment of John Barrett (2006)

Too much confidence was placed in clinical judgements unsupported by evidence and rigorous analysis. Ways of working did not facilitate effective discussion and challenge of clinical views. There was a tendency to emphasise unduly the desirability of engaging John Barrett rather than intervening against his wishes to reduce risk. There was insufficient regard for legal and good practice requirements. (NHS, 2006: 9)

The panel found that the team misjudged the essential balance between managing risk and allowing liberty to John Barrett. Too much liberty was given to John Barrett, in spite of indications both immediate and historical that John Barrett was high risk and 'hard to read.' (NHS, 2006: 398)

Making decisions

One pragmatic attempt to construct a framework for analysis of these dilemmas is to use Ackoff's three classes (Gammack et al., 2007). As a systems thinker Ackoff recognised that 'better solutions to problems can be found by appreciating the whole system and finding a perspective beyond the narrow focus of a single part or discipline' (Gammack et al., 2007: 212). This is illustrated in Box 12.2.

For a team the task is to attempt to structure the situation and variables to reduce mess to problems and ultimately problems to puzzles. This may occur in small steps over time.

Teams fail when they lack the leadership to tackle these issues, or lack the means of communication within the team and throughout the system. They either avoid making decisions or become paralysed by the complexity of the task. The unfortunate case presented in Box 12.3 is from a forensic community service dealing with a man who was hard to engage, and consistently did not believe he was in need of treatment. The extract is from the independent inquiry into his care and treatment. The inquiry was prompted by his murder of a stranger innocently cycling through a local park in 2004. John Barrett suffered from paranoid schizophrenia and had been conditionally discharged to the community by a tribunal in 2003, following detention with restriction order from a criminal court for seriously injuring three people with a knife in 2002.

Principles

One of the most successful attempts to produce clear guidance and legislation in the area of formal mental health treatment has been the Scottish example. The Millan Committee (Scottish Executive, 2001) was tasked with examining the ethical basis of compulsory treatment as part of the review of legislation. The ten principles in Box 12.4, that came from a recommendation of this committee, cover four distinct areas of medical ethics: justice (recommendations 1–4), autonomy (5–7), beneficence and non-malificence (meaning to seek to do good and to do no harm, respectively; 8–10). These admirable Scottish principles were quoted often in the consultation for the English legislative changes but the resulting five principles in the English Code of Practice failed to adopt them so clearly (Department of Health, 2008). Furthermore, these are *guiding* principles, limited in their enforcement, abstract in nature and, therefore, subject to interpretation.

Coercion and compulsion in assertive outreach

Team members (for personal or theoretical reasons) often hold very different views about when it is appropriate to strongly encourage an individual to accept treatment or to compel them to do so. It is crucially important in such instances that teams can debate issues openly and effectively, with a common framework to discuss the dilemmas. The literature on coercion in mental health and assertive outreach is developing rapidly and reflects this variance of opinion (Stovall, 2001; Sheehan & Molodynski, 2007). Those who object to any form of influence or coercion in mental healthcare, such as Thomas Szasz (2007), are now relatively isolated voices but serve an important purpose by reminding us of the power imbalances inherent in our relationships with those under our care. Most of those involved in the care of the severely mentally ill would accept that treatment will at times be non consensual; there can be few assertive outreach patients who have not been admitted under legal powers at some point. Increasing attention is rightly being placed upon patients' perceptions of coercion and the effects these may have upon the therapeutic relationship, engagement with services and clinical and social outcomes. The area is complex, with difficult terminology at times, but the hierarchy proposed by Szmukler & Appelbaum (2008) is clear and concise and has proved useful to the authors in their clinical practice (see Figure 12.1).

As can be seen, the hierarchy represents a range of interactions, those at the beginning of the hierarchy being quite common in day to day practice, the use of inducements, threats and compulsion becoming progressively less prevalent, as well as more problematic. The hierarchy can be further illustrated by considering Case study 12.1.

Box 12.4 Statement of principles from the Millan Committee. Reproduced under the terms of the Click-Use Licence.

1. Non discrimination
People with mental disorder should whenever possible retain the same rights and entitlements as those with other health needs.

2. Equality
All powers under the Act should be exercised without any direct or indirect discrimination on the grounds of physical disability, age, gender, sexual orientation, race, colour, language, religion or national or ethnic or social origin.

3. Respect for diversity
Service users should receive care, treatment and support in a manner that accords respect for their individual qualities, abilities and diverse backgrounds and properly takes into account their age, gender, sexual orientation, ethnic group and social, cultural and religious background.

4. Reciprocity
Where society imposes an obligation on an individual to comply with a programme of treatment and care, it should impose a parallel obligation on the health and social care authorities to provide appropriate services, including ongoing care following discharge from compulsion.

5. Informal care
Wherever possible, care, treatment and support should be provided to people with mental disorder without recourse to compulsion.

6. Participation
Service users should be fully involved, to the extent permitted by their individual capacity, in all aspects of their assessment, care, treatment and support. Account should be taken of their past and present wishes, so far as they can be ascertained. Service users should be provided with all the information necessary to enable them to participate fully. All such information should be provided in a way which renders it most likely to be understood.

7. Respect for carers
Those who provide care to service users on an informal basis should receive respect for their role and experience, receive appropriate information and advice, and have their views and needs taken into account.

8. Least restrictive alternative
Service users should be provided with any necessary care, treatment and support both in the least invasive manner and in the least restrictive manner and environment compatible with the delivery of safe and effective care, taking account where appropriate of the safety of others.

9. Benefit
Any intervention under the Act should be likely to produce for the service user a benefit which cannot reasonably be achieved other than by the intervention.

10. Child welfare
The welfare of a child with mental disorder should be paramount in any interventions imposed on the child under the Act.

Case study 12.1 Helen

Helen is a woman in her mid-30s who has been under the care of her local assertive outreach team for five years. She was diagnosed with schizophrenia when she was 21 and this resulted in her giving up her university course. She remains unhappy and angry about this loss. She lives alone,

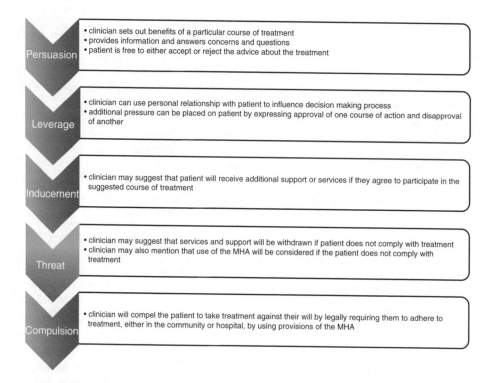

Figure 12.1   The hierarchy of treatment pressures. Adapted from Szmukler & Appelbaum, 2008.

but has two children who live with her parents in the next town. She has regular contact with the children mediated by her parents 'as long as things are going okay' in her mum's words. She does not work and relies heavily on her assertive outreach worker Claire and her parents for material support and help with housing and benefit issues. She has been out of hospital for two years and reasonably stable on oral antipsychotic medication but has been increasingly concerned about weight gain so has been reducing it. She has also been using some amphetamines to try to keep her weight down. When ill in the past Helen has been hostile and aggressive and has been detained against her will.

Persuasion – Claire is worried when she hears about the amphetamines and the reduction in her prescribed medication as Helen was admitted to hospital under similar circumstances last time. She talks with Helen and outlines the dangers of taking stimulants and not taking medication and that both of these will make a return of her illness more likely. She answers Helen's objections and questions as best as she can.

Leverage – The initial discussion has made no difference and Helen has now reduced her medication to a very low dose. She feels better because she is less sleepy and is keen to say so but Claire has noticed she is bit more irritable and is concerned. She talks again with Helen and entreats her to take the medication on the basis that she has known her for many years and wants the best for her. She tells Helen she would be very disappointed if she couldn't at least try and stop the drugs and take a reasonable amount of medication.

Inducement – A few days later Helen tells Claire that she has stopped the medication completely and 'feels great'. Prior to seeing her, Claire had a telephone call from Helen's mother expressing *concern about her and informing her that she was irritable with the children last weekend. The children had noticed and were asking if 'mummy was ok'. When Claire calls round to see Helen it is apparent that she may be deteriorating as she is now openly irritable. Claire is keen to engage her and keep some kind of relationship going. There is an education fair coming up later that week and she offers to take Helen as this forms part of the agreed goals. While talking to her about the possibility of going she explains to Helen that really she needs to be taking treatment if she is serious about trying to do a course as it would otherwise be hard for her to concentrate and hard for Claire to support her application. It may not be that the two are linked, but Helen's interpretation is that Claire will not help her unless she accepts medication again.*

Threat – *The situation continues to deteriorate, with Helen becoming more irritable. She had a bad argument with her mother in front of the children and Helen was unable to tolerate the education fair. Helen's mum telephones Claire and explains to her that she has told Helen she cannot see her children this weekend as 'she is not well enough and not accepting help'. Claire talks with Helen about the situation, but to no avail and contact with her children is suspended. Helen is very unhappy regarding what she sees as an unjustified restriction upon her by her mother.*

Compulsion – *Because Helen is so angry, she and Claire see a little less of each other and it becomes clear that Helen is using drugs more heavily and is acting more erratically. She avoids contact. Claire arranges a visit with a colleague and the doctor on the team but their combined efforts to encourage Helen to accept help fail. She is assessed as a risk to others as she is now openly hostile and this has lead to threatening behaviour with locals who have telephoned the police. Helen is subsequently legally detained by the team and admitted to her local psychiatric hospital.*

Many readers will recognise familiar elements in the case history above and indeed spend a significant proportion of their time dealing with similar issues. In this fictional case, as so often in real life, pressures are brought to bear by concerned families as well as by statutory services.

A study conducted in the US (Monahan et al., 2005) attempted to ascertain the prevalence of the use of 'leverage tools' in the care of those with mental health problems by statutory services or others giving support such as partners and families. In this case the phrase leverage tool refers to a mechanism by which a provider (often a community mental health service) attempts to improve treatment adherence in an individual by making support with such things as housing or finances contingent upon accepting treatment. They described leverage in four main areas as follows: outpatient commitment, the criminal justice system, finance and housing provision. They then interviewed 1000 psychiatric clinic attendees in five different parts of the US to ascertain their experiences. They concluded that leverage was ubiquitous in mental health services, with approximately half of patients experiencing at least one form of leverage at some point. They found associations with the factors described in Box 12.5.

It is immediately apparent that many of these factors are common amongst those under the care of assertive outreach teams, and indeed some are inclusion criteria.

Reflection point

In your experience to what extent does the assertive outreach style of working contribute to the use of coercion, and to what extent is this a product of the individual characteristics of people referred to assertive outreach teams?

Box 12.5   Factors associated with leverage

- Younger age (44 or below).
- Lower level of functioning, as defined by Global Assessment of Functioning (GAF) score of below the median.
- Multiple previous hospital admissions.
- Higher intensity outpatient use.
- Longer overall time in treatment.

In clinical practice it seems that many of those under the care of assertive outreach servcies find them responsive and supportive (Priebe et al., 2005), while a number describe the contact with the team as pressurising as it is hard to 'drop out'. There is little research evidence in this area, though a study by Moser & Bond (2009) found that the extent to which service users felt 'controlled' was not related to the fidelity of the assertive outreach team involved with their care, but was related to having a diagnosis of schizophrenia or misusing substances, suggesting that the service model is not inherently coercive and can respond in different ways to different perceived needs. Again, terminology and concepts here can be confusing and hard to reconcile. The clinical example in Case study 12.2 illustrates one form of what could be described as leverage.

Case study 12.2   Peter

Peter is a young man who has had a number of compulsory admissions to hospital with relapses of his psychotic illness. These are very distressing for him and usually involve the police and long periods of time in secure settings. Relapse has very often been associated with Peter stopping his medication and using drugs. Peter uses cocaine regularly but increases his use when becoming unwell. Peter is estranged from his family and has few contacts apart from those with his assertive outreach workers, who see him often and help him with most of his issues around money and accommodation. Peter finds it hard to manage his money and will often go without food, having spent it on drugs. He regularly comes into contact with the police and they will generally let the team know or drop him off at the base if they are more worried.

After his latest admission the team decides that there needs to be a change in approach to try to help Peter achieve more stability. Peter himself, having got better, wants to go home and get on with things but allows the team to have control over his finances. His rent and bills are all paid in advance and Peter gets a certain amount of cash each day to spend as he wishes. To get his money Peter comes to the team base to pick it up, and at the sametime will collect and take his antipsychotic medication and have a chat with the administrative staff or his worker. This arrangement works fairly well, with Peter being on medication more consistently and not running out of money as much. There are no more problems with unpaid bills or rent and he feels a bit better and more settled in himself, if irritated at times with the need to attend each day. He has not been admitted to hospital for nearly two years, the longest period that he (or anyone else) can remember.

This scenario, where an isolated and vulnerable indiviual is given substantial practical and emotional support by workers while being 'encouraged' to accept treatment, is common in assertive outreach services. It is important to be mindful that such interventions, while likely to be helpful in improving outcome, should be used judiciously and in an individualised way rather than as a regular response to need.

Community Treatment Orders

The highest form of treatment pressure in the heirarchy is compulsion, treatment being given under mental health laws (with their associated safeguards). Most states have well established legislation for compulsory hospital treatment and powers which can enforce treatment beyond the hospital walls are increasingly available internationally. In the UK, Community Treatment Orders (CTOs) have received a lot of attention in the course of their introduction in Scotland in 2005 and England and Wales in 2008.

The international research evidence relating to the use of CTOs is patchy and contradictory in parts, but it is clear that where available they are used and typically become part of standard mental healthcare delivery. There is substantial variation in their use between different regions and countries and even between different clinicians in one area. In England and Wales, it was 'predicted' by official sources that roughly 3–400 orders would be commenced in the first year, but in the first five months over 2000 were commenced (The NHS Information Centre for Health and Social Care, 2009). Anecdotal reports from clinicians suggest a wide variety of experience and it is too soon to say whether CTOs will prove effective in reducing morbidity and improving outcomes overall, but many believe they may be useful in particular cases. There are reports from clinicians in a number of areas that CTOs are already becoming an established part of practice in community care in assertive outreach teams in particular, especially in response to perceived risk to others or concerns from other agencies, such as child protection services.

There is a fear among some clinicians that the widespread use of CTOs will adversely affect patient–clinician relationships and may change the way services are organised and delivered. There are particular concerns that they may divert resources away from those accepting support voluntarily, leading to a situation where compulsion comes to be used as a criteria for resource allocation (Allen & Fox Smith, 2001). The latter appears to have been the case in some parts of the US, where compulsory treatment in the community has been widely used, with evidence that resource allocation is related to legal status. In at least one jurisdiction, those subject to orders were found to be more likely to receive housing, for example (Swartz et al., 2009). However, the opposite has been argued, with claims that if orders reduce hospital use they will 'free up' funding for community care, to the benefit of all (Swartz & Monahan, 2001) and the evidence from other jurisdictions is more reassuring, with CTOs becoming part of established practice without substantially changing patterns of service use (Preston et al., 2002).

Research in this field is legally and ethically complex. In terms of randomised controlled trials a Cochrane Review by Kisely et al. in 2005 found two studies both from the US, and concluded there was little evidence that CTOs were effective in any of the main outcome measures such as homelessness, mental state, readmission, social functioning or satisfaction with care. One of these studies (Swartz et al., 1999) did, however, find some benefit when the results were re-analysed to include only those kept on orders for at least six months and seen at least three times a month. With this group readmission rates were reduced by 57% and number of days in hospital by 20 over one year. The results were even more striking in those with a diagnosis of schizophrenia, with a 73% reduction in readmissions and 28 days less in hospital. There are valid criticisms of the fact that data was analysed retrospectively but the finidings are certainly intriguing and may be important. It may also be hard to generalise them to the UK as our societies and healthcare systems differ significantly but they are clearly suggestive of an effect.

Churchill et al. (2007) reviewed the international evidence of CTOs including non randomised studies, descriptive studies and stakeholder perceptions, concluding that the 'general quality of the empirical evidence is poor' (Churchill et al., 2007: 7) and that the evidence does not support a case for arguing the benefits or the harm of CTOs but that they 'may have a beneficial effect under certain circumstances and with certain groups of patients' (Churchill et al., 2007: 192).

A recent evaluation of one comprehensvely implemented and funded CTO programme in New York (Swartz et al., 2009) concludes that 'during Assisted Outpatient Treatment [CTO equivalent] there is a substantial reduction in the number of psychiatric hosptalizations and in days in the hospital if the person is hospitalised.' (Swartz et al., 2009: Executive Summary: vii). They also found that the programme reduces the likelihood of being arrested and found no evidence that the powers were disproportionately selecting African Americans. The authors correctly raise limitations about their data sources (Medicaid insurance claim records and, therefore, data were not available on ineligible people) and the applicability of the findings to other localities. Attempts are being made in the UK to replicate the results from the US and hopefully inform our use of compulsion in the community in the future (Burns & Dawson, 2009).

One benefit of compulsory treatment in the community is that it formalises and reinforces the community as the location for treatment not the hospital. The first person narrative in Box 12.6 likens this to a 'breath of fresh air'.

Box 12.6   A breath of fresh air

I've experienced mental health problems and I'm now in recovery. I've been in and out of hospital for twenty years or more and it's monotonous – all the time you spend there you are not really getting anywhere. I just felt really drugged up at the beginning – the medication made me feel very, very ill. You just feel like a cabbage, knackered, you can't sit up and everybody around you is sleeping.

I think because the law and supervision orders changed for people with mental health problems, they became more about promoting good health and discipline rather than control. You are put back into the community, plus I've never really been on any tablets in the community, it's always been a depot injection. It's very little; you don't feel like its taking control of your mind, you don't feel really tired or exhausted, or that you can't get by everyday. You don't feel deranged, or under the weather, or psychotic, you don't really feel negative, because the dose is very low, and it does help a lot. (Narrative Research Project. Scottish Recovery Network, 2005)

Conclusion

Assertive outreach patrols the hinterland between responding to private distress and the protection of the public. High profile tragedies continue to attract negative publicity and raise calls for the control of the mentally ill in society. Consumer groups and professional bodies remind us of the need for more collaborative working. As things stand there is no compelling evidence that the use of coercion or compulsion in community mental health-care improves important health and social outcomes. The balance between protecting (and even enhancing) the autonomy of those with severe mental illnesses and providing those who are reluctant with effective treatment has never seemed so delicate. The central issue, of balancing autonomy and care, is by no means a new one. Some of the earliest writings about mental healthcare in the UK contain similar (and just as impassioned) arguments relating to the 'care' of people in private madhouses.

It seems that the dilemma of self determination versus coercion will always be central in mental healthcare. The debate changes in nature according to service developments and in intensity due to alterations in the social and political climate. It is important for us to be mindful of our relationships with and effect upon others, both on an individual level and in terms of the way we plan and manage community mental health services. In these times of increasing financial austerity, tensions may increase if (as seems likely) services contract and our ability to provide individual support is diminished while our ability to compel becomes embedded in care systems.

References

Allen, M. & Fox Smith, V. (2001) Opening Pandora's Box: the practical and legal dangers of involuntary outpatient Commitment. *Psychiatric Services*, **52**, 342–346.

Burns, T. & Dawson, J. (2009) Community treatment orders: how ethical without experimental evidence? *Psychological medicine,* **39**, 1583–1586.

Churchill, R. (2007) *International Experiences of using Community Treatment Orders.* Institute of Psychiatry, Kings College University of London.

Department of Health (2007) *Mental Health Act.* Department of Health, London.

Department of Health (2008) *Code of Practice. Mental Health Act 1983.* Department of Health, London.

Gammack, J., Hobbs, V. & Pigott, D. (2007) *The Book of Informatics.* Thomson, Melbourne.

Graham, J.H. (2006) Community care or therapeutic stalking: two sides of the same coin? *Journal of Psychosocial Nursing & Mental Health Services*, **44**(8), 41–48.

Kisely, S., Campbell, L. & Preston, N. (2005) Compulsory community and involuntary outpatient treatment for patients with severe mental health disorders. *Cochrane database of Systematic reviews*, issue 3.

Macmillan, I. (2005) Targeting clients in community could amount to 'therapeutic stalking'. *Mental Health Practice*, Sep, **9**(1), 6.

Monahan, J., Redlich, A., Swanson, J., Clark Robbins, P., Appelbaum, P. & Petrila, J., et al. (2005) Use of leverage to improve adherence to psychiatric treatment in the community. *Psychiatric Services*, **56**, 37–44.

Morgan, S. & Ryan, P. (2004) Ethical Dilemmas. In: *Assertive Outreach: A strengths Approach to Policy and Practice*, (eds. P. Ryan & S. Morgan). pp. 73–96. Churchill Livingstone.

Moser, L.L. & Bond, G. (2009) Scope of agency control: assertive community treatment teams' supervision of consumers. *Psychiatric Services*, **60**(7), 922–928.

NHS (2006) *Report of the independent inquiry into the care and treatment of John Barrett*. National Health Service, London.

OPSI (1997) *Protection from Harassment Act 1997*. Office of Public Sector Information, London.

OPSI (2008) *Section 76 of the Criminal Justice and Immigration Act 2008*. Office of Public Sector Information, London.

Oshana, M. (2006) *Personal Autonomy in Society*. Ashgate Publishing, Aldershot.

Preston, N., Kisely, S. & Xiao, J. (2002) Assessing the Outcome of compulsory psychiatric treatment in the community; an epidemiological study in Western Australia. *British Medical Journal*, **324**, 1244.

Priebe, S., Watts, J., Chase, M. & Matanov, A. (2005) Processes of disengagement and engagement in assertive outreach patients: qualitative study. *British Journal of Psychiatry*, **187**, 438–443.

Scottish Executive (2001) *New Directions: Report on the Review of the Mental Health (Scotland) Act 1984*. Scottish Executive.

Scottish Recovery Network (2005) *A breath of fresh air*. http://www.scottishrecovery.net/Stories-from-the-narrative-research-project/.

Sheehan, K. & Molodynski, A. (2007) Compulsion and freedom in community mental health care. *Psychiatry*, **6**(9), 393–398.

Stovall, J. (2001) Is Assertive Community Treatment Ethical Care? *Harvard Review of Psychiatry*, **9**, 139–143.

Swartz, M.S., Swanson, J.W., Wagner, H.R., Burns, B.J., Hiday, V.A. & Borum, R. (1999) Can involuntary outpatient commitment reduce hospital recidivism? Findings from a randomized trial with severely mentally ill individuals. *American Journal of Psychiatry*, **156**(12), 1968–1975.

Swartz, M. & Monahan, J. (2001) Special section on involuntary outpatient commitment: introduction. *Psychiatric Services*, **52**, 323–324.

Swartz. M.S., Swanson, J., Steadman, H.J., Clark Robbins, P. & Monahan, J. (2009) *The New York State assisted Outpatient Treatment programme Evaluation*. Duke University school of medicine, North Carolina.

Szasz, T. (2007) *Coercion as Cure; a Critical History of Psychiatry*. Transaction, New Brunswick New Jersey.

Szmukler, G. & Appelbaum, P. (2008) Treatment pressures, leverage, coercion, and compulsion in mental health care. *Journal of Mental Health*, **17**(3), 233–244.

The NHS Information Centre for Health and Social Care (2009) *In-patients formally detained in hospitals under the Mental Health Act 1983 and patients subject to supervised community treatment: 1998–99 to 2008–09*. The NHS Information Centre for Health and Social Care, Leeds.

Williamson, T. (2002) Ethics of assertive outreach (assertive community treatment teams). *Current Opinion in Psychiatry*, **15**(5), 543–547.

Chapter 13

Targets, outcomes and service evaluation

Mike Firn

Introduction

The Department of Health target and reporting regime in England has been an effective driver to implementation of modern service structures (National Audit Office, 2007) but has been limited to outputs (teams and caseloads) and form (team characteristics) rather than outcomes (benefits to individuals and groups using the services). How can we apply more rounded metrics to routinely capture the benefits of assertive outreach, and keep us on the right track?

Contracts with purchasers have often set targets for the number of mental health professional to patient contacts that are to be achieved in a specific time period or team caseloads. These targets originated from 'cost and volume' agreements (Department of Health, 2007) between commissioning bodies and the mental health service providers. Such agreements may be a decade or more old. Furthermore, these agreements did not specify the nature of the contacts; hence targets do not bear relation to the processes of care, quality of service provided nor to the clinical outcome for the patient. If we as consumers were in a position to choose from local mental health services, as we can choose a maternity service or a school, how would we differentiate good from bad?

More sophisticated ways of measuring quality, efficiency and performance are now being pursued in many countries. Within the National Health Service (NHS) in England one of the main driving forces behind this change is payment by results (Department of Health, 2007). Experience from the United States (US) is that assertive community treatment (ACT) services are commissioned more rigorously from a range of independent providers using fidelity standards and outcome measures as well as the traditional activity based indicators such as frequency of visits. Although political priorities change there is no doubt that moving towards standard care pathways to manage care and cost, and routine outcome measures to determine cost versus benefits will be applied more rigorously in the future.

This chapter contrasts traditional command and control regulatory frameworks (Seddon, 2003) as a method of achieving high quality services with more sensitive and arguably more acceptable evaluation methods. To what extent can we move towards

Assertive Outreach in Mental Healthcare: Current Perspectives, First Edition. Edited by C. Williams, M. Firn, S. Wharne and R. Macpherson.

measures of value where quality is pulled from services by outcomes and satisfaction of people experiencing the service?

Consistent with other chapters, case studies and first person narratives will bring to life aspects of the discussion and evidence on outcomes. The chapter will cover available instruments, team examples from audit to evaluation and look to the future aspirations of payment by results policies.

The trouble with targets

> Social and political life is as rich and subtle as our own, and every bit as resistant to carica-
> ture by a single objective defined with a single measurement. If you want to summarise like
> this you have to accept the violence it can do to complexity. (Blastland & Dilnot, 2008: 88)

At best targets have limitations, at worst they distort decision making and behaviour to the detriment of health or social care outcomes. We are fortunate that assertive outreach services have not resorted to avoiding sicker patients to get better outcome results. In fact we pride ourselves on targeting those with the most complex needs and rightly so. In England at least, outcomes are not the national targets that are set. The basic set of targets have been the existence of a team, number of people receiving assertive outreach services measured by a snapshot of the team caseload and a set of service characteristics conforming to expert opinion of what is likely to provide better care and outcomes, for example small caseloads and seven day a week working (see Box 13.1).

Compliance or variance impacts on inspectorate ratings with multiple consequences (Healthcare Commission, 2008). Within these targets and associated guidance (VSMR, 2008; PIG, 2001) there are some get out clauses. As Firn (2007) observes:

> PIG guidance states: 'Assertive outreach services are best provided by a discrete, specialist
> team that has staff members whose sole (or main) responsibility is assertive outreach.' The
> guidance and VSMR fall short of stating that services must always be provided by a dedi-
> cated, self-contained team.

Box 13.1   English National Targets

Each locality is assigned a target number of teams and caseload based on weighted capitation to be reported centrally. In addition localities must self-report against their compliance with the following assertive outreach team characteristics:

1   A team approach (not intensive case management by individual members of community mental health teams).
2   A team caseload no larger than 12 service users for each member of staff.
3   A defined client group.
4   Planned long-term working with individuals.
5   Much of the work outside a service setting.
6   Evening and weekend availability with 24-hour access to an on-call system for service users on the team caseload. (VSMR 5214-Vital Signs Monitoring Returns, 2008)

Similarly the VSMR wording relating to out of hours working specifically uses evening and weekend *availability* and 24 hour *access*. This enables teams to consider local need and to make the best use of flexible working, non-resident on-call staff out of office hours, and protocols with local crisis resolution and home treatment services for assertive outreach service users.

These dilutions from strict fidelity can be legitimate and justifiable where they make the best use of resources to meet needs. An example of this might be pooling out of hours cover for small or dispersed assertive outreach populations. Other interpretations of targets are more spurious. Here we enter the realm of gaming and misrepresentation. Gaming is the alteration of behaviour to gain strategic advantage, misrepresentation includes creative accounting and fraud (NHS Centre for Reviews and Dissemination, 2003). Gaming becomes widespread as the honest manager fails to make a notional target and sees their neighbouring service hit their target by smoke and mirrors and be rewarded.

Case study 13.1

A locality has no true assertive outreach service. The locality counts a sub-set of patients in standard care as assertive outreach service users on the basis that they are typically getting frequent visits to an assertive outreach level. The locality reports that this 'service' uses the team approach based on a weekly care pathways meeting between standard care teams where complex clients are discussed.

Next time the honest manager will adopt the same gaming strategy and bad behaviour drives out the good (Blastland & Dilnot, 2008). And so it goes on up the chain as commissioners, service planners and politicians can 'demonstrate' how performance as measured is fine. We can see easily that the target was only ever going to tell us a small part of the complex picture and, through gaming, even that small part becomes illusory. Sometimes the target itself becomes a 'perverse incentive'. One example of best intentions becoming a blunt instrument is shown in Case study 13.2.

Case study 13.2

In one US State financial reimbursements (a very powerful kind of target) work against assertive community treatment teams reducing contact prior to discharge to a lower level of care. The State program has two billing rates for users of ACT services. The full rate can be billed for individuals receiving 6 visits per a month (of which 3 can be with carers) and a partial rate for those below this but above 1 visit per month. To prepare a service user for discharge means a loss of income to the team. To discharge quickly to the next level down challenges the confidence of the team and the service user. In this case the next level is intensive case management at 2–3 visits per month. As a result the ACT teams have not been discharging proactively and have generated a waiting list. Eventually they will not be serving those most in need. In this State there are over 70 ACT teams and over 4000 eligible 'slots' for ACT service users. The commissioning specification is derived from scores of 4–5 on the DACTS model fidelity scale (Teague et al., 1998) so these teams have high fidelity but low flexibility on finance driven items. (Personal communication, 2008)

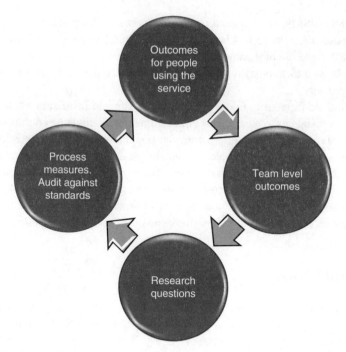

Figure. 13.1   Complementary process and outcome measure framework.

Who and what are measures for?

Figure 13.1 displays a framework of process and outcome measures to help articulate the levels of analysis. In reality the levels are complementary not discrete. Services that attempt to comprehensively answer all the levels will struggle with clinician compliance. It is better to have a small number of clear goals based on the aspirations of those experiencing the service and the information most informative for your service. We cannot, however, divorce ourselves from monitoring activity and quality proxies demanded by purchasers of mental health services and the inspectorates. One approach pursued for many years is to have a single IT solution which will generate well presented clinical records, care plans and data reports from simple routine clinician input. Sadly this remains elusive as the well publicised National Programme for Information Technology in England testifies in spiralling costs and increasingly disappointing progress (*Health Service Journal*, 2009).

Process measures

Case study 13.2 demonstrated the application of a crude process measure, namely frequency of contact. In assertive outreach the most widely quoted and used measure of processes of care and service organisation is the Dartmouth Assertive Community

---

Box 13.2   Process measures

Process measures ask the questions:

- Has assertive outreach been implemented faithfully and as planned?
- What are the strengths and weakness of our service?
- How does our service compare to accepted standards and other providers?

Treatment Scale or DACTS developed by Gregory Teague, Gary Bond and Bob Drake (Teague et al., 1998) and drawing its name from the Dartmouth Medical School in New Hampshire. The 28 criteria in the DACTS are extrapolated from model descriptions in the literature, expert opinion and previous attempts to capture fidelity such as the IFACT (McGrew et al., 1995). (See Box 13.2 for process measures.)

The Substance Abuse and Mental Health Services Administration (SAMHSA) have produced a publication (Assertive Community Treatment: Evaluating Your Program, 2008) which is freely available to download and includes a fully useable version of the DACTS together with a protocol and scoring sheet. We will, therefore, not reproduce the criteria items in this text but refer the reader to this reference.

The DACTS is generally accorded a level of empirical validity that it cannot live up to. Many of the criteria and scoring anchor points are described for an American setting and do not transfer well, for example, to the United Kingdom (UK). In item 8 in the human resources section teams score full marks, a 5 on the 1–5 rating scale, if they have two or more nurses for a team caseload of 100. This would be a particularly low number of professional nurses in a typical UK assertive outreach team where qualified nurses are more affordable and plentiful than the US. (Wright et al., PLAO, 1994). Nevertheless the IFACT and DACTS overall do have a modest predictive value, for example, with high scores for team organisation on IFACT being associated with reduced bed use, providing a tested link between process measures and outcomes (Burns et al., 2007). Burns and colleagues performed a particularly thorough meta-regression analysis of data from randomised controlled trials in intensive case management (ICM) and concluded that 'The effectiveness of intensive case management teams is increased as their organisation reflects the assertive community treatment model, but there is less evidence for the benefits of increased staffing levels' (Burns et al., 2007: 340).

National Institute for Health and Clinical Excellence (NICE) guidance for Schizophrenia (2009) provides a further set of standards based on evidence concerning clinical interventions of proven effectiveness. Teams should be familiar with the evidence base for pharmacological intervention strategies, whether maintenance versus intermittent dosage schedules, and for psycho-social interventions, and supported employment. Of particular relevance for assertive outreach populations is auditing the use of Clozapine for people with schizophrenia who have an inadequate or no response to treatment despite the sequential use of adequate doses of at least two different antipsychotic drugs (NICE, 2009).

Other commonly asked process measures include measures of engagement, whether individuals received a copy of their care plan, were involved in decisions about treatment and medication choice, or offered help with employment, direct payments or advance directives. For those of you who argue that engagement is an outcome in itself, there is merit in this but no one got better, or was employed or housed, purely by virtue of being engaged. To this extent it is a means to an end, or a means to an outcome.

Caution should be exercised in using negative outcomes such as critical incidents as a reliable marker of team performance, since major events involving harm are still rare and even two significant adverse events, such as suicide, falling in the same period cannot be independently attributed to team behaviour without further investigation. In the REACT study (Killaspy, 2006) three clients assigned to community mental health team care and one assigned to assertive community treatment committed suicide during the study period. Yet, because of the small numbers no statistical significance can be associated to this. A run of adverse events does correctly trigger scrutiny but until other information or consistent failures of the system are subsequently identified, should not trigger automatic criticism or speculative long-term changes in practice beyond the precautionary.

Implementing routine outcome measures

> Consumer outcomes are the bottom line for mental health services, like profit is in business. No successful businessperson would assume that the business was profitable just because employees worked hard. (Substance Abuse and Mental Health Services Administration, 2008: 4) (See Box 13.3 for outcome measures.)

Outcome measures are part of your quality assurance mechanism. By definition routine outcome measures require the serial application of standard instruments. Best practice guidance for routine outcome measures was produced by the National Institute for Mental Health in England (NIMHE) (2005). More recently this has been followed up by a compendium of outcome measurement tools and scales (NIMHE, 2008). In developing the guidance NIMHE used four pilot sites and three exemplar sites to understand the practical issued involved in implementing measures routinely. The pilot sites implemented four measures and studied collection over six months.

Box 13.3   Outcome measures

Outcome measures ask the questions:

- Has this individual got better as a result of the care and treatment provided by assertive outreach?
- Overall have the users of the assertive outreach service shown aggregate improvements over time since referral?

We also need to be prepared to answer the questions:
Would this person, or group, have got better over time with no intervention, with primary care or standard secondary care, or have the gains shown resulted from other agencies?

Two clinician rated measures of morbidity and social functioning:

- FACE – Functional Analysis of Care Environments.
- HoNOS – Health of the Nation Outcome Scale.

Two rated by individuals in receipt of services:

- CUES – Carer and User Expectations of Services.
- MANSA – service user rated quality of life scale.

This experience led to conclusions determining successful implementation at both clinical team and more strategic levels in the organisation:

- Gaining stakeholder support including having a senior driver within the organisation.
- Costs associated with training staff in the technical aspects of rating and supporting service users in self rating.
- Integrating rating points within the care pathway processes of care, for example, anchoring and synchronising within CPA reviews.
- Feeding back outcome data in a timely and relevant manner.
- IT systems and infrastructure issues.

> The national outcomes pilot has highlighted the importance of building incentives into outcome measurement at all levels in order to engage service users, carers, clinicians and managers for successful implementation. The most effective means of building positive incentives is to help them develop an understanding of the benefits of outcome measurement and how these benefits evolve over time. (NIMHE, 2005: 8)

Mannion & Dawson (2001) draw similar conclusions about the need for credible and relevant measures, supported by training, and with effective and timely clinician feedback mechanisms. When measures are owned more by commissioners or managers than by clinicians, patients and carers, then compliance will be a major issue. Whilst commissioners in England are typically requiring fairly basic matched pairs of outcomes measurements, for example HoNOS score on admission and discharge, many providers are struggling to achieve 25% compliance (personal communication (National Clinical Outcomes in Mental Health Group, 2009)).

Kisely et al., in Canada (2008) showed that effective presentation of data that could be feedback to clinicians showing changes for individual and aggregated team level data were factors in achieving high levels of HoNOS completion.

Gilbody (2003) surveyed 500 randomly sampled working age adult consultant psychiatrists in the UK about measuring outcome in psychiatric practice:

> Twenty-six responses specifically related to the HoNOS, whereas no other measure was mentioned specifically by name. Comments were largely critical (n = 21), and related to: time to complete (n = 16); inadequate psychometric properties (n = 8); the lack of additional information that it adds to the routine clinical assessment (n = 5); the lack of enthusiasm amongst staff (n = 7). Positive comments (n = 7) included the fact that it could be completed by non-clinicians (n = 4), and that it acted as a useful aide memoire in clinical decision making (n = 3). (Gilbody, 2003: 49)

Case study 13.3

Hitch (2007) describes the process by which one assertive outreach service in South London selected and implemented the use of routine outcome measures. The multi-disciplinary team worked together to draw up a short list of outcome measures. The team then met to rate the measures for relevance to assertive outreach, user friendliness and sensitivity. Measures were randomly allocated to members of the team to test them out and then votes were cast to select measures covering several dimensions. The team ended up with a consensus to implement five measures routinely on top of their organisation's risk assessment tool. Case managers would repeat the measures at every major review, typically six months and update them at times of major change such as admission.

HoNOS
Camberwell Assessment of Need Short Appraisal Schedule (CANSAS)
Drug Attitude Inventory (DAI–10 item)
Engagement Scale (Hall et al., 2001)
Drug Use Screen (DUS) and Alcohol Use Screen (AUS)

The team recognised that HoNOS and CANSAS overlapped in several domains but that CANSAS added useful quality of life information.

Individual and team level outcomes

SAMHSA (2008) recommends that teams monitor a core set of outcomes reflecting the primary goals of assertive outreach.

- Psychiatric or substance abuse hospitalization.
- Incarceration.
- Housing stability.
- Independent living.
- Competitive employment.
- Educational involvement.
- Stage of substance abuse treatment.

The SAMHSA toolkit suggests that teams limit themselves to simple ratings rather than adding in complexity that would be more suitable for research questions. They give the positive example of:

Did the consumer hold a competitive job in this quarter? Rather than the more challenging:

How many hours during this quarter did the consumer work competitively? SAMHSA suggests, initially at least, limiting measures to those than can be collected from team members, rather than from individuals and families experiencing the service. However, subjective satisfaction, experience of service and patient reported quality of life are undeniably important outcomes.

Especially where individuals and families are informants they need to be involved in designing and field testing the questions and language in outcome measures. The flexible availability of independent advocates or researchers is also necessary as an aide to completion, assisting those with concentration, literacy, cultural, language and other needs. Postal satisfaction and experience questionnaires are not effective for assertive outreach. One large mental health provider has several years of comparable data on the satisfaction and experience of those receiving services using such best practice (Perkins & Nell, 2009). Data is collated and reports provided to teams with follow up from operational managers, and established user and carer representatives. The outcome in question here is primarily satisfaction and acceptability of services.

Service user quotes from these local evaluation surveys typically talk about experience of services and process. The following are from people receiving assertive outreach:

> I feel part of my treatment. I am given choices and I get on well with the nurses.

> I have received a huge amount of support both for my addiction problems and the fact that I'm bi-polar. I have found it amazing how much support is available.

> We have staff that come in once a day and I have the emergency staff numbers and helplines.

Service user aspirations become the outcome goals, in this case relating to quality of life:

> If I succeed then I should be with my friends, go out a lot with my friend and go to the cinema.

For service users, homes, jobs and friends are cited as goals more typically than medical goals, such as fewer symptoms.

Case study 13.4   Assertive outreach team example

Gloucester and Forest of Dean assertive outreach team in England implemented routine outcome measures in 2003 (MacPherson et al., 2007). In one six month period they were able to demonstrate changes within the following simple and meaningful items, which tracked over time can guide service response.
Unmet need:

Reduced patient-rated unmet need.
No change in staff rated unmet need.

Engagement measures:

No change.

Accommodation changes:

4 moved to independent living, 3 to supported accommodation,
3 became homeless and 2 went to prison.

Medication changes:

10 people started Clozapine.
9 people stopped depot antipsychotics.

Employment status:

16 people started regular daytime activity.
0 stopped.

The recovery star is an outcome measurement tool with a highly visual interface that is engaging for clinicians and service users alike (The Mental Health Providers Forum and Triangle Consulting, 2008). The tool measures and displays ten recovery orientated areas of life, each self-rated according to meaningful anchor points on a 1–10 scale: 1 relates to being stuck and 10 to self-reliance. Each category explains in everyday language what it might be like at each increment, described as a step on a ladder, so the service user and their assertive outreach worker can agree where they are presently. Scores are displayed on the star shaped scale in Figure 13.2. The recovery star has been designed for use in a number of mental health and social care settings by service users and their key workers

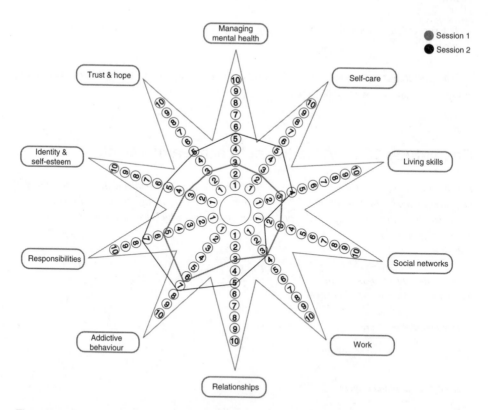

Figure 13.2   Example recovery star score sheet. Joy MacKeith Sara Burns, copyright Triangle Consulting and Mental Health Providers Forum.

together. It is compatible with working towards recovery for people receiving assertive outreach services. The service user quote below illustrates the utility of this tool:

> You can see the progress you've made. It's visual, powerful. Some people can't understand from written reports, but can understand this.

Further recovery oriented outcome measures and provider self-assessment instruments that may be useful in an assertive outreach context are published and comprehensively introduced in a compendium of recovery measures which is also available online (Human Services Research Institute, 2005).

Research questions

> A recurrent criticism of measurement in schizophrenia research is that symptom suppression is overemphasised as the sole criterion measure of treatment effectiveness, to the neglect of other endpoints, such as the quality of life and subjective experience of the patient. (Collins, et al. (1991) in Gilbody, 2003: 27)

Typically BPRS (Overall & Gorham 1962) and the PANSS (Kay et al., 1987) are used to measure symptomatic changes and untypically in medication trials is the patient ever asked whether they subjectively feel better.

The complexity, reliability, feasibility and validity of capturing patient based outcomes have been discussed throughout this chapter. These obstacles become more daunting in the world of scientific peer reviewed research. Reliable outcome measures with reliable psychometric properties for publication may not be acceptable to those receiving services in routine settings. For example, one quality of life measure (Lehman, 1983) regularly used in research and designed for people with severe and enduring mental health problems took 40 minutes to complete. This and other shortcomings were later addressed by the Manchester Short Assessment of Quality of Life or MANSA (Priebe et al., 1999) with as few as 16 questions.

Satisfaction with services outcomes are often referred to in research as secondary outcomes, after the primary outcomes of bed days or symptomatology have been analysed. These are sometimes unfairly characterised as 'hard' and 'soft' outcomes suggesting that consumer satisfaction is somehow of a lesser order, more shapeless and slippery.

Killaspy et al. (2006; 2009) in their UK randomised controlled trial of ACT versus standard care followed the format used in previous ACT studies. They asked the primary outcome question of the number of days spent as a mental health inpatient during the 18 month study period. Secondary outcome questions for the study covered a wide range including satisfaction with services, clinical and social functioning, quality of life, serious incidents, engagement, compliance with medication, use of the Mental Health Act and substance misuse.

This large well conducted trial demonstrated no significant differences between the ACT group and treatment as usual on any measure of hospitalisation. For the secondary measures ACT recipients were better engaged, less likely to be lost to follow up and more satisfied with services. ACT was the more expensive service in terms of staff costs, with small case loads and 2–3 times higher face to face contact activity. Given the absence of 'hard' primary outcome benefits of ACT the authors speculated on the cost effectiveness of ACT versus standard care. With staffing and inpatient beds being the most costly elements of services they concluded that these outcomes showed that ACT was not cost effective, or that satisfaction and engagement would need to be valued extremely highly for it to be considered so.

Can the implementation of routine outcome measures improve services and outcomes?

NIMHE guidance (2005) is cautiously optimistic in its assessment of the utility of routine outcome measurement:

> Collecting outcomes data alone has limited value, it is only when it is interpreted and translated into positive changes in practice that it will yield improvements in the quality of services (NIMHE, 2005: 9)

Others cast doubt on whether there is any evidence to suggest that the use of outcome measures has any impact on actual outcomes or even in changing clinical practice processes or improvements to the quality of care. Using both a survey of UK psychiatrists and a systematic review of the effectiveness of routine outcome measurement on quality of care, Gilbody et al. (2003) drew disappointing conclusions:

> UK psychiatrists gave few examples of positive experiences or knowledge of routinely collected outcomes data being used in the planning or improvement of clinical services. (Gilbody et al., 2003: 87)

> There is little evidence to support the potential for routine outcome measures to improve the quality of mental healthcare. (Gilbody et al., 2003: 8)

A similar conclusion is reached by Prabhu et al. (2008) in Australia reviewing their use of routine measures in an outreach setting:

> HoNOS scores reflected positive changes in patients and were useful as a global overview, but did not tap into process issues that are more clinically meaningful. (Prabhu, 2008: 195)

Slade and colleagues (2006) tackled this question head on with an ingenious randomised controlled trial to test the link between the use of routine outcome measures and improved outcome for service users. Patients were recruited from eight standard community mental health teams in London. Participants were paired with a staff member who was working most closely with them and both completed baseline and seven month follow up measures using patient and staff versions of scales. The 101 intervention arm staff and patients additionally received a battery of three outcome assessments sent out by post monthly for the six months between baseline and follow up interviews.

After three and then six months each intervention group pair received identical feedback from the outcome measures including coloured graphs and text showing changes over the months, and highlighting any areas of disagreement between the staff-rated and patient-rated measures. This rigorous but short study showed no advantage for intervention participants in outcomes concerning unmet need, quality of life or the secondary measures of mental health problem severity, symptoms and social disability. Yet, the intervention patients did have fewer and shorter hospitalisations compared to those who did not have the monthly outcome measurement and feedback. The authors conclude that routine outcome assessment was not shown to be effective since the mechanism hypothesised could not be shown to have operated through their analysis of the subjective measures or by self-report and looking at changes to care plans. The mechanism supposed that staff and patients would be prompted to modify the process and content of care by the completion of focussed assessments and the consideration of feedback given on progress, which in turn would lead to better outcomes. The findings on admission are intriguing. The authors discuss these findings but do not reach a conclusion. Staff received more information about the intervention patients perhaps prompting them to offer more support in avoiding admission. Frequency of contact for the intervention and standard care patients was not reported.

Conclusion

Implementing outcome measures routinely is recommended, inspected and makes common sense. Measurement helps signal and interpret the fruits of our labours for affirmative or corrective action. There are dangers of simply implementing 'rituals of verification' which satisfy inspectorates and flatter our clinical aspirations. There are risks of systematic implementation eating into face to face clinician time, but also risks in not doing so, of being unable to demonstrate effectiveness at different levels. As an intensive and, therefore, relatively expensive service, assertive outreach teams need to demonstrate continued effectiveness on so called 'hard' and soft' outcomes, and be clear about true outcomes and mere processes. They also have to manage their reputation in an increasingly competitive and finance driven system.

We all know we should be evaluating and focusing more on outcome locally. Yet, it is the minority of assertive outreach teams in England that are routinely and comprehensively applying outcome measurement as part of a quality assurance system. We know this from holding practitioner meetings and workshops via the National Forum for Assertive Outreach. Teams report their activity but struggle with reporting outcome data beyond hospitalisation. Even with hospitalisation they will know current use but not be clear on trends, have historical comparisons or be robustly linking service delivery changes to bed use patterns. Some have tried to collate routine outcome measures and they have withered after only partial implementation for some of the reasons shown here. Others have never collected beyond bed use or readmission rates.

Without measurement how will we, our service users and commissioners, know if our considerable endeavours are helpful? A reimbursement system of payment by results will be a sharp stick to drive on the implementation of outcome measures but as we have seen establishing a valid metric is elusive. Whether or not we will be successful in getting measures relevant to true service user goals remains to be seen.

References

Blastland, M. & Dilnot, A. (2008) *The Tiger that Isn't. Seeing through the world of numbers*. Profile Books, London.

Burns, T., Catty, J., Dash, M., Roberts, C., Lockwood, A. & Marshall, M. (2007) Use of intensive case management to reduce time in hospital in people with severe mental illness: systematic review and meta-regression. *British Medical Journal*, **335**(7615), 336–340.

CSIP (2006) *Measuring Health and Social Care Outcomes in Mental Health*. Care Services Improvement Partnership, Leeds.

Collins, E.J., Hogan, T.P. & Himansu, D. (1991) Measurement of therapeutic response in schizophrenia. *Schizophrenia Research*, **5**, 249–253.

Curtis, R. & Beevor, A. (1995) Health of the Nation Outcome Scales (HoNOS) In: *Measurement for Mental Health: contributions from the College Research Unit*, (ed. J. Wing). pp. 33–46. Royal College of Psychiatrists, London.

Department of Health (2007) Payment by Results. Background and History. http://www.dh.gov.uk/en/Policyandguidance/Organisationpolicy/Financeandplanning/NHSFinancialReforms/DH_077259.

Firn, M. (2007) Assertive outreach: has the tide turned against the approach? *Mental Health Practice*, **10**, 7.

Gilbody, S.M., House, A.O. & Sheldon, T.A. (2003) *Outcomes Measurement in Psychiatry. A Critical Review of Outcomes Measurement in Psychiatric Research and Practice*. NHS Centre for Reviews and Dissemination, University of York.

Healthcare Commission (2008) *The Annual Health Check 2008/09: Assessing and Rating the NHS*. Commission for Healthcare Audit and Inspection.

Hitch, D. (2007) Outcome measures in assertive outreach: one team's journey towards a system of implememntation. *Mental Health Practice*, **10**(7), 28–31.

Human Services Research Institute (2005) *Measuring the Promise: A Compendium of Recovery Measures* Volume II. http://www.tecathsri.org

Kay, S.R., Opler, L.A. & Lindenmayer, J.P. (1987) The Positive and Negative Syndrome Scale (PANSS): rationale and standarisation. *British Journal of Psychiatry*, **155**, (Suppl 7), 59–67.

Killaspy, H., Bebbington, P., Blizard, R., Johnson, S., Nolan, F. & Pilling, S., et al. (2006) The REACT study: randomised evaluation of assertive community treatment in north London. *British Medical Journal*, **332**, 815–20.

Kisely, S., Campbell, L.A., Robertson, H., Crossman, D., Martin, K. & Campbell, J. (2008) Routine measurement of mental health service outcomes: Health of the Nation Outcome Scales in Nova Scotia. *Psychiatric Bulletin*, **32**(7), 248–250.

Lehman, A.F. (1983) The well being of chronic mental patients: assessing their quality of life. *Archive of General Psychiatry*, **40**, 369–373.

Macpherson, R., Gregory, N., Slade, M. & Foy, C. (2007) Factors associated with changing patient need in an assertive outreach team. *International Journal of Social Psychiatry*, **55**, 389–396.

Mannion, R. & Goddard, M. (2001) Impact of published clinical outcomes data: case study of NHS hospital trusts. *British Medical Journal*, **323**, 260–264.

Mental Health Providers Forum (2008) *Mental Health Recovery Star, User and Organisation Guides*. Developed by Joy MacKeith & Sara Burns of Triangle Consulting with the Mental Health Providers Forum, London. http://www.mhpf.org.uk/recoveryStarResources.asp

National Audit Office (2007) *Helping People through Mental Health Crisis: The role of Crisis Resolution and Home Treatment Services*. The Stationery Office, London.

NIMHE (2005) *Outcome Measures Implementation. Best Practice Guidance*. National Institute for Mental Health in England, Leeds.

Overall, J.E. & Gorham, D.L. (1962) "The Brief Psychiatric Rating Scale", *Psychological Reports*, **10**, 799–812.

Perkins, R. & Nell, R.D. (2009) *The experience of using inpatient and community mental health services*. Unpublished reports 2006–2009. South West London and St George's Mental Health NHS Trust.

Prabhu, R. & Oakley Browne, M. (2008) The use of the Health of the Nation Outcome Scale in an outreach rehabilitation program. *Australasian Psychiatry*, **16**(3), 195–199.

Priebe, S., Huxley, P., Knight, S. & Evans, S. (1999) Application and results of the Manchester Short Assessment of Quality of Life. *International Journal of Social Psychiatry*, **45**, 7–12.

Seddon, J. (2003) *Freedom from Command and Control: A Better way to Make the Work Work.* Vanguard Education.

Slade, M., McCrone, P., Kuipers, E., Leese, M., Cahill, S. & Parabiaghi, A., et al. (2006) Use of standardised outcome measures in adult mental health services: randomised controlled trial. *British Journal of Psychiatry*, **189**, 330–336.

Substance Abuse and Mental Health Services Administration (2008) *Assertive Community Treatment: Evaluating Your Program*. DHHS Pub. No. SMA-08-4344, Rockville, MD: Center for Mental Health Services, Substance Abuse and Mental Health Services Administration, U.S. Department of Health and Human Services. http://www.samhsa.gov/shin

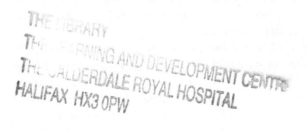

Chapter 14

Funky mental health

Steve Morgan and Sue Jugon

Warning: the following chapter should only be read by those with an open mind, and a challenging disposition!

Introduction

If you spend so many of your waking hours, and some anxious restless nights, devoted to working in mental health, are you right to expect at least some joy, fun, excitement, productive challenge and even intrinsic reward from your complex interactions with service users and colleagues? Our managed, regulated, monitored and audited system is intended to ensure consistent good practice, but it is arguable whether it contributes anything towards producing a motivated workforce through its relentless pursuit of numbers and targets. A sea of fidelity scales, outcome measures, policy initiatives, service protocols and templates, research based models, and increasing mountains of paperwork may be a satisfying representation of service delivery for the academics and managers, but largely feels unconnected to the pursuit of genuine creative person-centred practice for practitioners, or service users for that matter.

The *strengths approach* to assertive outreach was fully articulated by Ryan & Morgan (2004), and in a review of their book (replicated in *Practice Based Evidence*, 2009) the approach was likened to 'the Funky Business of mental healthcare'; providing practitioners with a different perspective from the mire of mechanistic, risk averse, box-ticking required by most organisations. The book places a strong emphasis on creative collaboration, true team working and the need to be anchored by the well-being of the people we serve.

Continuing the theme of this book review, *funky mental health* should be seen primarily as working with and around the rules. It is about how different people may look at the same thing but see something different. A small proportion of all practitioners are exceptional in their ability to reflect on situations, think creatively about complex interactions and manage the demands placed on them organisationally without losing their vision of person-centred practice as the most important goal. A small proportion of all practitioners are exceptionally poor, shouldn't by rights be inflicted upon service users,

Assertive Outreach in Mental Healthcare: Current Perspectives, First Edition. Edited by C. Williams, M. Firn, S. Wharne and R. Macpherson.

but organisational systems and teams can be cursed by an inability to offload them. The large majority of practitioners are good people wanting to do good work, but they become easily paralysed by their narrow interpretation of policies and outcome measures within the wider perceived context of a blame culture. They unintentionally prioritise a focus on what might go wrong before considering the challenges and often risk-taking demands of a genuine person-centred approach. The ultimate losers will always be the service users, though you wouldn't necessarily believe this from the incredible spin the management machine can often place on its own contradictory demands of services.

Funky mental health is not about ignoring the rules or breaking the rules in any illegal way. Buckingham & Coffman (2005) talk about 'First, break all the rules', but only as a challenge to see and do things differently in order to gain the most positive and successful outcomes from identifying and working with anyone's individual talents.

Rules are generally guidelines, not usually immovable impositions or rigid barriers. Assertive outreach has been established specifically to find ways of working with people for whom the traditional rules of community mental health have proved less workable. So, by definition these rules, or norms, have failed to bring about anyone's desired outcomes (neither service user or service provider). In this instance do we give practitioners more time to do more of the same thing, in the hope of re-shaping the service user to better fit the pattern of service delivery? This undeniably represents a 'service-centred' approach to practice, and often includes punitive responses towards the service users and their needs. Or, do we give practitioners the permission to create new ways of engaging and working alongside the service users in creative and flexible ways (i.e. a more person-centred approach)?

Funky working needs a vision

In some instances funky mental health should produce the 'I can't believe you do that' response from the majority of the good practitioners. It starts with a clear underpinning vision that can be returned to and checked against at any stage of a team's development or experience of significant challenges. The vision should be about how we develop and sustain a 'team' that can incorporate the maximum range of qualities in a small group of practitioners so they may be made available to the diverse range of people who naturally make up the client group. It is about a clear underpinning philosophy, and an eagerness to reflect, individually and collectively, on the personal values that influence our every decision; including the big questions of why we do this type of work, what we feel about the people who need services and how we intend to best work with them. It is about people who have a healthy respect for how work and personal lives inter-relate, not about rigid nine-to-five demarcations. It is about genuine flexible responses to needs, rather than the rigidity of extended shift patterns. It is about being challenged to think, and being aware of the rewards of the intrinsic value of thinking through a challenge. In the world of funky mental health there is a more healthy developed appreciation of how much we become a part of service users' lives; but also going one step further, seeing how service users become an important part of our lives if we have a belief in the value of the work we are doing.

What do the exceptional few do?

As a starting point, funky mental health is about the default thought processes – the majority of people accept the traditional processes and structures as evidence-based gospel, but the few start by asking why, analysing what the intentions and outcomes are, and thinking of the best ways of achieving them that uphold the essential goal of genuine person-centred practice. For the perplexed majority, funky mental health may look loose, uncoordinated and unstructured; they will instantly see the faults – but these are the faults when processing a different way of doing things through your own traditional parameters of thinking. For example, the monthly business meeting is a widely adapted means of gathering many people together to share masses of information of variable value and interest, very little of which sticks and influences what people do. The funky mental health lead will use different means or levels of communication for different messages and priorities – vitally important practice-changing initiatives or training will be accommodated by setting aside specific team time for the purpose. It is about using precious time resources in the most efficient and effective ways, not a one-size-fits-all solution.

However, funky mental health is not about trading on the passion of people who want to do good work through exploitation of their time and commitment. The exceptionally good practitioners know what they will do and what they will not do in the name of a service that has no real understanding or interest in their motivations. They are clear about who they serve – the service users and carers, not the policy makers and remote risk-averse managers. They are also able to reflect on the narrow-sightedness of service structures designed by people who do not understand the true meaning of translating their own policy measures into practice. For example, an exceptional practitioner knows that flexibility is not always offered by rigidly implementing a two-shift system across a twelve hour day. There is a need for people to be seen outside of a traditional nine-to-five working day, but blindly extending staff availability could create an artificial demand just because the people are available, which is not necessarily the same as a real need. Exceptional practitioners adjust their own work schedules and priorities to meet the real needs as they arise. They will take back the time in equally flexible ways. Shift patterns designed to meet a perceived need out-of-hours can just as likely result in staff sitting in offices doing paperwork rather than seeing people. Peak-time demands for face-to-face contacts can then become pressured as practitioners are involved in service-centred meetings, or are less on the ground to accommodate the extended hours of opening.

It is also about the environment

The ability to deliver funky mental health will be influenced as much by the working environment as it is by the structures and systems we put in place. The team approach is about whole team thinking, not just a range of people in face-to-face contacts with service users. Nobody having their own office and specially personalised workspace, and more time sat at the table facing each other (not away from each other) underpin the sense of team. The manager trades the 'open door continuous interruptions' for the closer belonging to the team.

Underpinned by a 'team'

The vision is constantly revisited by asking ourselves: what is the team? We need to research and fact-find what makes good teams click (e.g. no more than eight or communication begins to fragment), and developing sub-teams to differentiate the importance of the whole team approach to deliver best services for service users. We need to think about how we sell the concept of team to most service users from the outset (i.e. what the gains are). Crucially, most of the client group have impoverished social networks, so meeting a range of people through the team is one way of building social networks with people who understand the condition more sensitively (acknowledging that most service users do not ultimately want their relationships to be largely with professionals).

Can local effectiveness be centrally legislated?

Infidelity to the model is not the exact message, but it will suffice to challenge the more conventional rigidity of thinking that underpins supposed good practice in many good practitioners. Funky mental health does not ignore the research, but it does adopt a healthy focus in trying to process the research through a local practice-based perspective, rather than allowing it to rigidly prescribe local practice in ways that often do not fit as well as in the original research programmes.

We need to be asking different questions in this more advanced phase of service development, where assertive outreach has established its ability to meet a need that other service configurations will struggle to work with. We need to stop trying to just replicate the same research questions that have repeatedly occupied the interest of the national and international academic community. We need to ask locally what contributes to making assertive outreach more or less effective? Is it staff attitudes and values? Is it the way we implement a 'team approach'? Is it greater attention to identifying and working with service user 'strengths'? Is it greater attention applied to involving service users in the development of their own support plans? We have a new national public service agenda focused on the concept of *personalisation*, and assertive outreach services already have a lot of local experience to contribute to the development and implementation of the new agenda.

Ultimately, funky mental health should be more about giving good people the freedom to find good local solutions to their identified problems. We need to permit more and prescribe less – prescribe the outcome not the journey. The international business literature is full of messages about setting the parameters, but then giving people freedom to explore their expertise in order to find their own solutions (Pfeffer & Sutton, 2006; Buckingham, 2007). If we motivate people we get more from them, if we prescribe every step of the way we produce people who think less about what they are doing.

A Day in the life

What does normal everyday practice look like? In a field such as assertive outreach, or even mental health in general, that becomes a very difficult question to answer. The remainder of this chapter will outline examples that contribute to what a day could look like in a team that is constantly thinking about what it does and how it needs to develop and sustain its good practice. The following is based on examples of practice that are or have happened in Assertive Outreach (North) Northamptonshire, based in offices in Kettering, England.

8.56 a.m. – morning handover

Handover is a critical function of communication that supports good team working. With exceptions, the two sub-teams are already getting into place ready to start a 9.00 a.m. meeting. The issue of punctuality is deeply embedded into the culture of the service from when it was a small pilot team, and any visitors or new staff are made aware of this. Late-comers have no opportunity to interrupt the flow of the meeting, as time is precious and focused, and the quality of communication and listening is owned by everyone who arrives with a relatively empty diary for the day ahead. Staff with near-full diaries are doing their own thing, not functioning as a true team. Allocation of tasks for the day is shared amongst those present on the day, and will be planned at the end of handover.

Not all assertive outreach teams develop such a focused daily handover. If you do not operate sub-teams to enact a whole team approach the numbers are likely to be prohibitive to focused discussion of the whole caseloads. Some will opt to split the team caseload into sections across the week, with a traffic light system for additional priorities. Some will opt for more individual caseload diaries with agreed space held open each day to just share out the immediate demands or crises. Whatever the system that is adopted, the practice development question is how closely have you analysed and monitored the amount of time and effectiveness of the time spent in meetings across a whole week. Most teams fall into a system, and will defend it to the hilt without ever giving sufficient attention to how they are using time. Furthermore, the more a group of individuals adopt their own caseloads the less they are functioning in a team approach, and the less benefit they and the service users gain from the shared responsibilities for continuing the challenging work uninterrupted at times when annual and sick leave intervene. (See Box 14.1 for an evaluation of handovers.)

Box 14.1   Evaluating how handovers function

The external *Practice Based Evidence* initiative has regularly involved focused observation and statistical evaluation of the ways in which sub-team handovers manage the following elements:

- Timing and focus of discussions.
- Reflecting a whole team approach.
- Identifying strengths.
- Identifying and managing risks.
- The range of bio-psycho-social and practical interventions.
- Links with other services, teams and agencies.
- The ratio of long-term planning and responding to immediate crises.

White lightening

How many light-bulbs does it take to change an assertive outreach team? Answer: one – 'the white-board'; which illuminates most assertive outreach team offices to differing degrees, depending on its location or vantage point, and more importantly on its functional usefulness within the team. Its importance is often so significant and central to the functioning of the team, its very existence is often taken for granted. The white-board is a *working tool*, with the capability of facilitating improved communications within a team, and contributing to the overall effectiveness of team working in practice. It could be argued that an effective white-board is the equivalent of a part-time member of staff in terms of the resource it offers to a team. The communication angle is not just provided by the focus of attention driven by the needs of a team meeting; even outside of team meetings informal observation of individual practitioners in highly functioning teams shows they make frequent conscious and sub-conscious references to the white-board as they go about the tasks of the day.

How the white-board is structured in layout and content may vary from team to team. The 'team' involvement in the design will promote a greater sense of ownership, which can sharply influence its usefulness and impact on team functioning. It is clearly recognised throughout the team that keeping the white-board up-to-date is an essential collective function of the team. This is especially important if the white board is to perform an essential support to groups of people who spend so much of their working time outside of the office. It becomes one of the most indispensable tools for facilitating good lines of communication and creative collaborations.

Where the white-board becomes a harbour of static information it is less likely to be changed or up-dated; it is less likely to be used to convey messages in creative ways; and it is less likely to be something that team members spend much time noticing, even if it has a commanding size and place within the office environment. For these reasons, some teams have subsequently abandoned the use of white-boards, or still use them but very ineffectively.

The following are two of many examples of how the white-board has been used in Kettering in a way that sheds light on daily practice issues:

1. A member of staff had developed a concern about the appropriateness of one particular service user being on the assertive outreach team caseload. In some of the daily handover meeting discussions, when the person's name was duly raised the majority of the team took it for granted that the stability being reported was a good reflection of their substantial input (and to a great degree it was); but the mention of instigating gradual disengagement garnered little support at this stage. The concerned member of staff chose to make a creative use of the white-board, and wrote up the service user's whereabouts day-to-day on the board (in a different colour pen to most information). The visual message was a powerful communication to the team that they were having difficulty getting time from the service user to meet up, and of the high functioning and widening social network the person was developing. This triggered the need for a fuller team discussion of how to plan for gradual and positive disengagement, reinforcing to the person their positive progress and sustainable supports, while leaving open the possibility of contacting the team in the event of future needs. This person soon became inactive on the team caseload.

2. During an individual clinical supervision session, a member of staff expressed how pleased they felt with their own marked improvement in managing to complete essential paperwork with the involvement of the specific service users. Previously, *administration* had been seen as a last minute rush to the detriment of effective service user consultation. In a previous supervision session, this member of staff had identified an opportunity for personal practice development focused on advanced planning for care programme approach (CPA) reviews with the service users. This effort had been positively acknowledged by some service users expressing their feelings of being more involved in the process through holding prior discussions.

When reflecting on what had influenced personal development, the practitioner responded with 'I know this sounds amazing but it's the white-board, with the visual register of outpatient appointments and CPA review dates.' This enlightenment provided not only a boost for the morale and confidence of the individual staff member, but also a reminder of the supportive prompting role that the white-board could offer to the team as a whole.

The impact of this *working tool* on the daily functioning of teams is likely to be variable. If it only becomes a whereabouts board, it depends on the safety consciousness of the whole team to fill it in whenever they leave the office; and it becomes the domain of the office administrator. In reality, these are much smaller white-boards, often to be found in reception/administrator sections of the office. *The* white-board is an altogether more domineering entity, but still subject to the active use by all team members. It can still become a screen for static information leading to a more dormant level of function within the team's daily life cycle. Its potential to illuminate the team should not be bound by any restrictions other than local creativity and desire of all team members.

9.49 a.m. – doing the work

When handover is complete and tasks are allocated it is time for a quick cup of coffee in the office, a cigarette outside on the street, and the visits and phone calls to begin. The remainder of this morning will outline examples of the creative and flexible work carried with and for service users. On this particular day the afternoon will largely be devoted to the periodic *practice based evidence* focus on team reflection and practice development, so visits are more restricted in time than would be the case for the vast majority of days.

Pimp my crib

A homeless person with a dual diagnosis and chaotic lifestyle pattern is being offered a tenancy, but the place is a completely empty shell. The staff member following up the offer is concerned the service user will not cope with the stress of an empty place, and could lose the tenancy unless it is partly furnished with the basics this morning. The process of applying for grants would be time-consuming, so the task becomes more challenging at a perceived high risk time with the person being in a place of his own for the first time. First thoughts are to ask his manager for the cash to buy stuff this morning. Based on a good interpersonal relationship, the manager is able to reply 'bugger off, what do you think I am, a cash-point?' She encourages him to think creatively and see what he can do, possibly through contacts with colleagues as well. He uses known contacts, informal chats and trading on the anxiety about the task, resulting in a range of people coming up with the goods to the point of achieving a near fully furnished flat in less than half a day. Flush with success, and with knowledge of co-workers talents, the staff member even plans to ask some of his female colleagues at handover the next day to do some crystals and feng shui (as something that might respond well to the service user's interests), also providing a calming influence at a time of stressful change.

Who put the 'out' into outpatients?

The service is unencumbered by the need to have outpatient clinics. 'Out' means wherever, and the consultant psychiatrist working with the team tries not to keep a fully booked diary, so he can respond to needs and review people where it suits them. Time spent around the office is not seen as wasted, it is for catching up on phone calls and being available to respond to immediate needs.

Today the courts require an in-depth report about a service user with a history of sexual abuse. When asked where they would like to meet to discuss the report the service user requested to meet in McDonalds. This initially caused more issues for the workers about the need for a highly sensitive and confidential set of enquiries to be discussed in a public space in order to compile the report. The result was the service adapting to the service user's personal wishes, and a highly complex report was discussed and produced in a public place leading up to and across a shared lunch.

Service user becomes their own care coordinator

From the morning handover one of the long-standing service users has requested a specific visit from one member of staff. Contrary to the frequently claimed criticism of the team approach presenting reluctant people with too many workers, this person has evolved their relationship with the team to the level where he is able to identify the qualities, interests and skills of different team members, and to request the best person to meet his specific identified needs in the moment. In effect, he has developed his own strengths assessment of the team, and applies it to his best advantage. Furthermore, the team sees this as a fabulous way to be responding to people in a person-centred way, rather than creating an issue about the service user putting demands on the team that they cannot meet. On this occasion he has identified someone he wants to talk through issues about his housing. During the last year he has identified different members of staff to provide calming reassurance through a court appearance, supporting his education about internet information around psychosis, and the person he wants to accompany the consultant psychiatrist when he has met up to review his medical and medication issues at home. (See Box 14.2 on developing the service.)

Taking the sting out of the call

A specific service user has felt pressured this morning by two bills arriving in the post totalling more than £1000. She has not felt particularly supported by another service provider who was supposed to help with this kind of problem, leading to verbal disagreements. The other service provider rings assertive outreach (north) to report the distress and seek help. The worker who takes the call just before he is due out on another visit asks for the service user to be put onto the phone. During the conversation the other service provider is heard in the background saying their phone should only be used for emergencies, to which the service user instantly replies 'this is an emergency I am talking about my medication.' The assertive outreach worker says to the service user he can see the funny side of the situation and how well she is managing it, particularly in keeping the phone call going under pressure from the other service provider. He offers to try rearranging his plans for this morning, and will phone her back on her mobile. Another worker in the office immediately offers to switch plans to enable this issue to be resolved; particularly based on the conversation that had ensued in morning handover earlier. The whole team approach enables flexible working to meet service user needs with a minimum of fuss about precious personal caseloads and over-flowing diaries.

1.14 p.m. – team reflection and practice development

On this day most of the team are able to bring lunch back into the office to share a communal experience before the planned team reflection and practice development session with the external practice based evidence facilitation. Team reflection focuses on a more flexible free-flowing review of elements of the service vision and methods underpinning good team working. Practice development takes a specific element of practice, and offers the team an opportunity to think creatively about ways of developing and implementing it into routine practice.

This is not 'yet another meeting' that takes time out from busy practitioners. It is a relatively frequent session that is booked in advance in response to needs identified at other times in the team's usual functioning. In a world of funky mental health practitioners are encouraged to see 'reflection' and 'development' of practice as potential creative and enjoyable elements of team working that they can all contribute to and own. As such, anybody in the team can raise an issue that is slipping or problematic, either openly in the office or through their own supervision. For example, in recent morning handover meetings the issue seems to be emerging that links with the crisis team are working inconsistently. There are different opinions within the assertive outreach service as to whether this is more about assertive outreach or more about the procedures followed by the crisis team. It is agreed that this would be an important issue for reflection as a service before looking at potential practice development solutions between the assertive outreach and crisis teams. Time is booked in advance to enable most or all staff to be involved, and consideration is given to whether an external person with the right expertise might facilitate the session. (See Box 14.2 on developing the service.)

Box 14.2   Developing the service

Team reflection is predominantly about asking the questions that underpin the vision, the model of practice and the ethical dilemmas that any assertive outreach service should regularly debate. For example:

- Are we really doing assertive outreach, or are we a community mental health team by another name?
- Are we keeping to a vision of strengths-working, and do we still understand what this approach has to offer in delivering genuine person-centred practice?
- How do we respond to the ethical dilemmas of the work, such as people's rights to refuse a service, and degrees of negotiation and coercion used?

Practice development focuses on opportunities to implement creative and flexible ways of achieving best practice. For example:

- Developing a 'strengths approach' (Morgan, 2008).
- Creative ways of achieving the principles of CPA (Morgan et al., 2009).
- Gradual disengagement and personal community integration.
- Reasoned and structured approach to positive risk-taking (Morgan, 2004).
- Links with other services.

An example of a 'team reflection' session would start with a challenging question from a practice based evidence perspective: *So you think you are team?* As an introduction, the facilitator suggests that most of us work in teams – or do we? We claim to work in teams; we may belong to something called a team; we define our role as being a part of such-and-such team. But do we really work as a team; and if so, how?

The session may explore what being in a team is all about (e.g. needs or identity linked to a group), and define the boundaries that help us to manage the work we do. There is the value of having someone we can 'talk shop with' without having to go through lengthy boring explanations. We have people we can share a problem with, find a solution or just collectively share the 'rest of the world against us' type of script if it feels constructive. In the case of assertive outreach the whole issue of the team approach and whether it helps or hinders the service user needs regular thoughtful reflection. Whether we are actually doing it is a further cause for regular investigation, and if so, how are we sure? Can we identify the evidence from analysis of our service user contact statistics and evaluation of handover discussions?

In the literature on the subject, the idea is that service user dependency on one service provider is not a good thing. Inevitably workers move on, and the service user has the frustrating experience of going back almost to square one, to recount the failures of their life history to yet another stranger. Dependency on a service or team is seen to be healthier than dependency on one person. It allows for a wider degree of skill and expertise to be offered to meet your individual needs, and it will enable people to cope more successfully with changes of service personnel. Not to say, the benefits enjoyed by the workers through greater support and shared responsibility for a wide range of people, rather than the burden of feeling like you carry sole responsibility for the outcomes of a single caseload.

In conclusion, such a session may arrive at an understanding that a team approach is not just about function. It is about different personalities gelling with each other, in a way that recognises their individuality, and that they are even better for being able to respect and work with each others' strengths and personal qualities. In the original pilot team a small group of people were identified as the 'soul sister' providing the drive, the 'earth mother' as the conscience, the 'heartbeat', the 'dynamo', the 'rock' and the 'organiser'. All contribute equally to the effective working of a 'team'. A good team recognises differences of approach, ideas and individuality. It celebrates and works with these differences, rather than suppressing them. It instils all its work with a 'can do' attitude – thinking the unthinkable, and then doing it. Much of this style of working requires smaller size of teams. A true 'team approach' is not something that can be easily achieved with groups of 12, 15, 20 or more people (Onyett, 2003). How many service users can any of us hold significant amounts of detail about in our heads?

4.01 p.m. – administration hour

Agreed by the team as an important time for tying-up the loose ends of the day through necessary phone calls and form-filling; for the identified 'buddy' in each sub-team to set up the white-board with available information for the following day; and to put a dent into the never-ending mountain of paperwork associated with all parts of the job. As most members of the team are likely to be present, it can also be the best time for a range of information-sharing, though the constant noise of a busy open-plan office and regular interruptions can be detrimental to concentration on focused pieces of work. The easiest solution is the offices of the service lead and the consultant psychiatrist being open and available for anyone in the team to use as quieter space if negotiated.

6.29 p.m. – real flexibility and response to needs

A home visit has been agreed by one member of staff to meet with a carer who works during the day. This visit has been negotiated based on a real need, and on the vitally important role the carer is playing in the support of the specific service user they are a father to. The expectations are that the meeting will be fraught with anxieties from the carer's position, and part of an on-going level of support that focuses on long-term gains rather than instant fixes. The team have identified that there is no need for a two-person visit, but the worker doing the visit has made plans to phone the sub-team 'buddy' at 7.15 p.m.

7.00 p.m. – a daily phone conversation

A team member accepts a phone call from a service user for a few minutes, who wishes to tell her about the football on Sky TV this evening or a film he intends to watch. It has long been recognised that this is the service user's best way of managing the most psychotic part of his day. Genuinely service user focused work is about real needs, and often can mean doing the little bit extra for a very good reason that becomes integrated by the funky mental health practitioner into their routine without thought of intrusion. In this instance, a staff member's family and social network become aware of the routine, and accept it as a part of the rich tapestry of human interactions. A situation develops whereby the service user is known for his specific interests by a wider network of people who never meet him. Issues of confidentiality are addressed by no information being discussed with these other people other than the sport and film interests and any other low key normal conversation.

The service user has always understood this contact to have its boundaries, and he will only talk about anything to do with psychotic experiences with the staff member. This is genuine flexible responsiveness, rather than the rigid prescription of a shift-based system; it meets a clearly identified need in a social way, rather than generating artificial levels of need through a bureaucratic system that talks about person-centred care, then responds with service-centred solutions.

7.11 p.m. – a call to the 'buddy'

The home visit has gone better than expected, with the carer reflecting on how much they value the support of the assertive outreach service in comparison to the infrequent contact and lack of information they experienced in a nine-to-five appointment system prior to the involvement of assertive outreach. The worker goes home with a feeling of satisfaction to be shared with the team in the following morning's handover meeting – the buddy turns off the phone for another day.

Conclusions

The practice of a funky mental health approach is not without its challenges and difficulties; not the least of which will be some staff members within any team who just don't get it. There is no accounting for the lack of reflection and fixed mindsets that will regularly be encountered, and even denied or defended by those practicing them. For some, the opportunity to reflect on, think about and creatively develop their practice is nothing more than a hindrance to just getting on with all the pressures they experience in a busy and demanding job. There is also no substitute for a good consistent moan to some people. This is not to say they do not do good work; but the amount of energy expended on negative feeling and expressions of emotion takes away from time that could be devoted to more constructive management of the challenges, but also serves to demotivate others subject to the whining and claims to have done it all before.

The individuals who practice funky mental health are a lucky few – predominantly reflective and ethical people, they understand how to achieve a level of enjoyment out of their work, it being an intrinsic part of their life interwoven with other elements of who they are. They encounter a majority of people who are eternally trying to find reasons to separate what they do at work from who they are as people outside of demarcated work hours. They understand that the less you integrate the more you fragment, and a fragmented life is the basis for further dissonance. However, these practitioners or team managers are not naïve enough to allow themselves to be exploited by the considerable demands of a system more equipped to grind down excellence for the sake of uniform bureaucratic mediocrity. They understand the system better than most, because they reflect on and analyse what is going on around them, and think about the sometimes hidden motives and connections in the games people play.

In the real world of person-centred practice funky mental health is about 'permission' to think and do things differently, rather than a 'prescription' of how things are expected to be done. Traditional expected ways can be fine, in some circumstances, but don't have to be the usual way in all circumstances. Can funky mental health apply outside of assertive outreach? Yes, in the funky world of trying to recapture all that is interesting, motivating and exciting about working in mental health – assertive outreach could be seen as providing a guiding light for other areas of practice to adapt into their functions and responsibilities.

Whether that will be understood from a higher level policy and management perspective is another question altogether.

References

Buckingham, M. (2007) *Go Put Your Strengths to Work*. Simon & Schuster, London.

Buckingham, M. & Coffman, C. (2005) *First, Break all the Rules*. Simon & Schuster, London.

Morgan, S. (2004) Positive risk-taking: an idea whose time has come. *Health Care Risk Report*, **10**(10), 18–19.

Morgan, S. (2008) Strengths assertive outreach: a review of seven practice development programmes. *Mental Health Review Journal*, **13**(2), 40–46.

Morgan, S., Wetherell, A. & Wetherell, R. (2009) *The Art of Co-ordinating Care: A Handbook of Best Practice for Everyone Involved in Care and Support*. OLM-Pavilion, Brighton.

Onyett, S. (2003) *Teamworking in Mental Health*. Palgrave Macmilan, Basingstoke.

Pfeffer, J. & Sutton, R.I. (2006) *Hard Facts, Dangerous Half-Truths & Total Nonsense*. Harvard Business School Press, Boston.

Practice Based Evidence (2009) The 'Strengths Approach' section at: http://www.practicebased evidence.com

Ryan, P. & Morgan, S. (2004) *Assertive Outreach: A Strengths Approach to Policy and Practice*. Churchill Livingstone, Edinburgh.

Index

Assertive Outreach in Mental Healthcare: Current Perspectives, First Edition. Edited by C. Williams, M. Firn, S. Wharne and R. Macpherson.
© 2011 Blackwell Publishing Ltd. Published 2011 by Blackwell Publishing Ltd.